Injury & Trauma Sourcebook

Learning Disabilities Sourcebook, 3rd Edition

Leukemia Sourcebook

Liver Disorders Sourcebook

Medical Tests Sourcebook, 4th Edition

Men's Health Concerns Sourcebook, 3rd Edition

Mental Health Disorders Sourcebook, 4th Edition

Mental Retardation Sourcebook

Movement Disorders Sourcebook, 2nd Edition

Multiple Sclerosis Sourcebook

Muscular Dystrophy Sourcebook

Obesity Sourcebook

Osteoporosis Sourcebook

Pain Sourcebook, 3rd Edition

Pediatric Cancer Sourcebook

Physical & Mental Issues in Aging Sourcebook

Podiatry Sourcebook, 2nd Edition

Pregnancy & Birth Sourcebook, 3rd Edition

Prostate & Urological Disorders Sourcebook

Prostate Cancer Sourcebook

Rehabilitation Sourcebook

Respiratory Disorders Sourcebook, 2nd Edition

Sexually Transmitted Diseases Sourcebook, 4th Edition

Sleep Disorders Sourcebook, 3rd Edition

Smoking Concerns Sourcebook

Sports Injuries Sourcebook, 4th Edition

Stress-Related Disorders Sourcebook, 2nd Edition

Stroke Sourcebook, 2nd Edition

Surgery Sourcebook, 2nd Edition

Thyroid Disorders Sourcebook

Transplantation Sourcebook

Traveler's Health Sourcebook

Urinary Tract & Kidney Diseases & Disorders Sourcebook, 2nd Edition

Vegetarian Sourcebook

Women's Health Concerns Sourcebook, 3rd Edition

Workplace Health & Safety Sourcebook

Worldwide Health Sourcebook

Teen Health Series

Abuse & Violence Information for Teens

Accident & Safety Information for Teens

Alcohol Information for Teens, 2nd Edition

Allergy Information for Teens

Asthma Information for Teens, 2nd Edition

Body Information for Teens

Cancer Information for Teens, 2nd Edition

Complementary & Alternative Medicine Information for Teens

Diabetes Information for Teens, 2nd Edition

Diet Information for Teens, 3rd Edition

Drug Information for Teens, 3rd Edition

Eating Disorders Information for Teens, 2nd Edition

Fitness Information for Teens, 2nd Edition

Learning Disabilities Information for Teens

Mental Health Information for Teens, 3rd Edition

Pregnancy Information for Teens, 2nd Edition

Sexual Health Information for Teens, 3rd Edition

D0966814

Stress Information for Teens

Suicide Information for Teens, 2nd Edition

Tobacco Information for Teens, 2nd Edition

Disabilities

SOURCEBOOK

Second Edition

Health Reference Series

Second Edition

Disabilities
SOURCEBOOK

Basic Consumer Health Information about Disabilities That Affect the Body, Mind, and Senses, Including Birth Defects, Hearing and Vision Loss, Speech Disorders, Learning Disabilities, Psychiatric Disorders, Degenerative Diseases, and Disabilities Caused by Injury and Trauma, Such as Amputation, Spinal Cord Injury, and Traumatic Brain Injury

Along with Facts about Assistive Technology, Physical and Occupational Therapy, Maintaining Health and Wellness, Special Education, Legal, Financial, Education, and Insurance Issues, a Glossary of Related Terms, and Resources for Additional Help and Information

Edited by
Amy L. Sutton

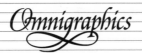

155 W. Congress, Suite 200, Detroit, MI 48226

Bibliographic Note
Because this page cannot legibly accommodate all the copyright notices, the Bibliographic
Note portion of the Preface constitutes an extension of the copyright notice.

Edited by Amy L. Sutton

Health Reference Series

Karen Bellenir, *Managing Editor*
David A. Cooke, MD, FACP, *Medical Consultant*
Elizabeth Collins, *Research and Permissions Coordinator*
Cherry Edwards, *Permissions Assistant*
EdIndex, Services for Publishers, *Indexers*

* * *

Omnigraphics, Inc.
Matthew P. Barbour, *Senior Vice President*
Kevin M. Hayes, *Operations Manager*

* * *

Peter E. Ruffner, *Publisher*

Copyright © 2011 Omnigraphics, Inc.

ISBN 978-0-7808-1222-2

Library of Congress Cataloging-in-Publication Data

Disabilities sourcebook : basic consumer health information about
disabilities that affect the body, mind, and senses ... / edited by Amy L.
Sutton. -- 2nd ed.
     p. cm. -- (Health reference series)
  Includes bibliographical references and index.
  Summary: "Provides basic consumer health information about physical,
cognitive, emotional, and sensory disabilities, along with facts about
assistive technologies and other tools and services to foster independence,
and guidance for families on educational, legal, and financial concerns.
Includes index, glossary of related terms, and other resources"-- Provided
by publisher.
  ISBN 978-0-7808-1222-2 (hardcover : alk. paper) 1. People with
disabilities--United States--Handbooks, manuals, etc. 2. People with mental
disabilities--United States--Handbooks, manuals,etc. I. Sutton, Amy L.
  RA644.6.D57 2011
  362.2--dc23
                                                              2011038653

Table of Contents

Visit www.healthreferenceseries.com to view *A Contents Guide to the Health Reference Series*, a listing of more than 16,000 topics and the volumes in which they are covered.

Preface xiii

Part I: Introduction to Disabilities

Chapter 1—What Is a Disability? 3

Chapter 2—Statistics on People with Disabilities
in the United States 7

Chapter 3—Myths and Facts about People
with Disabilities 19

Chapter 4—Aging and Disabilities 23

Chapter 5—Communicating with and about People
with Disabilities 27

Chapter 6—A Guide for Caregivers of People
with Disabilities 31

Chapter 7—Abuse and People with Disabilities 43

    Section 7.1—Bullying 44

    Section 7.2—Abuse of Children with
    Intellectual Disabilities 48

    Section 7.3—People with Disabilities
    and Sexual Violence 53

Part II: Types of Disabilities

Chapter 8—Overview of Birth Defects 61

Chapter 9—Cerebral Palsy 65

Chapter 10—Cleft Lip and Palate 69

Chapter 11—Cystic Fibrosis 77

Chapter 12—Inherited Disorders of Metabolism 81

Chapter 13—Muscular Dystrophy 89

Chapter 14—Spina Bifida 93

Chapter 15—Sensory Disabilities 97

   Section 15.1—Hearing Loss 98

   Section 15.2—Vision Loss 102

   Section 15.3—Deaf-Blindness 111

Chapter 16—Speech Disorders 121

   Section 16.1—Aphasia 122

   Section 16.2—Apraxia 124

Chapter 17—Intellectual and Cognitive Disabilities 127

   Section 17.1—Down Syndrome 128

   Section 17.2—Fetal Alcohol Spectrum
       Disorders 130

   Section 17.3—Head Trauma in Infants
       (Shaken Baby Syndrome) 132

Chapter 18—Learning Disabilities 133

   Section 18.1—Dyscalculia 134

   Section 18.2—Dyslexia 138

   Section 18.3—Dysgraphia 142

   Section 18.4—Dyspraxia 147

   Section 18.5—Executive Functioning
       Problems 149

   Section 18.6—Information Processing
       Disorders 155

Chapter 19—Autism Spectrum Disorders 157

Chapter 20—Attention Deficit Hyperactivity Disorder 161

Chapter 21—Psychiatric Disability and
Mental Disorders 165

Chapter 22—Degenerative Diseases That Cause
Disability 169

Section 22.1—Alzheimer Disease 170

Section 22.2—Amyotrophic Lateral
Sclerosis 172

Section 22.3—Arthritis 175

Section 22.4—Multiple Sclerosis 179

Section 22.5—Parkinson Disease 183

Chapter 23—Disability Caused by Injury
and Trauma 189

Section 23.1—Amputation and
Limb Loss 190

Section 23.2—Back Pain 193

Section 23.3—Spinal Cord Injury:
Understanding Paralysis,
Paraplegia, and
Quadriplegia 196

Section 23.4—Traumatic Brain Injury 200

Part III: Technologies and Services That Help People with Disabilities and Their Families

Chapter 24—What Is Assistive Technology? 207

Chapter 25—Mobility Aids: From Canes to Wheelchairs 211

Chapter 26—Home Use Devices and Modifications 219

Section 26.1—What Are Home Use
Medical Devices? 220

Section 26.2—Adapting Your Living
Space to Accommodate
Your Disability 225

Chapter 27—Technology for People with
Intellectual Disabilities 231

Chapter 28—Devices for Improving Communication
    and Hearing 237

    Section 28.1—Captions for Deaf and
              Hard-of-Hearing Viewers 238

    Section 28.2—Cochlear Implants 242

    Section 28.3—Hearing Aids 245

    Section 28.4—Other Hearing Assistive
              Technology 249

    Section 28.5—Profoundly Paralyzed
              Communicate with
              Brain-Computer Interface 253

Chapter 29—Therapy to Aid Communication 255

    Section 29.1—Speech-Language Therapy 256

    Section 29.2—Augmentative and
              Alternative Communication 260

Chapter 30—Low Vision Devices and Services 267

    Section 30.1—Living with Low Vision 268

    Section 30.2—Reading and Vision Loss 270

    Section 30.3—What Is Braille? 277

    Section 30.4—Web-Braille 280

    Section 30.5—Low Vision Aids for
              Computer Users 282

Chapter 31—Occupational and Physical Therapy 287

    Section 31.1—Occupational Therapy
              for People with Disabilities 288

    Section 31.2—Physical Therapy for
              People with Disabilities 290

Chapter 32—Art and Music Therapy 293

    Section 32.1—The Benefits of Art
              Therapy for People with
              Disabilities 294

    Section 32.2—Music Therapy Helps
              People with Disabilities 296

Chapter 33—Service Animals and People with Disabilities 299

Chapter 34—Finding Accessible Transportation 305

    Section 34.1—Adapting Motor
        Vehicles for People
        with Disabilities 306

    Section 34.2—Assistance and
        Accommodation for
        Air Travel 311

Chapter 35—Family Support Services 315

    Section 35.1—Understanding Respite
        Care 316

    Section 35.2—Adult Day Care 327

Part IV: Staying Healthy with a Disability

Chapter 36—Nutrition and Weight Management Issues
    for People with Disabilities 333

    Section 36.1—Nutrition and Disability 334

    Section 36.2—Nutrition for Swallowing
        Difficulties 341

    Section 36.3—Overweight and Obesity
        among People with
        Disabilities 343

Chapter 37—Physical Activity for People with Disabilities 347

    Section 37.1—Exercise Guidelines 348

    Section 37.2—Yoga for People with
        Disabilities 352

Chapter 38—Personal Hygiene for People with Disabilities 363

    Section 38.1—Dental Care 364

    Section 38.2—How to Bathe Someone
        with a Disability 365

Chapter 39—Bowel and Bladder Problems Associated
    with Disability 369

Chapter 40—Pressure Sores: What They Are and
    How to Prevent Them 377

Chapter 41—Managing Pain 381

Chapter 42—Coping with Depression and Anxiety 385

Chapter 43—Health Insurance Concerns............................. 389

    Section 43.1—Facts about Health
                Insurance That People
                with Disabilities Need
                to Know 390

    Section 43.2—Affordable Care Act for
                Americans with Disabilities 392

    Section 43.3—Medicare and Nonelderly
                People with Disabilities 395

    Section 43.4—Medicaid and Children's
                Health Insurance Program 399

Chapter 44—Dealing with Hospitalization 403

Chapter 45—Rehabilitation: Options for People
            with Disabilities...................................... 407

Chapter 46—Choosing a Long-Term Care Setting.................... 425

Part V: Special Education for Children with Disabilities

Chapter 47—Balancing Academics and Disability 431

Chapter 48—The Parent's Role in the Education Process........ 435

Chapter 49—Laws about Educating Children with
            Disabilities 439

    Section 49.1—Individuals with
                Disabilities Education
                Act (IDEA) 440

    Section 49.2—No Child Left Behind Act......... 441

    Section 49.3—Section 504 of the
                Rehabilitation Act 445

Chapter 50—Evaluating Children for Disability 447

Chapter 51—Early Intervention Services 459

Chapter 52—Individualized Education Programs (IEPs)......... 469

Chapter 53—Supports, Modifications, and
            Accommodations for Students............................. 475

Chapter 54—Transitioning Students with Disabilities
to Higher Education and Adulthood.................... 481

Part VI: Legal, Employment, and Financial Concerns for People with Disabilities

Chapter 55—A Guide to Disability Rights Laws 487

Chapter 56—Questions and Answers about the
Americans with Disabilities Act 495

Chapter 57—Housing and Safety Issues for People
with Disabilities.. 501

Section 57.1—The State of Housing for
People with Disabilities 502

Section 57.2—Disability Rights in
Housing.................................... 507

Section 57.3—Understanding the Fair
Housing Amendments Act 511

Section 57.4—Homelessness among
People with Disabilities 517

Section 57.5—Fire Safety for People
with Disabilities and
Their Caregivers...................... 519

Section 57.6—Disaster Preparedness
for People with Disabilities
and Special Needs 521

Chapter 58—Employees with Disabilities............................... 525

Section 58.1—Why Work Matters to
People with Disabilities 526

Section 58.2—In the Workplace:
Reasonable Accommodations
for Employees with
Disabilities............................... 528

Section 58.3—Job Accommodation
Situations and Solutions.......... 529

Section 58.4—Accommodations for
Employees with Psychiatric
Disabilities............................... 532

Chapter 59—Social Security Disability Benefits 535

Chapter 60—Tax Benefits and Credits for People
    with Disabilities... 539

Chapter 61—Preparing for the Future:
    End-of-Life Planning 545

    Section 61.1—Frequently Asked
        Questions about
        End-of-Life Care 546

    Section 61.2—Wills, Advance Directives,
        and Other Documents
        Associated with
        End-of-Life Planning................ 548

Part VII: Additional Help and Information

Chapter 62—Glossary of Terms Related to Disabilities 573

Chapter 63—Directory of Organizations That Help
    People with Disabilities...................................... 577

Chapter 64—Directory of Organizations for Athletes
    with Disabilities... 597

Chapter 65—Finding Financial Help for Assistive Devices 603

Index.. 629

Preface

About This Book

More than 54 million Americans—about one in five U.S. citizens—experience physical, cognitive, emotional, or sensory disabilities that impair functioning and interfere with daily activities. Although most people with disabilities lead healthy, productive lives, having a disability may increase the risk for illness or injury and interfere with educational goals or employment. In addition, people with more severe disabilities may require help with activities of daily living, such as dressing, bathing, and meal preparation, or even need part- or full-time nursing care.

Disabilities Sourcebook, Second Edition offers people with disabilities and their caregivers basic information about birth defects, hearing and vision loss, speech disorders, intellectual and cognitive disabilities, learning disabilities, and other types of impairment caused by chronic illness, injury, and trauma. It discusses assistive technology, home use devices, mobility aids, therapies, and services that foster independence. Information about the importance of nutrition, exercise, personal hygiene, and pain management is also provided. For parents of children with disabilities, the book offers facts about special education, including early intervention services, individualized education programs, and classroom supports. Legal, employment, and financial concerns for people with disabilities are also discussed. The book concludes with a glossary of related terms and directories of resources for additional help and information.

How to Use This Book

This book is divided into parts and chapters. Parts focus on broad areas of interest. Chapters are devoted to single topics within a part.

Part I: Introduction to Disabilities discusses the prevalence of physical, cognitive, emotional, and sensory impairments. It identifies common barriers that people with disabilities face in mainstream society, such as access to housing, employment, and education, and it offers tips on communicating with and caring for people with disabilities. Abuses sometimes encountered by people with disabilities are also discussed.

Part II: Types of Disabilities identifies the symptoms, diagnosis, and treatment of the most common forms of disabling conditions, including birth defects, sensory disabilities, speech disorders, intellectual and cognitive disabilities, learning disabilities, psychiatric disabilities, degenerative diseases, and disabilities caused by injury and trauma.

Part III: Technologies and Services That Help People with Disabilities and Their Families provides information about devices, therapies, and supports that help people with disabilities attend school, engage in work, and enjoy recreational activities. Facts about mobility aids such as canes and wheelchairs, home use medical devices, communication and hearing aids, and low vision devices are discussed, and information about speech, occupational, physical, and recreational therapies is provided.

Part IV: Staying Healthy with a Disability discusses strategies for maintaining physical health and emotional wellness in people who have disabilities. Patients and caregivers will find information on healthy eating, weight management, and physical activity, as well as tips on managing bowel and bladder problems, pressure sores, pain, depression, and anxiety. The part concludes with an explanation of health insurance concerns, tips on dealing with hospitalization and rehabilitation, and considerations when choosing a long-term care setting.

Part V: Special Education for Children with Disabilities identifies laws that support the education of children with disabilities, such as the Individuals with Education Act (IDEA), the No Child Left Behind Act, and Section 504 of the Rehabilitation Act. Facts about evaluating children for disability, early intervention services, individualized education programs (IEPs), and supports, modifications, and accommodations for students are also included.

Part VI: Legal, Employment, and Financial Concerns for People with Disabilities describes disability rights laws that protect people with disabilities from discrimination, such as the Americans with Disabilities Act (ADA) and the Fair Housing Amendments Act. It also discusses housing and safety issues for people with disabilities and addresses employment and workplace concerns, Social Security disability benefits, and difficult decisions near the end of life.

Part VII: Additional Help and Information provides a glossary of important terms related to disabilities. A directory of organizations that help people with disabilities and their families is also included, along with a list of summer camps for children with disabilities, a list of organizations for athletes with disabilities, and resources for finding financial help for assistive devices.

Bibliographic Note

This volume contains documents and excerpts from publications issued by the following U.S. government agencies: ADA National Network; Administration on Aging (AOA); Centers for Disease Control and Prevention (CDC); Federal Emergency Management Agency (FEMA); Internal Revenue Service (IRS); National Cancer Institute (NCI); National Heart, Lung, and Blood Institute (NHLBI); National Highway Traffic Safety Administration (NHTSA); National Institute of Arthritis and Musculoskeletal and Skin Diseases (NIAMS); National Institute of Child Health and Human Development; National Institute of Dental and Craniofacial Research (NIDCR); National Institute of Mental Health (NIMH); National Institute of Neurological Disorders and Stroke (NINDS); National Institute on Aging (NIA); National Institute on Deafness and Other Communication Disorders (NIDCD); National Institutes of Health (NIH); Office of Disability Employment Policy (ODEP); U.S. Bureau of the Census (BOC); U.S. Department of Education (ED); U.S. Department of Health and Human Services (HHS); U.S. Department of Homeland Security (DHS); U.S. Department of Housing and Urban Development (HUD); U.S. Department of Justice (DOJ); U.S. Department of Labor (DOL); U.S. Department of State (DOS); U.S. Equal Employment Opportunity Commission (EEOC); U.S. Fire Administration (FA); U.S. Food and Drug Administration (FDA); U.S. Library of Congress (LOC); U.S. Social Security Administration (SSA); and Walter Reed Army Medical Center (WRAMC).

In addition, this volume contains copyrighted documents from the following organizations: A.D.A.M., Inc.; Access Living; Access Media Group, LLC; AgingCare, LLC; Alzheimer's Association; American Academy of Family Physicians; American Academy of Physical Medicine and

Rehabilitation; American Foundation for the Blind; American Geriatrics Society; American Speech-Language-Hearing Association; Amputee Coalition; Arc of the United States; ARCH National Respite Network and Resource Center; Council for Exceptional Children; Easter Seals; Family Caregiver Alliance; International Dyslexia Association; Job Accommodation Network; Henry J. Kaiser Family Foundation; National Center for Learning Disabilities, Inc.; National Center on Physical Activity and Disability; National Consortium on Deaf-Blindness; National Dissemination Center for Children with Disabilities; National Hospice and Palliative Care Organization; National Multiple Sclerosis Society; Nemours Foundation; Oregon Department of Human Services; Rehabilitation Institute of Chicago; United Spinal Association; and the University of Montana Rural Institute Research and Training Center on Disability in Rural Communities.

Full citation information is provided on the first page of each chapter or section. Every effort has been made to secure all necessary rights to reprint the copyrighted material. If any omissions have been made, please contact Omnigraphics to make corrections for future editions.

Acknowledgements

Thanks go to the many organizations, agencies, and individuals who have contributed materials for this *Sourcebook* and to medical consultant Dr. David Cooke and prepress service provider WhimsyInk. Special thanks go to managing editor Karen Bellenir and research and permissions coordinator Liz Collins for their help and support.

About the Health Reference Series

The *Health Reference Series* is designed to provide basic medical information for patients, families, caregivers, and the general public. Each volume takes a particular topic and provides comprehensive coverage. This is especially important for people who may be dealing with a newly diagnosed disease or a chronic disorder in themselves or in a family member. People looking for preventive guidance, information about disease warning signs, medical statistics, and risk factors for health problems will also find answers to their questions in the *Health Reference Series*. The *Series*, however, is not intended to serve as a tool for diagnosing illness, in prescribing treatments, or as a substitute for the physician/patient relationship. All people concerned about medical symptoms or the possibility of disease are encouraged to seek professional care from an appropriate health care provider.

A Note about Spelling and Style

Health Reference Series editors use *Stedman's Medical Dictionary* as an authority for questions related to the spelling of medical terms and the *Chicago Manual of Style* for questions related to grammatical structures, punctuation, and other editorial concerns. Consistent adherence is not always possible, however, because the individual volumes within the *Series* include many documents from a wide variety of different producers and copyright holders, and the editor's primary goal is to present material from each source as accurately as is possible following the terms specified by each document's producer. This sometimes means that information in different chapters or sections may follow other guidelines and alternate spelling authorities. For example, occasionally a copyright holder may require that eponymous terms be shown in possessive forms (Crohn's disease *vs.* Crohn disease) or that British spelling norms be retained (leukaemia *vs.* leukemia).

Locating Information within the Health Reference Series

The *Health Reference Series* contains a wealth of information about a wide variety of medical topics. Ensuring easy access to all the fact sheets, research reports, in-depth discussions, and other material contained within the individual books of the *Series* remains one of our highest priorities. As the *Series* continues to grow in size and scope, however, locating the precise information needed by a reader may become more challenging.

A Contents Guide to the Health Reference Series was developed to direct readers to the specific volumes that address their concerns. It presents an extensive list of diseases, treatments, and other topics of general interest compiled from the Tables of Contents and major index headings. To access *A Contents Guide to the Health Reference Series*, visit www.healthreferenceseries.com.

Medical Consultant

Medical consultation services are provided to the *Health Reference Series* editors by David A. Cooke, MD, FACP. Dr. Cooke is a graduate of Brandeis University, and he received his M.D. degree from the University of Michigan. He completed residency training at the University of Wisconsin Hospital and Clinics. He is board-certified in Internal Medicine. Dr. Cooke currently works as part of the University of Michigan Health System and practices in Ann Arbor, MI. In his free time, he enjoys writing, science fiction, and spending time with his family.

Our Advisory Board

We would like to thank the following board members for providing guidance to the development of this *Series*:

- Dr. Lynda Baker, Associate Professor of Library and Information Science, Wayne State University, Detroit, MI

- Nancy Bulgarelli, William Beaumont Hospital Library, Royal Oak, MI

- Karen Imarisio, Bloomfield Township Public Library, Bloomfield Township, MI

- Karen Morgan, Mardigian Library, University of Michigan-Dearborn, Dearborn, MI

- Rosemary Orlando, St. Clair Shores Public Library, St. Clair Shores, MI

Health Reference Series *Update Policy*

The inaugural book in the *Health Reference Series* was the first edition of *Cancer Sourcebook* published in 1989. Since then, the *Series* has been enthusiastically received by librarians and in the medical community. In order to maintain the standard of providing high-quality health information for the layperson the editorial staff at Omnigraphics felt it was necessary to implement a policy of updating volumes when warranted.

Medical researchers have been making tremendous strides, and it is the purpose of the *Health Reference Series* to stay current with the most recent advances. Each decision to update a volume is made on an individual basis. Some of the considerations include how much new information is available and the feedback we receive from people who use the books. If there is a topic you would like to see added to the update list, or an area of medical concern you feel has not been adequately addressed, please write to:

Editor
Health Reference Series
Omnigraphics, Inc.
155 W. Congress, Suite 200
Detroit, MI 48226
E-mail: editorial@omnigraphics.com

Part One

Introduction to Disabilities

Chapter 1

What Is a Disability?

Disability has been defined in many ways. In general, a disability is a feature of the body, mind, or senses that can affect a person's daily life. Many Americans experience disability first hand.

- Some people are born with a disability.

- Some people get hurt or sick and have a disability as a result.

- Some people develop a disability as they age.

- Some people have a disability that lasts a short time. Other people have a disability that lasts a lifetime.

Today, over 54 million—or one in five—people living in the United States have at least one disability. Based on what we know about disability, the reality is that you or someone you care about will have a disability at some point.

With good health habits and access to health care, many disabilities can be delayed or even prevented.

Excerpted from "To Improve the Health and Wellness of Persons with Disabilities," by the Department of Health and Human Services (HHS, www.hhs.gov), published on the Centers for Disease Control and Prevention's website (www.cdc.gov), 2005. Reviewed by David A. Cooke, MD, FACP, July 23, 2011.

Who Are People with Disabilities?

Anyone of any age can have a disability. People of all races and ethnicities can have disabilities. People with disabilities live throughout the United States, in towns, cities, and rural areas.

People with disabilities go to school and attend places of worship. They also vote, marry, have children, work, and play. To do all these things, people with disabilities need health care and health programs for the same reasons anyone else does—to stay well, active, and a part of the community.

The chance of having a disability goes up with age, from less than 10% for people 15 years of age or younger, to almost 75% for people 80 or older. Anyone can have a disability:

- An infant can be born with hearing loss.
- A child can become paralyzed by an injury from a car crash.
- A young adult can have depression or another mental illness.
- A woman in her early 30s can have multiple sclerosis.
- A man in midlife can develop type 2 diabetes.
- An older adult can lose her sight from glaucoma.

Different kinds of disabilities affect people in different ways. And the same disability can affect each person differently.

Health Care for People with Disabilities

People with disabilities need health care and health programs for the same reasons anyone else does—to stay well, active, and a part of the community. Being healthy means the same thing for all of us—getting and staying well so we can lead full, active lives. That means having the tools and information to make healthy choices, and knowing the risk factors for illness. For people with disabilities, it also means knowing that problems related to a disability can be treated. These problems can include pain, depression, and a greater risk for certain illnesses. To be healthy, people with disabilities require health care that meets their needs as a whole person, not just as a person with a disability. People with or without disabilities can stay healthy by learning about and living healthy lifestyles.

To make sure you are getting the best possible health care, do the following:

4

- Know your body and how you feel when you're well and when you're not.

- Talk openly with your health care professional about your concerns.

- Find out who the best health care professionals are in your area to meet your needs.

- Check to be sure you can get into your health care professional's office and that he or she has the staff and equipment you need.

- Think through your concerns before you visit your health care professional.

- Bring your health records with you.

- Take a friend with you, if you're concerned you might not remember all your questions and all the answers.

- Get it in writing. Write down, or have someone write down for you, what is said by the health care professional.

- Ask for help finding more information.

What Health Care Professionals Can Do

All health care professionals should do the following:

- Give each patient—including people with disabilities—the information needed to live a long and healthy life.

- Listen and respond to the patient's health concerns. Give each patient the information needed to prevent or treat a health concern—even if the patient does not ask for it.

- Communicate clearly and directly with the patient. If the patient does not understand your questions or instructions, repeat what you have said, use other words, or find another way to provide the information.

- Take the time needed to meet the patient's health care needs.

Among nonelderly people with disabilities, 25% reported they had difficulty finding a health care professional who understood their disability. Many training and continuing education programs for health care professionals are now focusing on training them to understand disabilities.

Getting Needed Care and Services

Sometimes, we take things for granted—like being able to open a door, climb stairs, fill out a form, or see or hear someone. For people with disabilities, getting health care can be difficult because of lack of access.

Access can include parking spaces close to entrances, well-placed ramps or curb cuts, and doors that are wide and easy to open so that people with disabilities can get into buildings. Once inside, people with disabilities need access to counters that are low enough to reach, print that is large enough to read, and equipment that is easy to use.

People with disabilities face many challenges, including the following:

- Mobility

- Accessibility

- Social barriers

- Communication

Offices, parks, health care facilities, schools, or any other public spaces should be built to meet the needs of all of the people who will use the space. Health care professionals should be able to communicate with all of the people who see them. This means making sure of the following points of access:

- Parking spaces are close to entrances.

- Front entrances have ramps and curb cuts.

- Doors, inside and out, are wide and easy to open.

- Accessible routes connect all features and service areas.

- Floor spaces are free of equipment and other barriers.

- Counters and service windows are low enough for everyone to reach.

- Restrooms and dressing rooms are accessible.

- Alarm systems can be seen and heard.

- Staff and health care professionals can use or access sign language.

- Print materials and signs are in large print for people with low vision.

- Raised lettering and Braille are used on signs, such as those on elevators.

Chapter 2

Statistics on People with Disabilities in the United States

Americans with Disabilities

Recent public policy in the United States concerning disability has focused on improving the socioeconomic conditions for people with disabilities. Increasing access to employment opportunities by reducing discrimination and providing public services are the centerpieces of the New Freedom Initiative, which renewed the government's commitment to the Americans With Disabilities Act of 1990 (ADA). For years, the ADA has mandated that people with disabilities be afforded legal protections and provided with essential public services. In addition to these provisions, the ADA provides a definition for people with disabilities, in part, as those who have "a physical or mental impairment that substantially limits one or more major life activities." Other federal laws that offer guidance on issues affecting people with disabilities include the Rehabilitation Act of 1973, the Individuals With Disabilities Education Act, the Fair Housing Amendments Act of 1988, and the Telecommunications Act of 1996.

Highlights

- Of the 291.1 million people in the population in 2005, 54.4 million (18.7 percent) had some level of disability and 35.0 million (12.0 percent) had a severe disability (see Table 2.1).

This chapter includes text excerpted from "Americans With Disabilities, 2005," a report by the U.S. Census Bureau (www.census.gov), December 2008, and text excerpted from "Developmental Disabilities Increasing in US," by the Centers for Disease Control and Prevention (CDC, www.cdc.gov), June 14, 2011.

- Of people 6 years and older, 11.0 million people (4.1 percent) needed personal assistance with one or more activities of daily living (ADLs) or instrumental activities of daily living (IADLs).

- Among the population 15 years and older, 7.8 million people (3.4 percent) had difficulty seeing words or letters in ordinary newspaper print, and 1.8 million of these people reported being unable to see.

- An estimated 7.8 million people aged 15 and older (3.4 percent) had difficulty hearing a normal conversation, and 1.0 million of them reported being unable to hear.

- Of the population aged 21 to 64, 28.1 million people (16.5 percent) had a disability, and 45.6 percent of this group was employed. The employment rate was 30.7 percent for people with a severe disability, compared with rates of 75.2 percent for people with a non-severe disability and 83.5 percent for people with no disability.

- Among people aged 65 and older, 18.1 million people (51.8 percent) had a disability. About 12.9 million people 65 years and older (36.9 percent) had a severe disability.

Disability Prevalence

Of the 291.1 million people in the 2005 population of the United States, 54.4 million, or 18.7 percent, reported some level of disability (see Table 2.1). Among this population, 35.0 million (12.0 percent of all people) reported a severe disability. Both the number and percentage of people with any disability was higher in 2005 than in 2002—51.2 million people and 18.1 percent in 2002. The number and percentage of people with a severe disability was also higher in 2005 than in 2002. Of people aged 6 and older, approximately 11.0 million people (4.1 percent) reported needing assistance with one or more ADLs or IADLs—not statistically different from those in 2002.

As age increases, so does the prevalence of disability. As shown in Figure 2.1, the disability rate for each age group was higher than the rates for the younger age groups, with people 80 years and older having the highest incidence of disability at 71.0 percent. At a rate of 30.1 percent, people aged 55 to 64 were nearly three times as likely to have a disability as people aged 15 to 24 (10.4 percent). An increase in the likelihood of severe disability was also seen in successively older age groups, ranging from 3.6 percent for the population under 15 years to 56.2 percent for the population 80 years and older. Transitions into nursing facilities amongst older people with disabilities, and subsequently

(Numbers in thousands)

Category	Number		Percentage	
	Estimate	90-percent C.I. (±)[1]	Estimate	90-percent C.I. (±)[1]
All ages	**291,099**	**497**	**100.0**	**(X)**
With a disability	54,430	936	18.7	0.3
Severe disability	34,953	779	12.0	0.3
Aged 6 and older	**266,752**	**803**	**100.0**	**(X)**
Needed personal assistance with an ADL or IADL	10,999	456	4.1	0.2
Aged 15 and older	**230,391**	**1,047**	**100.0**	**(X)**
With a disability	49,073	898	21.3	0.4
Severe disability	32,776	757	14.2	0.3
Difficulty seeing	7,794	386	3.4	0.2
Severe difficulty seeing	1,783	186	0.8	0.1
Difficulty hearing	7,809	386	3.4	0.2
Severe difficulty hearing	992	139	0.4	0.1
Aged 21 to 64	**170,349**	**1,212**	**100.0**	**(X)**
With a disability	28,145	708	16.5	0.4
Employed	12,836	491	45.6	1.3
Nonsevere disability	9,435	423	5.5	0.2
Employed	7,099	369	75.2	2.0
Severe disability	18,710	587	11.0	0.3
Employed	5,737	332	30.7	1.5
No disability	142,204	1,219	83.5	0.4
Employed	118,702	1,191	83.5	0.4
Aged 65 and older	**35,028**	**780**	**100.0**	**(X)**
With a disability	18,133	578	51.8	1.2
Severe disability	12,943	493	36.9	1.1

(X) Not applicable.

[1] A 90-percent confidence interval is a measure of an estimate's variability. The larger the confidence interval in relation to the size of the estimate, the less reliable the estimate. For further information on the source of the data and accuracy of the estimates, including standard errors and confidence intervals, go to <www.census.gov/sipp/sourceac/S&A04W1toW7(S&A-7).pdf>.

Source: U.S. Census Bureau, Survey of Income and Program Participation, June–September 2005.

Table 2.1. Selected Disability Measures by Selected Age Groups: 2005 (Numbers in Thousands)

out of the population universe, may lessen the magnitude of increases in disability prevalence for older populations as 97.3 percent of people in nursing facilities had a disability, and the median age of this population was 83.2 years.

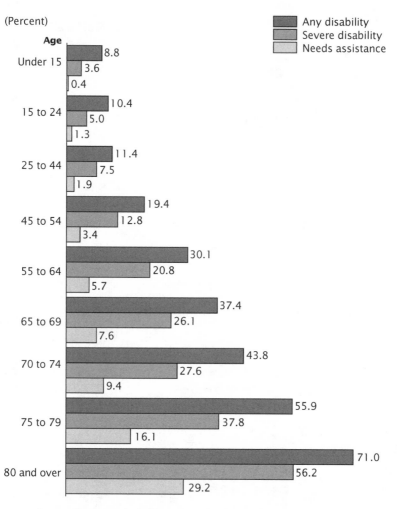

Note: The need for assistance with activities of daily living was not asked of children under 6 years.

Source: U.S. Census Bureau, Survey of Income and Program Participation, June–September 2005.

Figure 2.1. *Disability prevalence and the need for assistance by age: 2005 (percent).*

Differences in disability were also present when looking at prevalence by sex, race, and Hispanic origin. Blacks had a higher prevalence of disability (20.5 percent) than Asians (12.4 percent) and Hispanics (13.1 percent) and were not statistically different from non-Hispanic Whites (19.7 percent). The prevalence of disability among Asians was not statistically different from that of Hispanics. With a disability rate of 20.1 percent, females were more likely to have a disability than males (17.3 percent). Furthermore, the percentage with a disability for females was higher than that of males for each race group and Hispanics.

Blacks also had the highest rate of severe disability at 14.4 percent, compared with non-Hispanic Whites at 12.4 percent and Asians at 7.6 percent. Hispanics had a severe disability rate of 8.7 percent. Severe disability was more prevalent among females (13.4 percent) than males (10.6 percent). Like the overall disability rate, the percentage of females with a severe disability was higher than that of males for each race group and Hispanics.

Many of the differences between the disability rates by race and Hispanic origin can be attributed to differences in the age distributions of their populations. For example, Hispanics are predominantly younger than non-Hispanic Whites—roughly 6 percent of Hispanics are 65 years or older compared with 15 percent of non-Hispanic Whites. Likewise, higher disability rates for females are associated with proportionally larger groups of older women than older men—there are almost 6 million more females than males aged 65 and older.

Specific Measures of Disability

Limitations in seeing, hearing, and speaking: An estimated 6.4 percent of people 15 years old or over (14.7 million people) had difficulty seeing, hearing, or having their speech understood. About 7.8 million reported difficulty seeing the words and letters in ordinary newsprint, even when wearing glasses or contacts (if normally worn). Of this group, 1.8 million reported being unable to see printed words at all or were blind. About 7.8 million people reported difficulty hearing a normal conversation, even when wearing a hearing aid (if normally worn); an estimated 1 million reported deafness or being unable to hear conversations at all. About 2.5 million reported difficulty having their speech understood.

Roughly 4.3 million people reported using a hearing aid, of whom 1.8 million indicated having difficulty hearing even when using the hearing aid.

Upper and lower body limitations: Of people aged 15 and older, 27.4 million (11.9 percent) had difficulty with ambulatory activities of the lower body. About 22.6 million people (9.8 percent) had difficulty walking a quarter of a mile; 12.7 million were not able to perform this activity. About 21.8 million people (9.4 percent) had difficulty climbing a flight of stairs; 7.4 million of them were not able to do it at all. Roughly 3.3 million people (1.4 percent) used a wheelchair or similar device and 10.2 million (4.4 percent) used a cane, crutches, or walker to assist with mobility.

Roughly 19.0 million people (8.2 percent) aged 15 and older experienced difficulty with certain upper body physical tasks. An estimated 15.9 million people (6.9 percent) had difficulty lifting a 10-pound bag of groceries; 7.6 million were not able to do it at all. About 7.1 million people (3.1 percent) had difficulty grasping objects like a glass or pencil; 687,000 of them were not able to do it at all.

In addition to these physical tasks, the survey asked about difficulty performing other tasks that were not included in the disability definition. About 22.5 million people had difficulty moving a large object like a chair, 23.9 million had difficulty standing for an hour or longer, 9.9 million had difficulty sitting for an hour or longer, 27.4 million had difficulty crouching, and 11.7 million had difficulty reaching overhead.

Personal assistance: People with disabilities were asked about difficulty performing ADLs or IADLs and whether any assistance from another person was needed in order to perform the activities. ADL limitations included difficulty getting around inside the home, getting into or out of a bed or chair, taking a bath or shower, dressing, eating, and getting to or using the toilet. IADL limitations included difficulty going outside the home alone, managing finances, preparing meals, performing light housework, taking prescription medications, and using the telephone.

An estimated 8.5 million people aged 15 and older (3.7 percent) had difficulty with one or more ADL limitations, of whom 4.5 million needed the assistance of another person to help perform the activity or activities. Roughly 13.7 million people (5.9 percent) had difficulty with one or more IADL limitations, and 10.3 million of them needed assistance. Together, about 10.8 million people (4.7 percent) needed personal assistance with one or more ADLs or IADLs.

Cognitive, mental, and emotional functioning: People who had difficulty with cognitive, mental, or emotional functioning accounted for 7.0 percent of the population 15 years and older, or 16.1

million people. Of this group, 9.6 million reported one or more selected conditions that include a learning disability, mental retardation, Alzheimer disease, senility, dementia, and other mental or emotional conditions. About 8.4 million reported one or more selected symptoms that interfere with daily activities, which include frequently being depressed or anxious, trouble getting along with others, trouble concentrating, and trouble coping with stress. In addition, 5.1 million people reported difficulty managing finances.

Employment limitations: Among people aged 16 to 64, 13.3 million, or 7.0 percent, reported difficulties finding a job or remaining employed due to a health-related condition. Not included in the disability definition was a question asking if the respondents were limited in the kind or amount of work they could do because of a physical, mental, or other health condition, to which about 22.7 million people (11.9 percent) reported that they had this limitation. The survey then followed up with a question about whether they were prevented from working, to which 13.3 million people (6.9 percent) responded in the affirmative.

Disability domains: The many types of functional and activity limitations can be categorized into three disability domains—communication, mental, and physical. About 28.3 million people, or 12.3 percent of the population aged 15 and older, had disabilities in one domain—2.7 million in communication, 20.8 million in physical, and 4.9 million in mental. Of the 14.7 million people who had disabilities in two domains, 7.3 million had disabilities in communication and physical, 710,000 had disabilities in communication and mental, and 6.7 million had disabilities in physical and mental. About 4.7 million people had disabilities in all three domains. Roughly 1.3 million people had disabilities not categorized into a domain.

Economic Characteristics

Poverty status: Among people aged 25 to 64 with a severe disability, 27.1 percent were in poverty, compared with 12.0 percent for people with a nonsevere disability and 9.1 percent for people with no disability. Among people aged 65 and older, the poverty rate was 10.1 percent for people with a severe disability, 8.5 percent for people with a nonsevere disability, and 6.6 percent for people with no disability.

Program participation: For the population aged 25 to 64, program participation through cash assistance, food stamps, and subsidized housing programs was more prevalent among people with a severe disability than people with a nonsevere disability and people with no disability. Fifty-seven percent of people with a severe disability received some form of public assistance, compared with 16.3 percent of people with a nonsevere disability and 7.3 percent of people with no disability.

At 21.6 percent, people with a severe disability were about three times as likely to receive food stamps as people with a nonsevere disability (6.9 percent) and six times as likely as people with no disability (3.6 percent). The percentage of people with a severe disability residing in public or subsidized housing (12.1 percent) was also higher than percentages for people with a nonsevere disability and people with no disability— 3.1 percent and 1.8 percent, respectively.

Employment: Fewer than half (45.6 percent) of people with a disability between the ages of 21 and 64 were employed at the end of the interview period. People with a nonsevere disability were less likely to be employed than people with no disability, 75.2 percent and 83.5 percent, respectively. People reporting a severe disability were the least likely to be employed (30.7 percent). For people with no disability, 62.9 percent worked full-time, while 48.1 percent of those with a nonsevere disability and 15.6 percent of those with a severe disability worked fulltime. More than two-thirds (69.3 percent) of people with a severe disability were not employed, compared with 24.8 percent of people with a nonsevere disability and 16.5 percent of people with no disability.

Employment also varied by specific disability type. At 59.1 percent, people with difficulty hearing were more likely to be employed than people with difficulty seeing, at 40.8 percent. Of people with one or more ADL limitations, 19.5 percent were employed, not statistically different from 22.2 percent of people with an IADL limitation. People with a disability in one domain were more likely to be employed (51.5 percent) than people with a disability in two domains (40.0 percent) and about twice as likely as people with a disability in three domains (25.1 percent).

Monthly earnings and family income: Median monthly earnings were $1,458 for people with a severe disability, $2,250 for people with a nonsevere disability, and $2,539 for people with no disability. The median monthly earnings for people with difficulty seeing was $1,932, lower than the median monthly earnings for people with difficulty hearing at $2,252.24. People who needed assistance with an ADL had median monthly earnings of $1,412, not statistically different from the median monthly earnings for people who needed assistance with an IADL. For people with a disability in one domain, the median monthly earnings were $2,000—higher than that of people with a disability in two domains ($1,766) and people with a disability in three domains ($1,210). People with a severe disability had a median monthly family income of $2,182, compared with $3,801 for people with a nonsevere disability and $4,669 for people with no disability. People with difficulty hearing had a higher median monthly family income ($3,162) than people with difficulty seeing ($2,188). The median monthly family income for people with a disability in one domain was $3,049, higher than $2,252 for people with a disability in two domains and $1,743 for people with a disability in three domains.

Children

Disability is categorized differently for children than for adults, primarily due to differences in the types of functions and activities in which they participate. For children under 3 years old, disability is based on whether the child has a developmental delay or has difficulty moving his or her arms or legs. Disability status for children 3 to 5 years old considers whether they have a developmental delay or have difficulty walking, running, or playing. Those with difficulty with these activities are considered to have a disability. In 2005, parents reported 228,000 children under 3 years old (1.9 percent) with a disability and 475,000 children 3 to 5 years old (3.8 percent) with a disability.

For children 6 to 14 years old, the definition of disability is broader, including communication-related difficulties, mental or emotional conditions, difficulty doing regular schoolwork, difficulty getting along with other children, difficulty walking or running, use of some assistive devices, and difficulty with ADLs. Of the 36.4 million children 6 to 14 years old, 4.7 million (12.8 percent) had a disability and 1.6 million (4.4 percent) had a severe disability.

Of the specific aspects of disability for children 6 to 14 years old, difficulty doing regular schoolwork was the most prevalent at 7.0 percent (2.5 million children). About 5.8 percent of children had one or more selected developmental conditions. These children included 2.8 percent with a learning disability; 0.5 percent with mental retardation; 1.0 percent with some other developmental disability, such as autism or cerebral palsy; and 2.9 percent with some other developmental condition that required therapy or diagnostic services.

About 0.8 percent of children in this age group had difficulty seeing, 0.7 percent had difficulty hearing, and 2.0 percent had difficulty having their speech understood. About 748,000 children (2.1 percent) had difficulty walking or running, and 263,000 children (0.7 percent) had difficulty with an ADL.

Developmental Disabilities Increasing in the United States

Researchers from the Centers for Disease Control and Prevention (CDC), in collaboration with researchers from the Health Resources and Services Administration (HRSA), have published a new study in [the June 2011 issue of] *Pediatrics*: "Trends in the Prevalence of Developmental Disabilities in U.S. Children, 1997–2008." Prevalence refers to the number of people who have these conditions during the time period of the study. This number includes all those who may have been diagnosed in prior years, as well as in the current year. People who no longer have the condition are not included in the prevalence figure for that year.

This study determined the prevalence of developmental disabilities in U.S. children and in selected populations for a 12-year period (see Table 2.2).

Table 2.2. Developmental Disabilities in Children Aged 3–17 Years

Any developmental disability	13.87%
Learning disability	7.66%
ADHD	6.69%

Note: These figures represent the percentage of children in this age group, 1997-2008.

Main Findings from This Study

Data from the study showed that developmental disabilities (DDs) are common: About one in six children in the United States had a DD in 2006–2008. These data also showed that prevalence of parent-reported DDs has increased 17.1% from 1997 to 2008.

This study underscores the increasing need for health, education and social services, and more specialized health services for people with DDs.

The prevalence of any DD in 1997–2008 was 13.87%:

- Prevalence of learning disabilities was 7.66%.

- Prevalence of attention deficit hyperactivity disorder (ADHD) was 6.69%.

- Prevalence of other developmental delay was 3.65%.

- Prevalence of autism was 0.47%.

16

The researchers found the following over the last 12 years (see Table 2.3):

- Prevalence of DDs has increased 17.1%—that's about 1.8 million more children with DDs in 2006–2008 compared to a decade earlier.

- Prevalence of autism increased 289.5%.

- Prevalence of ADHD increased 33.0%.

- Prevalence of hearing loss decreased 30.9%.

In addition, data from this study showed the following:

- Males had twice the prevalence of any DD than females and more specifically had higher prevalence of ADHD, autism, learning disabilities, stuttering/stammering, and other DDs.

- Hispanic children had lower prevalence of several disorders compared to non-Hispanic white and non-Hispanic black children, including ADHD and learning disabilities.

Table 2.3. Specific Developmental Disabilities in U.S. Children Aged 3–17 Years

Disability	Percent Change between 1997–1999 and 2006–2008
Any developmental disability	17.1%*
ADHD	33.0%*
Autism	289.5%*
Blind/unable to see at all	18.2%
Cerebral palsy	–
Moderate to profound hearing loss	-30.9%
Learning disability	5.5%
Intellectual disability	-1.5%
Seizures, past 12 months	9.1%
Stuttered or stammered, past 12 months	3.1%
Other developmental delay	24.7%*

Source: Centers for Disease Control and Prevention, National Center for Health Statistics, NHIS 1997–2008. * = Statistically significant trend over four time periods (1997–1999, 2000–2002, 2003–2005, and 2006–2008).

- Non-Hispanic black children had higher prevalence of stuttering/stammering than non-Hispanic white children.

- Children insured by Medicaid had a nearly two-fold higher prevalence of any DD compared to those with private insurance.

- Children from families with income below the federal poverty level had a higher prevalence of DDs.

To better understand why the prevalence has increased, future research should focus on understanding the influence of increases in the prevalence of known risk factors, changes in acceptance and awareness of conditions, and benefits of early intervention services.

About Developmental Disabilities and This Study

Developmental disabilities are a diverse group of severe chronic conditions that are due to mental and/or physical impairments. People with developmental disabilities have problems with major life activities such as language, mobility, learning, self-help, and independent living. Developmental disabilities begin any time during development up to 22 years of age and usually last throughout a person's lifetime.

For this study, researchers aimed to determine the prevalence of DD in U.S. children overall and in certain populations from 1997–2008. Researchers analyzed responses from the 1997–2008 National Health Interview Surveys. A total of 119,367 children ages 3–17 were included in the study. Parents or legal guardians were asked if their child had any of the following conditions: ADHD, autism, blindness, cerebral palsy, moderate to profound hearing loss, intellectual disability, learning disorders, seizures, stuttering/stammering, and other developmental delay.

Reference

Boyle CA, Boulet S, Schieve L, Cohen RA, Blumberg SJ, Yeargin-Allsopp M, Visser S, Kogan MD. Trends in the Prevalence of Developmental Disabilities in US Children, 1997–2008. *Pediatrics*. 2011.

Chapter 3

Myths and Facts about People with Disabilities

Everybody's fighting some kind of stereotype, and people with disabilities are no exception. The difference is that barriers people with disabilities face begin with people's attitudes—attitudes often rooted in misinformation and misunderstandings about what it's like to live with a disability.

Myth 1: People with disabilities are brave and courageous.

Fact: Adjusting to a disability requires adapting to a lifestyle, not bravery and courage.

Myth 2: All persons who use wheelchairs are chronically ill or sickly.

Fact: The association between wheelchair use and illness may have evolved through hospitals using wheelchairs to transport sick people. A person may use a wheelchair for a variety of reasons, none of which may have anything to do with lingering illness.

Myth 3: Wheelchair use is confining; people who use wheelchairs are "wheelchair-bound."

Fact: A wheelchair, like a bicycle or an automobile, is a personal assistive device that enables someone to get around.

"Myths and Facts About People with Disabilities," © Easter Seals (www.easter seals.com). All rights reserved. Reprinted with permission. This document is undated. Reviewed by David A. Cooke, MD, FACP, May 5, 2011.

Myth 4: All persons with hearing disabilities can read lips.

Fact: Lip-reading skills vary among people who use them and are never entirely reliable.

Myth 5: People who are blind acquire a "sixth sense."

Fact: Although most people who are blind develop their remaining senses more fully, they do not have a "sixth sense."

Myth 6: People with disabilities are more comfortable with "their own kind."

Fact: In the past, grouping people with disabilities in separate schools and institutions reinforced this misconception. Today, many people with disabilities take advantage of new opportunities to join mainstream society.

Myth 7: Non-disabled people are obligated to "take care of" people with disabilities.

Fact: Anyone may offer assistance, but most people with disabilities prefer to be responsible for themselves.

Myth 8: Curious children should never ask people about their disabilities.

Fact: Many children have a natural, uninhibited curiosity and may ask questions that some adults consider embarrassing. But scolding curious children may make them think having a disability is "wrong" or "bad." Most people with disabilities won't mind answering a child's question.

Myth 9: The lives of people with disabilities are totally different than the lives of people without disabilities.

Fact: People with disabilities go to school, get married, work, have families, do laundry, grocery shop, laugh, cry, pay taxes, get angry, have prejudices, vote, plan, and dream like everyone else.

Myth 10: It is all right for people without disabilities to park in accessible parking spaces, if only for a few minutes.

Fact: Because accessible parking spaces are designed and situated to meet the needs of people who have disabilities, these spaces should only be used by people who need them.

Myth 11: Most people with disabilities cannot have sexual relationships.

Fact: Anyone can have a sexual relationship by adapting the sexual activity. People with disabilities can have children naturally or through adoption. People with disabilities, like other people, are sexual beings.

Myth 12: People with disabilities always need help.

Fact: Many people with disabilities are independent and capable of giving help. If you would like to help someone with a disability, ask if he or she needs it before you act.

Myth 13: There is nothing one person can do to help eliminate the barriers confronting people with disabilities.

Fact: Everyone can contribute to change. You can help remove barriers by:

- understanding the need for accessible parking and leaving it for those who need it;
- encouraging participation of people with disabilities in community activities by using accessible meeting and event sites;
- understanding children's curiosity about disabilities and people who have them;
- advocating a barrier-free environment;
- speaking up when negative words or phrases are used about disability;
- writing producers and editors a note of support when they portray someone with a disability as a "regular person" in the media;
- accepting people with disabilities as individuals capable of the same needs and feelings as yourself, and hiring qualified disabled persons whenever possible.

Chapter 4

Aging and Disabilities

Disability among Older Americans Continues Significant Decline

Chronic disability among older Americans has dropped dramatically, and the rate of decline has accelerated during the past 2 decades, according to a new analysis of data from the National Long-Term Care Survey (NLTCS). The study, published in the November 28, 2006 print edition of the *Proceedings of the National Academy of Sciences (PNAS)*, found that the prevalence of chronic disability among people 65 and older fell from 26.5 percent in 1982 to 19 percent in 2004/2005. The findings suggest that older Americans' health and function continue to improve at a critical time in the aging of the population.

The study was funded by the National Institute on Aging (NIA), a component of the National Institutes of Health (NIH). A caregiving component of the survey was supported by the Office of the Assistant Secretary for Planning and Evaluation. All are part of the U.S. Department of Health and Human Services. Kenneth G. Manton, PhD, and colleagues at Duke University conducted the research.

This chapter contains text from "Disability Among Older Americans Continues Significant Decline," by the National Institute on Aging (NIA, www.nia.nih.gov), part of the National Institutes of Health, December 1, 2006, and text excerpted from "A Profile of Older Americans: 2009," by the Administration on Aging (AOA, www.aoa.gov), 2009.

In addition to a drop in the percentage of older Americans reporting disability, the analysis found that the average annual rate of the decline has accelerated. The decline in disability averaged 1.52 percent annually over the 22-year time span, but the rate of change shifted gradually from 0.6 percent in 1984 to 2.2 percent in 2004/2005.

"This continuing decline in disability among older people is one of the most encouraging and important trends in the aging of the American population," says NIA Director Richard J. Hodes, MD.

The report is an eagerly anticipated update of the last assessment of NLTCS data in 2001. "The challenge now is to see how this trend can be maintained and accelerated especially in the face of increasing obesity," says Richard Suzman, PhD, director of NIA's Behavioral and Social Research Program. "Doing so over the next several decades will significantly lessen the societal impact of the aging of the baby-boom generation."

The analysis also showed that from 1982 to 2004/2005, the following occurred:

- Chronic disability rates decreased among those over 65 with both severe and less severe impairments, with the greatest improvements seen among the most severely impaired. The researchers note that environmental modifications, assistive technologies, and biomedical advances may be factors in these declines.

- The proportion of people without disabilities increased the most in the oldest age group, rising by 32.6 percent among those 85 years and older.

- The percentage of Medicare enrollees age 65 and older who lived in long-term care institutions such as nursing homes dropped dramatically from 7.5 percent to 4.0 percent. The emergence of assisted-living options, changes in Medicare reimbursement policies, and improved rehabilitation services may have fueled this decrease in institutionalization.

If they continue as anticipated, the downward trends in chronic disability rates among older adults could help bolster the Medicare program's fiscal health, the researchers suggest.

Funded through a cooperative agreement between the NIA and Duke University, the NLTCS is a periodic federal government survey of approximately 20,000 Medicare enrollees.

Reference: Manton, K.G., Gu, X., & Lamb V.L. (2006). Change in chronic disability from 1982 to 2004/2005 as measured by long-term changes in function and health in the U.S. elderly population. *PNAS,* 103(48); 18374–9.

A Profile of Older Americans: Disability and Activity Limitations in Older Adults

Some type of disability (i.e., difficulty in hearing, vision, cognition, ambulation, self-care, or independent living) was reported by 38% of older persons in 2008. Some of these disabilities may be relatively minor but others cause people to require assistance to meet important personal needs. Almost 37% of older persons reported in 2005 a severe disability and 16% reported that they needed some type of assistance as a result. Reported disability increases with age. Fifty-six percent of persons over 80 reported a severe disability and 29% of the over 80 population reported that they needed assistance. There is a strong relationship between disability status and reported health status. Among those 65+ with a severe disability, 64% reported their health as fair or poor. Among the 65+ persons who reported no disability, only 10% reported their health as fair or poor. Presence of a severe disability is also associated with lower income levels and educational attainment.

In another study which focused on the ability to perform specific activities of daily living (ADLs), over 25% of community-resident Medicare beneficiaries over age 65 in 2007 had difficulty in performing one or more ADLs and an additional 14.6% reported difficulties with instrumental activities of daily living (IADLs). By contrast, 83% of institutionalized Medicare beneficiaries had difficulties with one or more ADLs and 67% of them had difficulty with three or more ADLs. [ADLs include bathing, dressing, eating, and getting around the house. IADLs include preparing meals, shopping, managing money, using the telephone, doing housework, and taking medication.] Limitations on activities because of chronic conditions increase with age. The rate of limitations on activities among persons 85 and older are much higher than those for persons 65–74.

It should be noted that (except where noted) the figures in the preceding text are taken from surveys of the noninstitutionalized elderly. Although nursing homes are being increasingly used for short-stay post-acute care, about 1.3 million elderly are in nursing homes (about half are age 85 and over). These individuals often have high needs for care with their ADLs and/or have severe cognitive impairment due to Alzheimer disease or other dementias.

Chapter 5

Communicating with and about People with Disabilities

Words

Positive language empowers. When writing or speaking about people with disabilities, it is important to put the person first. Group designations such as "the blind," "the retarded," or "the disabled" are inappropriate because they do not reflect the individuality, equality, or dignity of people with disabilities. Further, words like "normal person" imply that the person with a disability isn't normal, whereas "person without a disability" is descriptive but not negative. Table 5.1 shows examples of positive and negative phrases.

Actions

Etiquette considered appropriate when interacting with people with disabilities is based primarily on respect and courtesy. The following text includes tips to help you in communicating with persons with disabilities.

General Tips for Communicating with People with Disabilities

- When introduced to a person with a disability, it is appropriate to offer to shake hands. People with limited hand use or who

From "Communicating with and about People with Disabilities," by the Office of Disability Employment Policy (ODEP, www.dol.gov/odep), U.S. Department of Labor, August 2002. Reviewed by David A. Cooke, MD, FACP, May 5, 2011.

27

Table 5.1. Affirmative and Negative Phrases

Affirmative Phrases	Negative Phrases
person with an intellectual, cognitive, developmental disability	retarded; mentally defective
person who is blind, person who is visually impaired	the blind
person with a disability	the disabled; handicapped
person who is deaf	the deaf; deaf and dumb
person who is hard of hearing	suffers a hearing loss
person who has multiple sclerosis	afflicted by MS
person with cerebral palsy	CP victim
person with epilepsy, person with seizure disorder	epileptic
person who uses a wheelchair	confined or restricted to a wheelchair
person who has muscular dystrophy	stricken by MD
person with a physical disability, physically disabled	crippled; lame; deformed
unable to speak, uses synthetic speech	dumb; mute
person with psychiatric disability	crazy; nuts
person who is successful, productive	has overcome his/her disability; is courageous (when it implies the person has courage because of having a disability)

wear an artificial limb can usually shake hands. (Shaking hands with the left hand is an acceptable greeting.)

- If you offer assistance, wait until the offer is accepted. Then listen to or ask for instructions.

- Treat adults as adults. Address people who have disabilities by their first names only when extending the same familiarity to all others.

- Relax. Don't be embarrassed if you happen to use common expressions such as "See you later," or "Did you hear about that?" that seem to relate to a person's disability.

- Don't be afraid to ask questions when you're unsure of what to do.

Tips for Communicating with Individuals Who are Blind or Visually Impaired

- Speak to the individual when you approach him or her.

- State clearly who you are; speak in a normal tone of voice.

- When conversing in a group, remember to identify yourself and the person to whom you are speaking.

- Never touch or distract a service dog without first asking the owner.

- Tell the individual when you are leaving.

- Do not attempt to lead the individual without first asking; allow the person to hold your arm and control her or his own movements.

- Be descriptive when giving directions; verbally give the person information that is visually obvious to individuals who can see. For example, if you are approaching steps, mention how many steps.

- If you are offering a seat, gently place the individual's hand on the back or arm of the chair so that the person can locate the seat.

Tips for Communicating with Individuals Who Are Deaf or Hard of Hearing

- Gain the person's attention before starting a conversation (i.e., tap the person gently on the shoulder or arm).

- Look directly at the individual, face the light, speak clearly, in a normal tone of voice, and keep your hands away from your face. Use short, simple sentences. Avoid smoking or chewing gum.

- If the individual uses a sign language interpreter, speak directly to the person, not the interpreter.

- If you telephone an individual who is hard of hearing, let the phone ring longer than usual. Speak clearly and be prepared to repeat the reason for the call and who you are.

- If you do not have a Text Telephone (TTY), dial 711 to reach the national telecommunications relay service, which facilitates the call between you and an individual who uses a TTY.

Tips for Communicating with Individuals with Mobility Impairments

- If possible, put yourself at the wheelchair user's eye level.

- Do not lean on a wheelchair or any other assistive device.

- Never patronize people who use wheelchairs by patting them on the head or shoulder.

- Do not assume the individual wants to be pushed—ask first.

- Offer assistance if the individual appears to be having difficulty opening a door.

- If you telephone the individual, allow the phone to ring longer than usual to allow extra time for the person to reach the telephone.

Tips for Communicating with Individuals with Speech Impairments

- If you do not understand something the individual says, do not pretend that you do. Ask the individual to repeat what he or she said and then repeat it back.

- Be patient. Take as much time as necessary.

- Try to ask questions which require only short answers or a nod of the head.

- Concentrate on what the individual is saying.

- Do not speak for the individual or attempt to finish her or his sentences.

- If you are having difficulty understanding the individual, consider writing as an alternative means of communicating, but first ask the individual if this is acceptable.

Tips for Communicating with Individuals with Cognitive Disabilities

- If you are in a public area with many distractions, consider moving to a quiet or private location.

- Be prepared to repeat what you say, orally or in writing.

- Offer assistance completing forms or understanding written instructions and provide extra time for decision-making. Wait for the individual to accept the offer of assistance; do not "over-assist" or be patronizing.

- Be patient, flexible, and supportive. Take time to understand the individual and make sure the individual understands you.

Chapter 6

A Guide for Caregivers of People with Disabilities

[*Editor's Note:* Though this document specifically addresses caregivers of patients with multiple sclerosis, those caring for people with other types of chronic disabilities face caregiving and emotional issues similar to the ones described here.]

Caring for someone with a chronic illness like multiple sclerosis (MS) can be deeply satisfying. Partners, family, and friends can be drawn more closely together when they meet the challenges. But caregiving can also be physically and emotionally exhausting, especially for the person who is the primary caregiver. That person is most often a partner or spouse, but can also be a child, parent, or friend.

There are a wide range of caregiving activities, just as there are a wide range of abilities and disabilities among people with MS. Someone giving care to a person who has relatively few functional difficulties may be helping with injections of a disease-modifying drug and offering support in dealing with the medical team. Someone caring for a person with a more severe level of disability may be involved in daily activities like toileting, dressing, transferring, and feeding, as well as medical treatments. This text provides an overview of the issues that caregivers in most kinds of situations might face. Those caring for someone who is newly diagnosed or who has little disability may want to concentrate only on those sections relevant to their particular situation.

Excerpted from "A Guide for Caregivers: Managing Major Changes," © 2008 National Multiple Sclerosis Society (www.nationalmssociety.org). Reprinted with permission.

Throughout this text, the term caregiver is used to refer to the person primarily responsible for providing daily care to a person with MS. It may help to remember that the person giving care and the person receiving care are in this together. This text sometimes refers to them as carepartners. MS doesn't change the fact that important relationships are always a two-way street. The person with disabilities may need a great deal of assistance, but the needs and concerns of both partners must be addressed if the relationship is to remain healthy.

Practical Decisions

Most people with MS do not develop such severe disability that they require full-time, long-term care. But since there is no way to predict who will develop severe disability, it is wise to make contingency plans. This means investigating the kinds and costs of local long-term care options before a crisis occurs.

Financial and Life Planning

Financial and life planning for continued financial stability are essential and should be undertaken early. The process of long-term planning will help the carepartners feel more secure about their well-being, regardless of what the future brings. A book titled *Adapting: Financial Planning for a Life with Multiple Sclerosis* is available at www.nationalmssociety.org/FinancialPlanning or from your chapter.

Life planning includes an investigation of income tax issues, protecting existing assets, saving for future financial needs, and end-of-life planning. People should seek advice about insurance, employment rights, and state assistance, and discuss all options.

Carepartners need to understand the coverage provided by their medical insurance, including Medicare, Social Security benefits, and available private disability insurance. Some people may qualify for state programs such as public assistance, food stamps, or Medicaid. Hospital or clinic social workers are resources for good information regarding these programs.

Carepartners also need a clear understanding of the Americans with Disabilities Act (ADA) and other legislation that provide protections concerning transportation, recreation, and employment. A booklet outlining the basics of the ADA is available from the National MS Society.

Since each person's situation is unique and the laws pertaining to legal and financial issues vary from state to state, it is wise to seek the advice of professional planners and elder law attorneys who specialize in disability-related law. Professionals can help sort through the available options and explain the possible consequences of various choices.

Advance medical directives preserve a person's right to accept or reject medical treatment. They are essential tools for maintaining personal control in the event of incapacitating illness or disability. Medical directives come in two forms. Both are needed for complete protection: (1) a living will, in which the person outlines specific treatment guidelines to be followed by healthcare providers; (2) a health care proxy in which the person designates a trusted individual to make medical decisions if the person is unable to do so. Advance directive requirements, like other legal and financial issues, vary from state to state. They should be written with the help of an attorney who is familiar with the relevant state laws. An attorney is not needed for advance directives naming a health care proxy.

What Level of Care Is Needed?

Evaluating care needs should also be a joint effort. Ask your medical team to assess what treatments, adaptations, and other changes are necessary. For some, training in self-administering medical treatments, advice on coping with fatigue and occasional relapses, and some long-range financial planning will suffice. For others, at-home care is the best option. And sometimes a nursing home or assisted living center is the better choice for all concerned.

It's important to be realistic about what the person with MS needs, and what the caregiver can provide in terms of time, kinds of care, and financial responsibility. This is more easily said than done. Making changes—whether small or large—can be enormously difficult. Coming to terms with chronic illness and disability takes time and strength. Rational decision making can be sidetracked by anger, guilt, grief, confusion, or shame. Carepartners can benefit from speaking with a therapist, counselor, or other person outside the situation to get a clearer perspective.

Don't be afraid to ask for help. The cost of not asking for help may be very high for everyone involved.

At-Home Care

Even people with a significant level of disability can live at home successfully. There are usually a number of solutions to practical problems. For example, someone who cannot transfer from wheelchair to bed or bath can be moved using the proper kind of lift. People with disabilities can be more independent when a home has wide doorways and grab bars. When the caregiver works full-time and the person with MS needs some aid and companionship during the day, adult day programs may be an option. Caregiver burnout can be avoided when the carepartners make use of respite care, friends, and support groups.

Other Care Options

Providing care at home will be impossible for some people. There are different kinds of live-in facilities, including assisted living, nursing homes, and continuing care communities. Deciding what kind of facility is best will depend on individual needs and financial resources available.

The Cost of Care

All care options cost money—a situation that often coincides with a drop in the income earned by the person with MS. Researching possible resources begins with asking questions. Start with the staff at your chapter of the National MS Society or with a social worker at your hospital, social agency, or MS clinic.

Resources include local public agencies for people with disabilities such as independent living centers and agencies for senior citizens. (They often serve younger people with disabilities.) Some states have respite care and/or personal-care assistant programs for people who are not otherwise eligible for Medicaid.

Caring at Home

Adapting for Safety, Accessibility, and Comfort

Adaptations can increase safety, accessibility, and comfort for everyone. But before deciding to make major home renovations, ask a doctor for a referral to an occupational therapist (OT) for a home visit. OTs can suggest ways to keep the person with MS as independent as possible, ensure safety, and reduce the physical strain on the caregiver. Ramps, widened doorways, and renovations in the kitchen and bath can often solve accessibility problems. Not all changes involve major expense. The National MS Society has information about practical, low-cost modifications and can provide referrals to appropriate resources.

Sometimes the best choice involves moving to more accessible housing. Moving to a place that is near public transportation, stores, and other public facilities can give a person with disabilities more choices. It might also make it easier to hire necessary help.

Flexible Roles

Changes are not confined to doorways or light switches. Relationships are affected as well. People with severe MS lose independence. Caregivers have to take on more responsibilities. This shift can be a source of tremendous anxiety.

Inevitably, the caregiver and the person with MS will have different perspectives about the same issue—about adaptations, the severity of symptoms, the amount of assistance needed, or how best to schedule hired help. It might help to remember that MS affects everyone involved, but it affects everyone differently.

MS is extremely changeable and unpredictable. People experience attacks and remission, loss, and recovery or partial recovery of abilities. One day a person with MS can dress alone, the next day the person can't. The caregiver has to take and then give back responsibility for tasks all the time.

Carepartners will need to rethink tasks and family schedules in order to ensure the smooth running of the household. For example:

- Household tasks such as general cleaning, shopping, cooking, laundry, child care, and transportation
- Care-related tasks such as dressing, bathing, eating, toileting, exercising, transportation, doctor visits, and taking medication
- Daily activities such as work, recreation, entertainment, exercise, hobbies, private time, and religious activities

Plan to re-evaluate schedules and task assignments as needs and circumstances change. And make sure to schedule personal time for everyone in the household.

Helping with Daily Activities

If a task seems impossibly difficult or stressful, there is probably an easier way to do it. The medical team can provide tips and techniques for bathing, dressing, toileting, and safe transfers. Other caregivers and the National MS Society are also good sources of advice and tips.

Roles and Gender Differences

Women and men who act as caregivers face the same day-to-day responsibilities, frustrations, and satisfactions. However, women caregivers may feel more comfortable than men caregivers, since caregiving has traditionally been viewed as a more feminine role.

Studies have found that many men who are caregivers report difficulty in discussing their problems and are more likely to suppress emotional reactions. They find it more difficult to ask for help and many do not use the resources available to caregivers. On the other hand, men may be more willing to participate in social and recreational activities that contribute to their overall well-being.

Some women are better at expressing their feelings and accessing supportive networks. But women caregivers are more likely to neglect their own health, and their need for outside activities. They tend to report more physical and emotional ailments than their male counterparts.

When a Child Is a Caregiver

Sometimes children assume major household and personal care responsibilities when a parent has disability due to MS. This is more likely to occur in single-parent households. While it is positive for children to take on household responsibilities, their needs must be carefully balanced with the amount and level of caregiving they are expected to do.

Children are not equipped to handle the stress of being a primary caregiver. They should never be responsible for a parent's medical treatments or daily functions such as toileting. Children under 10 can certainly handle some household chores. Young teenagers can take on more responsibility, but they also need to spend some time with their peers. Older teenagers and young adults may be competent caregivers, but they should not be expected to undertake long-term primary care. They have their own futures to attend to.

When a Parent Is a Caregiver

The return of an adult child to the home can be stressful for both the parents and the adult child. Often, this homecoming reproduces the earlier struggles that occurred before the child became independent. Parents probably have house rules that they want to have respected. But the adult child needs to be treated as an adult, and some house rules may presume the wrong kind of dependence.

As parents age, providing care will become more difficult. In time, one or both parents may become ill and require care themselves. Alternative care plans and living arrangements should be discussed with the adult child well before such a crisis occurs.

Family and Friends

Family and friends can be crucial members in a network of assistance but caregivers often report that it's hard to actually get their help. The first step is to tell friends and family that their help is needed and welcomed. Friends often worry that offering help might seem intrusive, especially when it looks as if things are being handled well.

Keep a list of projects, errands, and services that friends could do. Then, the next time someone offers to help in some way, it will be easy to oblige them. Give people specific, time-limited tasks. Asking a friend or relative to come by on Saturday for 3 hours in the afternoon so the caregiver can run errands is going to be more successful than asking them to stop by when they have a moment.

Hiring Help

People with disabilities need most help with daily care. Unfortunately, this kind of help is generally not covered by insurance plans. Unless one of the carepartners has a long-term care insurance policy with a home care provision, paid care will be limited to what the family can afford.

Doctors often refer to specific professional nurses and therapist agencies. However, it is often less expensive to hire home care aides and domestic assistants independently. Hiring capable, reliable, and trustworthy help will be easier if the needs and concerns of the person receiving care are discussed in advance. The person with MS should always be part of the interview process.

Other caregivers, the health-care team, and the National MS Society can be of help in locating reliable agencies that screen and refer potential candidates. They can also provide you with tips on how to find, interview, and train home care workers on your own.

Neighborhood teenagers are an underused source of low-cost help. Some schools require community service, and many teenagers would like part-time work. Ask the honors program advisor at the local public high school for names of interested students. Be willing to write recommendation letters for students who work for you and be ready to teach them something about MS and disability. Be prepared to pay at least the minimum wage.

Safety and Security

Leaving a person with significant disabilities home alone can be a frightening proposition for both partners. Advance planning and adaptation of the home can decrease these worries. Accessible peepholes in the front door, portable telephones with speed dial, automatic door openers, and "life-net" call systems that summon help in an emergency may provide security.

If there is no secure way to leave a person with a severe disability home alone, then don't do it! You must find help or alternatives.

Medical Issues

Management of MS and its symptoms will be easier if everyone involved learns as much about the disease as possible. For general information, contact the National MS Society. To get the best information about an individual, caregivers should rely first on the person with MS, and that person's medical professionals.

The Health-Care Team and Symptom Management

Many MS symptoms can be controlled by medications, management techniques, and rehabilitative therapies. The health-care team can advise carepartners about diet and routines that will regularize toileting and sleep habits. Although MS cannot yet be cured, symptoms can be managed.

For some people, the most frightening aspect of giving care to someone with a chronic disease is being responsible for treatments. This may involve keeping track of medications, administering injectable drugs, or performing intermittent urinary catheterization.

Caregivers can and should make appointments with health-care professionals to get information, advice, and training. Treatment plans can fail if the caregiver does not know the medical staff, does not understand why and how a procedure is done, or gets instructions that are impossible to carry out. If there are problems with carrying out a medical or treatment procedure, contact the health-care team and arrange for a followup training session. With proper training and a little experience, most caregivers end up feeling confident about this part of their role.

It Isn't Always MS

Both the person with MS and the caregiver need to remember that having MS doesn't protect anyone from the normal ills that can affect us. This is especially important for people with MS who see a neurologist for their medical care. Specialists may not suggest routine, preventive health exams like Pap smears or prostate exams.

Emotional Support

Handling Stress and Caregiver Burnout

Providing emotional support and physical care to someone with MS is often deeply satisfying, but it is sometimes distressing, and now and then simply overwhelming. The strain of balancing employment, child-rearing, increased responsibilities in the home, and the care of the ill person may lead to feelings of martyrdom, anger, and guilt.

One of the biggest mistakes caregivers make is thinking that they can—and should—handle everything alone. The best way to avoid burnout is to have the practical and emotional support of other people. Sharing problems with others not only relieves stress, but can give new perspectives on problems.

"Why Doesn't Anyone Ask How I Am?"

It is easy to feel invisible. Everyone's attention goes to the person with MS and no one seems to understand what the caregiver is going through. Many caregivers say no one even asks. Mental health experts say it's not wise to let feelings of neglect build up. Caregivers need to speak up and tell other people what they need and how they feel.

If this seems like disloyalty to a partner or family member, or a caregiver fears being labeled a complainer, reach out to support groups, religious advisors, or mental health counselors to learn constructive communication techniques.

Take Care of the Caregiver

Many caregivers neglect their own physical health, too. They ignore their ailments and neglect preventive health measures like exercise, diet, and regular medical examinations.

Many caregivers do not get 7 hours of sleep a night. If sleep is regularly disrupted because the person with MS wakes in the night needing help with toileting or physical problems, discuss the problems with a health-care professional.

The person with MS needs a healthy caregiver. Both partners need uninterrupted sleep.

Outside Activities

Researchers report that the emotional stress of caring has little to do with the physical condition of the person with MS or the length of time the person has been ill.

Emotional stress seems more related to how "trapped" caregivers feel in their situation. This, in turn, seems to be closely related to the satisfaction they have in their personal and social relationships, and the amount of time available to pursue their own interests and activities.

Successful caregivers don't give up enjoyable activities. Many organizations have respite care programs. Other family members are often willing—even pleased—to spend time with the person with MS. It may be possible to arrange respite care on a regular basis. Keep a list of people to ask on an occasional basis as well.

Two-Way Communication

Many emotional stresses are the result of poor communication. The caregiver should be able to discuss concerns and fears openly; the person receiving care isn't the only one who needs emotional support. Although collaboration isn't always easy or possible, working out long-term plans and goals together will help both carepartners to feel more secure.

The emotional and cognitive symptoms of MS are often more distressing than the physical changes. If memory loss, problems with problem solving, mood swings, or depression are interfering with open communication or disrupting daily activities, consult a health-care professional.

Effective Ways to Acknowledge Feelings

Ignoring a problem will not make it disappear. Anger, grief, and fear soon become guilt, numbness, and resentment. Some people find that talking about their concerns happens more easily when they schedule a regular time for conversation. Taking time out to collect feelings before presenting them for discussion will make it easier to speak clearly and calmly.

Handling Unpredictability

Living with MS means expecting the unexpected, making backup plans, and focusing on what can be done rather than what can't. The unpredictability of MS can be very stressful, but it can be managed.

When making plans for outings, for example, always include extra time for travel. Calling ahead to check out bathroom facilities and entranceways is wise. Buildings are not always accessible, even when they say they are. Don't make plans too complicated. And when plans fall through, have an alternative ready. If the night out is impossible, order in pizza.

A list of backup people who can be contacted for help at short notice is also useful.

Dependency and Isolation

Fear of dependency and isolation are common in the families of the chronically ill. The person with MS is increasingly dependent on the carepartner, and the carepartner needs others for respite and support. Many caregivers feel shame about being dependent on others. As a result, many don't ask for the help that they need. Anxieties are greatly reduced for carepartners who are able to develop personal and social support.

Anger

Anger is a common carepartner emotion. The situation feels—and is—unfair. Hurtful words might be spoken during a difficult task, doors might be slammed during a disagreement, shouting in frustration sometimes replaces conversation. Anger and frustration must be addressed and healthy outlets developed before angry encounters become physically or emotionally abusive.

Avoiding Abuse

Abusive behavior is never acceptable. But tensions can mount in the most loving of families. While circumstances that produce frustration and anger are often unavoidable, an emotionally damaging or physically aggressive response is not okay. If tensions are mounting, call for a time-out, and call for help.

Physical abuse usually begins in the context of giving or getting personal help—the caregiver might be too rough during dressing or grooming. The person with MS might scratch a carepartner during a transfer. Once anger and frustration reach this level, abuse by either partner may become frequent.

The dangers of physical abuse are obvious, but emotional abuse is also unhealthy and damaging. Continued humiliation, harsh criticism, or manipulative behaviors can undermine the self-esteem of either partner.

Family and social groups may provide support and counsel. Therapists and marriage counselors can help partners work out problems. The National MS Society can offer local referrals.

The majority of carepartners never experiences such levels of distress or become abusive. However, separation, divorce, or a nursing home is a healthier option than a corrosive relationship.

Sex and Intimacy

Carepartners who are also spouses or partners usually face changes in their sexual relationship. These changes can have physical or emotional causes. MS can interfere with both sex drive and function.

41

Problems can include decreased vaginal lubrication, numbness or painful sensations, decreased libido, erectile dysfunction, or problems reaching orgasm.

MS fatigue can interfere with sexual activity. Spasticity or incontinence problems can negatively affect sexual desire. Most of these symptoms can be managed, so it is a good idea to seek the help of a health-care professional.

In addition to MS-related functional problems, changes in roles may change the sexual relationship. Caregivers feel that they are performing a parental role, rather than being a lover or spouse, and this can dampen intimacy.

Sexuality does not have to disappear. Partners might begin by discussing what they find most rewarding about their intimate relationship. Many preconceived ideas of what sex should be prevent the satisfaction of actual needs and pleasures. Discussion could lead to the discovery of more imaginative sexual behaviors.

Open and honest communication about sexual needs and pleasures without fear of ridicule or embarrassment is the crucial first step. Counseling with a sex therapist can be helpful in this process.

Self-Help Groups

Self-help groups can provide an outlet for emotions and a source of much needed practical information. All National MS Society chapters have affiliated self-help groups for people with MS, and many have groups for caregivers as well. Religious and spiritual communities often provide support and guidance.

Many carepartners say it is difficult to find time to attend group meetings. They want to use their limited time for other things. The benefits of a group might be obtained through the internet. There are many useful online caregiver chat groups.

Chapter 7

Abuse and People with Disabilities

Chapter Contents

Section 7.1—Bullying 44

Section 7.2—Abuse of Children with
Intellectual Disabilities 48

Section 7.3—People with Disabilities
and Sexual Violence 53

Section 7.1

Bullying

Each day, 10-year-old Seth asked his mom for more and more lunch money. Yet he seemed skinnier than ever and came home from school hungry. It turned out that Seth was handing his lunch money to a fifth-grader, who was threatening to beat him up if he didn't pay.

Kayla, 13, thought things were going well at her new school, since all the popular girls were being so nice to her. But then she found out that one of them had posted mean rumors about her on a website. Kayla cried herself to sleep that night and started going to the nurse's office complaining of a stomachache to avoid the girls in study hall.

Unfortunately, the kind of bullying that Seth and Kayla experienced is widespread. In national surveys, most kids and teens say that bullying happens at school.

A bully can turn something like going to the bus stop or recess into a nightmare for kids. Bullying can leave deep emotional scars that last for life. And in extreme situations, it can culminate in violent threats, property damage, or someone getting seriously hurt.

If your child is being bullied, there are ways to help him or her cope with it on a day-to-day basis and lessen its lasting impact. And even if bullying isn't an issue right in your house right now, it's important to discuss it so your kids will be prepared if it does happen.

What Is Bullying?

Most kids have been teased by a sibling or a friend at some point. And it's not usually harmful when done in a playful, friendly, and mutual way, and both kids find it funny. But when teasing becomes hurtful, unkind, and constant, it crosses the line into bullying and needs to stop.

Bullying is intentional tormenting in physical, verbal, or psychological ways. It can range from hitting, shoving, name-calling, threats, and mocking to extorting money and treasured possessions. Some kids bully by shunning others and spreading rumors about them. Others use email, chat rooms, instant messages, social networking websites, and text messages to taunt others or hurt their feelings.

It's important to take bullying seriously and not just brush it off as something that kids have to "tough out." The effects can be serious and affect kids' sense of self-worth and future relationships. In severe cases, bullying has contributed to tragedies, such as school shootings.

Why Kids Bully

Kids bully for a variety of reasons. Sometimes they pick on kids because they need a victim—someone who seems emotionally or physically weaker, or just acts or appears different in some way—to feel more important, popular, or in control. Although some bullies are bigger or stronger than their victims, that's not always the case.

Sometimes kids torment others because that's the way they've been treated. They may think their behavior is normal because they come from families or other settings where everyone regularly gets angry, shouts, or calls names. Some popular TV shows even seem to promote meanness—people are "voted off," shunned, or ridiculed for their appearance or lack of talent.

Signs of Bullying

Unless your child tells you about bullying—or has visible bruises or injuries—it can be difficult to figure out if it's happening. But there are some warning signs. Parents might notice kids acting differently or seeming anxious, or not eating, sleeping well, or doing the things they usually enjoy. When kids seem moodier or more easily upset than usual, or when they start avoiding certain situations, like taking the bus to school, it might be because of a bully.

If you suspect bullying but your child is reluctant to open up, find opportunities to bring up the issue in a more roundabout way. For instance, you might see a situation on a TV show and use it as a conversation starter, asking "What do you think of this?" or "What do you think that person should have done?" This might lead to questions like: "Have you ever seen this happen?" or "Have you ever experienced this?" You might want to talk about any experiences you or another family member had at that age.

Let your kids know that if they're being bullied—or see it happening to someone else—it's important to talk to someone about it, whether it's you, another adult (a teacher, school counselor, or family friend), or a sibling.

Helping Kids

If your child tells you about a bully, focus on offering comfort and support, no matter how upset you are. Kids are often reluctant to tell adults about bullying because they feel embarrassed and ashamed that it's happening, or worry that their parents will be disappointed.

Sometimes kids feel like it's their own fault, that if they looked or acted differently it wouldn't be happening. Sometimes they're scared that if the bully finds out that they told, it will get worse. Others are worried that their parents won't believe them or do anything about it. Or kids worry that their parents will urge them to fight back when they're scared to.

Praise your child for being brave enough to talk about it. Remind your child that he or she isn't alone—a lot of people get bullied at some point. Emphasize that it's the bully who is behaving badly—not your child. Reassure your child that you will figure out what to do about it together.

Sometimes an older sibling or friend can help deal with the situation. It may help your daughter to hear how the older sister she idolizes was teased about her braces and how she dealt with it. An older sibling or friend also might be able to give you some perspective on what's happening at school, or wherever the bullying is happening, and help you figure out the best solution.

Take it seriously if you hear that the bullying will get worse if the bully finds out that your child told. Sometimes it's useful to approach the bully's parents. In other cases, teachers or counselors are the best ones to contact first. If you've tried those methods and still want to speak to the bullying child's parents, it's best to do so in a context where a school official, such as a counselor, can mediate.

Many states have bullying laws and policies. Find out about the laws in your community. In certain cases, if you have serious concerns about your child's safety, you may need to contact legal authorities.

Advice for Kids

The key to helping kids is providing strategies that deal with bullying on an everyday basis and also help restore their self-esteem and regain a sense of dignity.

It may be tempting to tell a kid to fight back. After all, you're angry that your child is suffering and maybe you were told to "stand up for yourself" when you were young. And you may worry that your child will continue to suffer at the hands of the bully.

But it's important to advise kids not to respond to bullying by fighting or bullying back. It can quickly escalate into violence, trouble, and someone getting injured. Instead, it's best to walk away from the situation, hang out with others, and tell an adult.

Here are some other strategies to discuss with kids that can help improve the situation and make them feel better:

- Avoid the bully and use the buddy system. Use a different bathroom if a bully is nearby and don't go to your locker when there is nobody around.

- Make sure you have someone with you so that you're not alone with the bully. Buddy up with a friend on the bus, in the hallways, or at recess—wherever the bully is. Offer to do the same for a friend.

- Hold the anger. It's natural to get upset by the bully, but that's what bullies thrive on. It makes them feel more powerful. Practice not reacting by crying or looking red or upset. It takes a lot of practice, but it's a useful skill for keeping off of a bully's radar. Sometimes kids find it useful to practice "cool down" strategies such as counting to 10, writing down their angry words, taking deep breaths or walking away. Sometimes the best thing to do is to teach kids to wear a "poker face" until they are clear of any danger (smiling or laughing may provoke the bully).

- Act brave, walk away, and ignore the bully. Firmly and clearly tell the bully to stop, then walk away. Practice ways to ignore the hurtful remarks, like acting uninterested or texting someone on your cell phone.

- By ignoring the bully, you're showing that you don't care. Eventually, the bully will probably get bored with trying to bother you.

- Tell an adult. Teachers, principals, parents, and lunchroom personnel at school can all help stop bullying.

- Talk about it. Talk to someone you trust, such as a guidance counselor, teacher, sibling, or friend. They may offer some helpful suggestions, and even if they can't fix the situation, it may help you feel a little less alone.

- Remove the incentives. If the bully is demanding your lunch money, start bringing your lunch. If he's trying to get your music player, don't bring it to school.

Reaching Out

At home you can lessen the impact of the bullying. Encourage your kids to get together with friends that help build their confidence. Help them meet other kids by joining clubs or sports programs. And find activities that can help a child feel confident and strong. Maybe it's a self-defense class like karate or a movement or other gym class.

And just remember: As upsetting as bullying can be for you and your family, lots of people and resources are available to help.

Section 7.2

Abuse of Children with Intellectual Disabilities

"Abuse of Children with Intellectual Disabilities," by Leigh Ann Davis, M.S.S.W., M.P.A. Reprinted courtesy of The Arc of the United States (www.thearc.org), Copyright 2009.

Are children with disabilities at higher risk of being abused?

Children with disabilities of any kind are not identified in crime statistic systems in the United States, making it difficult to determine their risk for abuse (Sullivan, 2003). A number of weak and small-scale studies found that children with all types of disabilities are abused more often than children without disabilities. Studies show that rates of abuse among children with disabilities are variable, ranging from a low of 22 percent to a high of 70 percent (National Research Council, 2001). Although the studies found a wide range of abuse prevalence, when taken as a whole, they provide consistent evidence that there is a link between children with disabilities and abuse (Sobsey, 1994).

One in three children with an identified disability for which they receive special education services are victims of some type of maltreatment (i.e., either neglect, physical abuse, or sexual abuse) whereas one in 10 nondisabled children experience abuse. Children with any type of disability are 3.44 times more likely to be a victim of some type of abuse compared to children without disabilities (Sullivan & Knutson, 2000).

Looking specifically at individuals with intellectual disabilities, they are four to 10 more times as likely to be victims of crime than others without disabilities (Sobsey et al., 1995). One study found that children with intellectual disabilities were at twice the risk of physical and sexual abuse compared to children without disabilities (Crosse et al., 1993).

Why are these children more likely to be abused?

According to researchers, disability can act to increase vulnerability to abuse (often indirectly as a function of society's response to disability rather than the disability in itself being the cause of abuse). For example, adults may decide against making any formal reports of abuse because of the child's disability status, making the abuse of those with disabilities easier for the abuser (Sullivan, 2003). Parents fear if they report abuse occurring in the group home, they may be forced to take their child out of the home with few options for other safe living arrangements. Often the abusers are parents or other close caregivers who keep the abuse secret and do not report out of fear of legal and other ramifications.

Children may not report abuse because they don't understand what abuse is or what acts are abusive. Communication problems that are inherent in many disabilities also make it difficult for children to understand and or verbalize episodes of abuse (Knutson & Sullivan, 1993). Those with limited speaking abilities have had no way to talk about or report abuse. Only recently have pictures demonstrating acts of abuse and sexual anatomy been added to communication boards to help non-communicative children and adults (or those with limited communication) report acts of abuse.

Are children with different types of disabilities more at risk for being abused?

A number of studies have found that different types of disabilities have differing degrees of risk for exposure to violence. For example, Sullivan (2003) reported that those with behavior disorders face greater risk of physical abuse, whereas those with speech/language disorders are at risk for neglect.

49

Sullivan & Knutson (1998) also found that out of all the types of disability, children with behavior disorders and children with intellectual disabilities were both at increased risk for all three forms of abuse (neglect, physical abuse, and sexual abuse) compared to those children with other types of disabilities (speech/language disorders, hearing impairments, learning disabilities, health impairments, and Attention Deficit Disorder).

There are no differences in which form of child maltreatment occurs the most often between disabled and nondisabled children. For both groups, neglect is the most prevalent, followed by physical abuse, sexual abuse, and emotional abuse (Sullivan & Knutson, 2000).

How can I tell if a child with disabilities is being abused?

Children with and without disabilities share similar indicators of abuse. Along with physical signs (bruises, broken bones, head injuries, or other outward marks) two primary indicators are reports from the child that abuse has occurred and changes in the child's behavior. Children with disabilities face greater risk of abuse going unnoticed if their behavior change can be attributed to their disability instead of the abuse. Also, children with intellectual disabilities may be viewed as easily suggestible or untrustworthy, especially when the report involves abuse that seems improbable. Any time abuse is suspected, it is the adult's responsibility to carefully monitor the child's behavior, ask the child about his or her safety, and follow through by reporting any suspected abuse. State laws vary regarding who is considered a mandated reporter, although usually professionals who have regular contact with children are included, such as teachers, physicians, dentists, speech pathologists, etc.

What are the consequences of being abused?

Consequences of abuse may be physical in nature, such as damage to the central nervous system, fractures, injury to internal organs of the abdomen, burns, malnutrition, and trauma to the head (such as in the case of Shaken Baby Syndrome). Other consequences reap havoc on the heart and in the mind of a child, with abuse resulting in long-term emotional trauma and behavioral problems.

Another possible consequence of being abused is to become disabled. Some children who had never had a disability before become disabled due to abuse. For example, a 1-year study of children with firearm injuries identified an 11.7% mortality rate and a 10% permanent disability rate. (Dowd et al., 1994).

How can I help prevent abuse of children with intellectual disabilities?

Encourage training and continuing education about violence against children with disabilities for those with disabilities themselves, their families, legal professionals, judges, prosecutors, victim advocacy agencies, Guardians ad Litem, public defenders, and police officers. Children with disabilities need early education about the risks of abuse and how to avoid it in a way that they can understand.

Parents can get to know all persons working with their child and observe interactions closely for any signs of abuse. Parents and other caregivers may be the abusers, so other adults in the child's life should also be able to identify possible abuse and know how to go about reporting the abuse.

Parents of children with disabilities and the organizations they are a part of (such as local chapters of The Arc or state Developmental Disability Councils) can form relationships with local victim assistance or child abuse agencies, share each other's expertise, and partner together in serving children with disabilities in their local communities.

Obtaining (or advocating for the funding of) family support programs, such as respite care, that have a direct impact on families with disabilities can help prevent abuse by giving families breaks from day-to-day caregiver responsibilities that can seem overwhelming.

What legislation exists to help children with disabilities?

Although there is no single public policy initiative that addresses abuse of children with disabilities, there have been some attempts to address the issue. The Crime Victims with Disabilities Awareness Act of 1998 mandated the inclusion of disability status in the U.S. National Crime Victim Survey. It also mandated that research be conducted to address crimes against individuals with disabilities, including children. See the report at www.nap.edu/catalog/10042.html.

The Child Abuse Prevention and Treatment Act (CAPTA) is a law that helps prevent children from being abused, including those with disabilities. Since 1974, this law has been part of the federal government's effort to help states and communities improve their practices in preventing and treating child abuse and neglect. CAPTA provides grants to states to support child protective services (CPS) and community-based preventive services, as well as research, training, data collection, and program evaluation. (See www.cwla.org for more information.)

Contact for More Information

Prevent Child Abuse America

Toll-Free: 800-244-5373
Website: www.preventchildabuse.org

To Report Abuse

Contact your local child protection or law enforcement agency. State laws vary regarding who is a mandated reporter. If you need assistance with reporting or have questions about reporting abuse, contact ChildHelp USA's 24-hour hotline at 800-4-A-CHILD (422-4453).

References

Crosse, S., Elyse, K. & Ratnofsky, A. (1993). *A report on the maltreatment of children with disabilities.* Washington, DC: National Center on Child Abuse and Neglect, U.S. Department of Health and Human Services.

Dowd, M.D., Knapp, J.P. & Fitzmaurice, L.S. (1994). Pediatric firearm injuries, Kansas City, 1992: A population-based study. *Pediatrics,* 94, 867–873.

Knutson, J. & Sullivan, P. (1993). Communicative disorders as a risk factor in abuse. *Topics in Language Disorders,* 13 (4), 1–14.

National Research Council (2001). *Crime victims with developmental disabilities: Report of a workshop.* Committee on Law & Justice. Joan Petersilia, Joseph Foote, and Nancy A. Crowell, editors. Commission on Behavioral and Social Sciences and Education. Washington, D.C: National Academy Press.

Sobsey, D. (1992). *Violence and abuse in the lives of people with disabilities: The end of silent acceptance?* Paul H. Brookes Publishing Co: Baltimore, MD.

Sobsey, D., Wells, D., Lucardie, R. & Mansell, S. (1995). *Violence & disability: An annotated bibliography.* Baltimore: Brookes Publishing.

Sullivan, P.M. (2003). *Violence against children with disabilities: Prevention, public policy, and research implications.* Conference Commissioned Paper for the National Conference on Preventing and Intervening in Violence Against Children and Adults with Disabilities (May 6-7, 2002), SUNY Upstate Medical University, NY.

Sullivan, P. & Knutson, J. (2000). Maltreatment and disabilities: A population-based epidemiological study. *Child Abuse & Neglect,* 24 (10), 1257–1273.

Sullivan, P. & Knutson, J. (1998). The association between child maltreatment and disabilities in a hospital-based epidemiological study. *Child Abuse & Neglect,* 22 (4), 271–288.

Section 7.3

People with Disabilities and Sexual Violence

"People with Intellectual Disabilities and Sexual Violence," by Leigh Ann Davis, M.S.S.W, M.P.A. Reprinted courtesy of The Arc of the United States (www.thearc.org), Copyright 2009.

What is sexual assault/sexual abuse?

Sexual assault is a crime of violence, anger, power, and control where sex is used as a weapon against the victim. It includes any unwanted sexual contact or attention achieved by force, threats, bribes, manipulation, pressure, tricks, or violence. It may be physical or non-physical and includes rape, attempted rape, incest and child molestation, and sexual harassment. It can also include fondling, exhibitionism, oral sex, exposure to sexual materials (pornography), and the use of inappropriate sexual remarks or language.

Sexual abuse is similar to sexual assault, but is a pattern of sexually violent behavior that can range from inappropriate touching to rape. The difference between the two is that sexual assault constitutes a single episode whereas sexual abuse is ongoing.

Sexual violence occurs in the home (sexual abuse of children, sexual assault by partners or relative), outside the home (in group homes or institutions), on the job, on transportation systems (while riding the bus or a taxi), and virtually anywhere.

How often do adults and children experience sexual violence?

Studies consistently demonstrate that people with intellectual disabilities are sexually victimized more often than others who do not have a disability (Furey, 1994). For example, one study reported that 25 percent of girls and women with intellectual disabilities who were referred for birth control had a history of sexual violence (Sobsey, 1994). Other studies suggest that 49 percent of people with intellectual disabilities will experience 10 or more sexually abusive incidents (Sobsey & Doe, 1991).

Any type of disability appears to contribute to higher risk of victimization but intellectual disabilities, communication disorders, and behavioral disorders appear to contribute to very high levels of risk, and having multiple disabilities (e.g., intellectual disabilities and behavior disorders) result in even higher risk levels (Sullivan & Knutson, 2000).

Children with intellectual disabilities are also at risk of being sexually abused. A study of approximately 55,000 children in Nebraska found that children with intellectual disabilities were 4.0 times as likely as children without disabilities to be sexually abused. (Sullivan & Knutson, 2000).

Women are sexually assaulted more often when compared to men whether they have a disability or not, so men with disabilities are often overlooked. Researchers have found that men with disabilities are twice as likely to become a victim of sexual violence compared to men without disabilities (The Roeher Institute, 1995).

Why is sexual violence so common among people with intellectual disabilities?

People with severe intellectual disabilities may not understand what is happening or have a way to communicate the assault to a trusted person. Others with a less severe disability may realize they are being assaulted, but don't know that it's illegal and that they have a right to say no. Due to threats to their well-being or that of their loved ones by the abuser, they may never tell anyone about the abuse, especially if committed by an authority figure whom they learn not to question. In addition, they are rarely educated about sexuality issues or provided assertiveness training. Even when a report is attempted, they face barriers when making statements to police because they may not be viewed as credible due to having a disability (Keilty & Connelly, 2001).

What risk factors contribute to the occurrence of sexual violence?

Some risk factors may include a feeling of powerlessness, communication skill deficits, and inability to protect oneself due to lack of instruction and/or resources. Individuals may live in over-controlled and authoritarian environments, contributing to the feeling of powerlessness over their situation. In addition, they are not given enough experiential opportunities to learn how to develop and use their own intuition (those who are taught can often detect between safe versus unsafe situations.)

Other factors include the caretaker's failure to 1) request information on the background of all those involved in the person's life, such as professionals, paraprofessionals, ancillary, and volunteer staff, 2) become familiar with the abuse-reporting attitudes and practices of the agency, and 3) assure there is a plan in place for responding to reports of abuse when they occur. Also, offenders are typically not caught and/or held accountable for these crimes, which allows abuse to continue.

Who is most likely to sexually assault?

As is the case for people without disabilities who experience sexual violence, perpetrators are often those who are known by the victim, such as family members, acquaintances, residential care staff, transportation providers, and personal care attendants. Research suggests that 97 to 99 percent of abusers are known and trusted by the victim who has intellectual disabilities. While in 32 percent of cases, abusers consisted of family members or acquaintances, 44 percent had a relationship with the victim specifically related to the person's disability (such as residential care staff, transportation providers, and personal care attendants). Therefore, the delivery system created to meet specialized care needs of those with intellectual disabilities contributes to the risk of sexual violence (Baladerian, 1991).

What are the effects of sexual violence on someone with intellectual disabilities?

Sexual violence causes harmful psychological, physical, and behavioral effects. The individual may become pregnant, acquire sexually transmitted diseases, bruises, lacerations, and other physical injuries. Psychosomatic symptoms often occur, such as stomachaches, headaches, seizures, and problems with sleeping. Common psychological consequences include depression, anxiety, panic attacks, low self-esteem, shame and guilt, irrational fear, and loss of trust. Behavioral difficulties include withdrawal, aggressiveness, and self-injurious and sexually inappropriate behavior (Sobsey, 1994).

What type of treatment or therapy is available for victims of sexual violence?

In the past the benefit of psychotherapy for people with intellectual disabilities was questioned, as well as the impact of sexual violence (whether or not it impacts people with intellectual disabilities as strongly as others without disabilities). Today, however, it is widely acknowledged that all people who experience sexual violence are affected and do require therapeutic counseling, even if they are non-verbal.

Locating a qualified therapist may be difficult since the person should be trained in child/adult sexual abuse and sexual assault treatment as well as intellectual disabilities. The therapist should also be trained in non-verbal mind-body healing modalities that do not require an intellectual processing component of the therapy. Payment for the therapy can be obtained through victim witness programs, community mental health centers or developmental disability centers.

How can sexual violence of people with intellectual disabilities be prevented?

The first step is recognizing the magnitude of the problem and facing the reality that people with intellectual disabilities are more likely to be assaulted sexually than those without disabilities. Also, societal attitudes must change to view victims with disabilities as having equal value as victims without disabilities, and giving them equal advocacy. Every sexual assault, regardless of who the victim is, must be taken seriously.

Secondly, sexual violence must be reported in order for repeat victimization to stop. While few people ever disclose sexual violence for a variety of understandable reasons, such non-disclosure promotes an environment ripe for continued victimization. Reporting can be increased by educating individuals with disabilities and service providers about sexual violence, improving the investigation and prosecution of this crime, and creating safe environments that allow victims to disclose.

In addition, employment policies must change to increase safety. For example, background checks on new employees should be conducted on a routine basis and those with criminal records should not be hired. Routine checks should consistently be conducted for current employees as well.

Sex education must be provided on a regular, ongoing basis, and self-determination and relationship-building skills taught so individuals with intellectual disabilities can learn how to develop safe relationships. Classes on sexual violence should be provided to teach individuals how to respond and protect themselves when they become sexual assault victims.

What should I do if I suspect sexual abuse/assault of someone I know?

All states have laws requiring professionals, such as case managers, direct care workers, police officers, and teachers to report abuse. Some states require the general public to report abuse as well. If you suspect a child is being sexually abused, contact your local child protective agency. If the person is an adult, contact adult protective services. These are also referred to as "Social Services," "Human Services," or "Children and Family Services" in the phone book.

You do not need proof to file a report. If you believe the person is in immediate danger, call the police. After a report is made, depending on how serious the abuse is, the incident is referred for investigation to the state social services agency (who handles civil investigations) or to the local law enforcement agency (who handles criminal investigations).

For more information on how you can help prevent sexual assault/ abuse, contact Prevent Child Abuse America at 800-555-3748 (200 S. Michigan Avenue, 17th Floor, Chicago, IL 60604) or visit their website at www.preventchildabuse.org and The Arc Riverside's CAN DO! Project at www.disability-abuse.com

References

Baladerian, N. (1991). Sexual abuse of people with developmental disabilities. Sexuality and Disability, 9(4), 323–335.

Furey, E. (1994). Sexual abuse of adults with mental retardation: Who and where. Mental Retardation, 32, 3, p. 173–180.

Keilty, J & Connelly, G. (2001). Making a statement: An exploratory study of barriers facing women with an intellectual disability when making a statement about sexual assault to police. Disability & Society, 16 (2), 273–291.

Sobsey, D. (1994). Violence and abuse in the lives of people with disabilities: The end of silent acceptance? Baltimore: Paul H. Brookes Publishing Co.

Sobsey, D. & Doe, T. (1991). Patterns of sexual abuse and assault. Sexuality and Disability, 9 (3), 243–259.

Sullivan, P.M. & Knutson, J.F. (1994). The relationship between child abuse and neglect and disabilities: Implications for research and practice. Omaha, NE: Boys Town National Research Hospital.

The Roeher Institute (1995). Harm's way: The many faces of violence and abuse against persons with disabilities in Canada.

Part Two

Types of Disabilities

Chapter 8

Overview of Birth Defects

What is a birth defect?

A birth defect is a problem that happens while the baby is developing in the mother's body. Most birth defects happen during the first 3 months of pregnancy.

A birth defect may affect how the body looks, works, or both. It can be found before birth, at birth, or any time after birth. Most defects are found within the first year of life. Some birth defects (such as cleft lip or clubfoot) are easy to see, but others (such as heart defects or hearing loss) are found using special tests (such as x-rays, CAT [computed tomography] scans, or hearing tests). Birth defects can vary from mild to severe.

Some birth defects can cause the baby to die. Babies with birth defects may need surgery or other medical treatments, but, if they receive the help they need, these babies often lead full lives.

What are the most common birth defects?

One of every 33 babies is born with a birth defect. A birth defect can affect almost any part of the body. The well-being of the child depends mostly on which organ or body part is involved and how much it is affected.

Excerpted from "Birth Defects: Frequently Asked Questions (FAQs)," by the National Center on Birth Defects and Developmental Disabilities (NCBDDD, www.cdc.gov/ncbddd), part of the Centers for Disease Control and Prevention, October 28, 2009.

Many birth defects affect the heart. About one in every 100 to 200 babies is born with a heart defect. Heart defects make up about one third to one fourth of all birth defects. Some of these heart defects can be serious, and a few are very severe. In some places of the world, heart defects cause half of all deaths from birth defects in children less than 1 year of age.

Other common birth defects are neural tube defects, which are defects of the spine (spina bifida) and brain (anencephaly). They affect about one of 1,000 pregnancies. These defects can be serious and are often life threatening. They happen less often than heart defects, but they cause many fetal and infant deaths.

Birth defects of the lip and roof of the mouth are also common. These birth defects, known as orofacial clefts, include cleft lip, cleft palate, and combined cleft lip and cleft palate. Cleft lip is more common than cleft palate. In many places of the world, orofacial clefts affect about one in 700 to 1,000 babies.

Some birth defects are common but rarely life threatening, though they often require medical and surgical attention. Hypospadias, for example, is a fairly common defect found in male babies. In babies with hypospadias, the opening of the urethra (where urine comes out) is not at the tip of the penis but on the underside. Treatment depends on how far away from the tip the opening is and can involve complex surgery. This defect is rarely as serious as the others listed in the preceding text, but it can cause great concern and sometimes has high medical costs. It rarely causes death.

These are only some of the most common birth defects. Two final points are worth noting. First, genetic conditions, though not mentioned so far, also occur often. Down syndrome, for example, is a genetic condition that affects about one in 800 babies, but it affects many more babies who are born to older women. Second, a woman who is pregnant may miscarry a baby (fetus) early, before it is time for the baby to be born. This often happens when the fetus has a severe birth defect. To know the true impact of birth defects and how often they occur, we not only need to look at babies born but also, if possible, look at all pregnancies.

What is my chance of having a baby with a birth defect?

In the United States, about 3% of babies are born with birth defects. Some women have a higher chance of having a child with a birth defect. Women over the age of 35 years have a higher chance of having a child with Down syndrome than women who are younger. If taken when a woman is pregnant, certain drugs can increase the chance of birth defects. Also, women who smoke and use alcohol while pregnant have a higher risk of having a baby with certain birth defects. Other women have a higher chance of having a baby with a birth defect because someone in their family had a similar birth defect. To learn more about your risk of having a baby with a birth defect, you can talk with a genetic counselor.

Also, to reduce your chances of having a baby with a birth defect, talk with your health care provider about any medicines that you take, do not drink alcohol or smoke, and be sure to take 400 micrograms of the B vitamin folic acid every day. It is the amount of folic acid found in most multivitamins.

Do genetic factors play a role in causing birth defects?

Yes, in some but not all cases. Changes in the genes can cause certain birth defects in infants. Genes tell each cell in the body how to combine with other cells to form parts of the body. For example, genes tell certain cells to make the heart, the kidneys, or the brain, and they tell other cells to make our physical features, like green eyes or brown hair. Genes also tell the cells how to work in the body. Genes give instructions for cells in our heart to beat, our stomach to digest food, our muscles to push and pull, and our brain to think.

Genes combine with many other genes to make chromosomes. Changes in single genes, groups of genes, or entire chromosomes can sometimes cause birth defects. These genetic changes might happen only in the infant, or they might pass down from one or both parents. Sometimes, there are other relatives in the family with the same birth defect, but not always.

Factors other than genetics can also increase the chance of having a baby with a birth defect. In some cases, the mother or baby has genes that are easily affected by factors outside the body that cause birth defects. In this case, genes and environment work together to cause a birth defect.

What causes birth defects?

We do not know what causes most birth defects. Sometimes they just happen and are not caused by anything that the parents did or didn't do. Many parents feel guilty if they have a child with a birth defect even if they did everything they could to have a healthy child. If you have a child with a birth defect, it might be helpful to talk with other parents who have had a child with the same condition. Sometimes the causes of birth defects are figured out after the baby is born. Whenever possible, it is important to know what you can do for a better chance of having a healthy child in the future. Some actions might increase the chances of having a baby with a birth defect.

Does smoking cause birth defects?

A woman who smokes while she is pregnant has a greater chance of having a premature (early) birth, a small baby, or a stillborn baby. If the mother smokes while pregnant, there is also an increased risk of the baby dying during the first year of life. Some types of birth defects have been linked to the mother's smoking. Birth defects that may be increased when the mother smokes include cleft lip, cleft palate, clubfoot, limb defects, some types of heart defects, gastroschisis (an opening in the muscles of the abdomen that allows the intestines to appear outside the body), and imperforate anus (there is no opening from the intestines to the outside of the body to allow stool or gas to be passed). Talk with your health care provider about ways to help you quit smoking if you are pregnant or can get pregnant.

Do illegal drugs cause birth defects?

Women who use illegal drugs, or street drugs, can have babies who are small, premature, or have other health problems, such as birth defects.

Women who use cocaine while pregnant are more likely to have babies with birth defects of the limbs, gut, kidneys, urinary system, and heart. Other drugs, such as marijuana and ecstasy, may also cause birth defects in babies.

Women should not use street drugs while they are pregnant. It is also important that women not use street drugs after they give birth because drugs can be passed through breast milk and can affect a baby's growth and development. Talk with your health care provider about ways to help you quit using street drugs before you get pregnant.

Chapter 9

Cerebral Palsy

Doctors use the term cerebral palsy to refer to any one of a number of neurological disorders that appear in infancy or early childhood and permanently affect body movement and muscle coordination but aren't progressive, in other words, they don't get worse over time. The term cerebral refers to the two halves or hemispheres of the brain, in this case to the motor area of the brain's outer layer (called the cerebral cortex), the part of the brain that directs muscle movement; palsy refers to the loss or impairment of motor function.

Even though cerebral palsy affects muscle movement, it isn't caused by problems in the muscles or nerves. It is caused by abnormalities inside the brain that disrupt the brain's ability to control movement and posture.

In some cases of cerebral palsy, the cerebral motor cortex hasn't developed normally during fetal growth. In others, the damage is a result of injury to the brain either before, during, or after birth. In either case, the damage is not repairable and the disabilities that result are permanent. New studies show links between abnormalities in the placenta (the after-birth) and cerebral palsy.

Children with cerebral palsy exhibit a wide variety of symptoms, including the following:

- Lack of muscle coordination when performing voluntary movements (ataxia)

Excerpted from "Cerebral Palsy: Hope Through Research," by the National Institute of Neurological Disorders and Stroke (NINDS, www.ninds.nih.gov), part of the National Institutes of Health, June 13, 2011.

- Stiff or tight muscles and exaggerated reflexes (spasticity)
- Walking with one foot or leg dragging
- Walking on the toes, a crouched gait, or a "scissored" gait
- Variations in muscle tone, either too stiff or too floppy
- Excessive drooling or difficulties swallowing or speaking
- Shaking (tremor) or random involuntary movements
- Difficulty with precise motions, such as writing or buttoning a shirt

The symptoms of cerebral palsy differ in type and severity from one person to the next, and may even change in an individual over time. Some people with cerebral palsy also have other medical disorders, including mental retardation, seizures, impaired vision or hearing, and abnormal physical sensations or perceptions.

Cerebral palsy doesn't always cause profound disabilities. While one child with severe cerebral palsy might be unable to walk and need extensive, lifelong care, another with mild cerebral palsy might be only slightly awkward and require no special assistance.

Cerebral palsy isn't a disease. It isn't contagious and it can't be passed from one generation to the next. There is no cure for cerebral palsy, but supportive treatments, medications, and surgery can help many individuals improve their motor skills and ability to communicate with the world.

What other conditions are associated with cerebral palsy?

Many individuals with cerebral palsy have no additional medical disorders. However, because cerebral palsy involves the brain and the brain controls so many of the body's functions, cerebral palsy can also cause seizures, impair intellectual development, and affect vision, hearing, and behavior. Coping with these disabilities may be even more of a challenge than coping with the motor impairments of cerebral palsy.

These additional medical conditions include:

- **Mental retardation:** Two thirds of individuals with cerebral palsy will be intellectually impaired. Mental impairment is more common among those with spastic quadriplegia than in those with other types of cerebral palsy, and children who have epilepsy and an abnormal electroencephalogram (EEG) or magnetic resonance imaging (MRI) are also more likely to have mental retardation.

- **Seizure disorder:** As many as half of all children with cerebral palsy have seizures. Seizures can take the form of the classic convulsions of tonic-clonic seizures or the less obvious focal (partial) seizures, in which the only symptoms may be muscle twitches or mental confusion.

- **Delayed growth and development:** A syndrome called failure to thrive is common in children with moderate-to-severe cerebral palsy, especially those with spastic quadriparesis. Failure to thrive is a general term doctors use to describe children who lag behind in growth and development. In babies this lag usually takes the form of too little weight gain. In young children it can appear as abnormal shortness, and in teenagers it may appear as a combination of shortness and lack of sexual development. In addition, the muscles and limbs affected by cerebral palsy tend to be smaller than normal. This is especially noticeable in children with spastic hemiplegia because limbs on the affected side of the body may not grow as quickly or as long as those on the normal side.

- **Spinal deformities:** Deformities of the spine—curvature (scoliosis), humpback (kyphosis), and saddle back (lordosis)—are associated with cerebral palsy. Spinal deformities can make sitting, standing, and walking difficult and cause chronic back pain.

- **Impaired vision, hearing, or speech:** A large number of children with cerebral palsy have strabismus, commonly called "cross eyes," in which the eyes are misaligned because of differences between the left and right eye muscles. In an adult, strabismus causes double vision. In children, the brain adapts to the condition by ignoring signals from one of the misaligned eyes. Untreated, this can lead to poor vision in one eye and can interfere with the ability to judge distance. In some cases, doctors will recommend surgery to realign the muscles. Children with hemiparesis may have hemianopia, which is defective vision or blindness that blurs the normal field of vision in one eye. In homonymous hemianopia, the impairment affects the same part of the visual field in both eyes. Impaired hearing is also more frequent among those with cerebral palsy than in the general population. Speech and language disorders, such as difficulty forming words and speaking clearly, are present in more than a third of those with cerebral palsy.

- **Drooling:** Some individuals with cerebral palsy drool because they have poor control of the muscles of the throat, mouth, and tongue. Drooling can cause severe skin irritation. Because it is socially unacceptable, drooling may also isolate children from their peers.

- **Incontinence:** A common complication of cerebral palsy is incontinence, caused by poor control of the muscles that keep the bladder closed. Incontinence can take the form of bed-wetting, uncontrolled urination during physical activities, or slow leaking of urine throughout the day.

- **Abnormal sensations and perceptions:** Some children with cerebral palsy have difficulty feeling simple sensations, such as touch. They may have stereognosis, which makes it difficult to perceive and identify objects using only the sense of touch. A child with stereognosis, for example, would have trouble closing his eyes and sensing the difference between a hard ball or a sponge ball placed in his hand.

How is cerebral palsy managed?

Cerebral palsy can't be cured, but treatment will often improve a child's capabilities. Many children go on to enjoy near-normal adult lives if their disabilities are properly managed. In general, the earlier treatment begins, the better chance children have of overcoming developmental disabilities or learning new ways to accomplish the tasks that challenge them.

There is no standard therapy that works for every individual with cerebral palsy. Once the diagnosis is made, and the type of cerebral palsy is determined, a team of health care professionals will work with a child and his or her parents to identify specific impairments and needs, and then develop an appropriate plan to tackle the core disabilities that affect the child's quality of life.

Chapter 10

Cleft Lip and Palate

Orofacial clefts are birth defects in which there is an opening in the lip and/or palate (roof of the mouth) that is caused by incomplete development during early fetal formation.

Cleft lip and cleft palate occur in about one or two of every 1,000 babies born in the United States each year, making it one of the most common major birth defects. Clefts occur more often in children of Asian, Latino, or Native American descent.

The good news is that both cleft lip and cleft palate are treatable. Most kids born with these can have surgery to repair these defects within the first 12–18 months of life.

About Oral Clefting

An orofacial cleft occurs when parts of the lip or palate do not completely fuse together during the first 3 months of pregnancy. A cleft lip may appear as a small notch in the edge of the lip only or extend into the nose. It may also extend into the gums.

A cleft palate may also vary in size, from a defect of the soft palate only to a complete cleft that extends through the hard palate. Because the lips and the palate develop separately, it is possible for a child to be born with a cleft lip only, cleft palate only, or both.

Most clefts can be categorized into three broad categories:

1. Cleft lip without a cleft palate
2. Cleft palate without a cleft lip
3. Cleft lip and cleft palate together

A cleft can occur on one side of the mouth (unilateral clefting) or on both sides of the mouth (bilateral clefting).

Cleft lip with or without cleft palate is generally more common among boys; however, cleft palate occurring alone is more common in girls than boys.

For the most part, because a cleft lip is visible it is often easier to identify than a cleft palate alone. A cleft lip may be detected through prenatal ultrasound; however, diagnosing a cleft palate this way is more difficult and it might not be seen.

Even if a cleft condition is detected during pregnancy, the diagnosis and extent of cleft lip and palate is confirmed by physical examination after the birth of the child.

Causes

Sometimes a cleft occurs as part of a syndrome, meaning there are birth defects in other parts of the body, too. Other times, it's genetic and runs in families—the risk may be higher for children whose sibling(s) or parents have a cleft or who have a history of cleft in their families. In these situations, both mothers and fathers can pass on a gene or genes that can contribute to the development of cleft lip or cleft palate.

Sometimes a cleft may be associated with environmental factors such as a woman's use of certain medications, exposure to cigarette smoke, or lack of certain vitamins while pregnant.

Most of the time, though, the cause isn't known.

Associated Problems

Cleft lip and palate can be associated with other problems, including feeding difficulties, middle ear fluid buildup and hearing loss, dental abnormalities, and speech difficulties.

Feeding Problems

Infants with a cleft lip alone usually have fewer problems feeding than those with a cleft palate. Feeding can be a big problem for a newborn baby with a cleft palate. Normally, the palate prevents food and liquids from entering the nose. The baby with an unrepaired cleft palate has difficulty sucking on a regular nipple and will usually require a special nipple and bottle along with proper positioning in order to feed. With these techniques, the caregiver will learn how to feed the baby before taking the baby home from the hospital. The child's doctor will carefully monitor the child's weight.

Middle Ear Fluid Buildup and Hearing Loss

Many children with cleft palate are prone to the buildup of fluid in the middle ear and/or ear infections caused by malfunction of the Eustachian tube. This fluid buildup behind the eardrum can cause hearing loss. For this reason, kids with cleft palate usually need small pressure equalization (PE) tubes placed in their eardrums to help them to drain the fluid and improve hearing. Kids with cleft palate should have their ears and hearing checked once or twice a year; more often if there is ear drainage or a child seems to be having difficulty hearing.

Dental Abnormalities

Children with a cleft lip and palate frequently have dental problems. These include small teeth, missing teeth, extra teeth (called supernumerary), or malpositioned teeth. They may have a defect in the gums or alveolar ridge (the bone that supports the teeth). Defects of the alveolar ridge can displace, tip, or rotate permanent teeth, or prevent permanent teeth from coming in properly.

Speech Difficulties

Kids with cleft lip have fewer speech problems than those with cleft palate. Approximately 15%–20% with cleft palate may have speech problems after repair of the cleft palate (palatoplasty). The most common is excess nasality or hypernasality. This happens because the palate that normally separates the nose from the mouth for most sounds does not close adequately. This condition makes it sound as if the person is talking through the nose.

Children with clefts also can have other types of speech problems unrelated to the cleft condition; for example, age-related errors such as saying "wed" instead of "red." Sometimes, the dental problems associated with the cleft will cause some sounds to be distorted, particularly "s," "sh," "ch," and "j" sounds.

A speech-language pathologist will carefully assess a child's speech and language skills. If your child does have a speech problem, the pathologist will identify the cause and recommend treatment.

Treatment

The complex needs of a child with cleft lip and cleft palate are best met by an interdisciplinary team of professionals from various specialities who work together. This is a standard of care that begins soon after the child's birth and continues to adulthood.

The members of the cleft lip and palate treatment team include [the following]:

- Geneticist

- Pediatrician

- Plastic surgeon

- Ear, nose, and throat physician (otolaryngologist)

- Oral surgeon

- Orthodontist

- Dentist

- Speech-language pathologist

- Audiologist

- Nurse

- Social worker

- Psychologist

- Team coordinator

The frequency of team visits will depend on the child's needs and can range from two to three times per year to once every 2 to 3 years. Which team members the child needs to see during a given visit will depend on his or her health needs, including psychosocial issues.

After each visit, a team report will be sent to the family and other professionals involved in the child's care. The team coordinator will help organize the visits with team members and other professionals.

Surgical Treatment for Cleft Lip and Cleft Palate

A cleft lip is usually repaired between the ages of 3 to 6 months. Some children who have very wide clefts of the lip may require a procedure such as lip adhesion or a device such as a molding plate to bring the parts closer together before the full lip repair. A child with a cleft lip that is repaired will have a scar on the lip under the nose. Surgery is performed in the hospital under general anesthesia.

A cleft palate is usually repaired between 9 and 12 months of age. By repairing the palate, the soft palate muscles from each side are connected to each other and the normal barrier between the mouth and nose created. Surgery for cleft palate is performed under general anesthesia and usually requires a 2-night stay in the hospital.

The goal of surgery is to create a palate that works well for speech. Some kids, however, will continue to sound nasal after cleft palate repair and some may become nasal due to natural growth changes or adenoid shrinkage.

In some cases, additional surgery may be needed to improve speech. This surgery is called a pharyngoplasty. It is often done when kids are in their early school years, but also can be done later.

As kids grow older, they might need additional surgeries, such as an alveolar bone graft, which is used to close the gap in the bone or gums near the front teeth. This provides stability for the permanent teeth and is usually done when kids are between 6 and 10 years old.

Other procedures might be options as kids get older. They may want to have their scars made less noticeable, improve the appearance of their nose and upper lip, or improve their bite with orthognathic surgery. These operations may improve speech and breathing, dental occlusion, and appearance. Your child's surgeon will talk with you about the timing and nature of these surgeries.

Dental and Orthodontic Treatment

The primary goal of dental care in kids with cleft lip and palate is to maintain healthy teeth and prevent cavities. Because of the various types of dental problems they may have, it is very important that they see their dentist regularly and keep their teeth clean by brushing and flossing regularly.

Orthodontic treatment is common in kids with cleft lip and palate and may begin as early as 6 years of age. Often orthodontic treatment involves various phases, typically starting with palatal expansion done to normalize the width of the palate. Later, braces are put on to place the teeth in their proper position. Your orthodontist will discuss timing of the phases of treatment with you.

Some kids with a cleft might be missing a permanent tooth, which can be replaced with a removable appliance or, in early adulthood, with a dental implant.

Speech Therapy

Expect to meet with the speech-language pathologist before your child's cleft palate surgery (about 7–9 months) to review the impact of the palate on speech and what to expect in speech development after surgery. An overview of treatment and ways to stimulate speech and language development will be discussed. After the cleft palate surgery, the speech-language pathologist will continue to closely monitor your child's speech and language and recommend therapy if needed.

Some kids with cleft palate will not require speech therapy after cleft palate repair. Others will have abnormal speech and will need intervention. After cleft palate repair, about 15–20% will have hypernasal speech and may require additional surgery or other forms of management to improve speech. Although surgery might improve nasality, it may not result in immediate correction of certain speech errors and speech therapy might be needed.

Some kids may require speech therapy for speech problems unrelated to the cleft. Whether or not your child will depends on the results of a detailed evaluation done by a certified speech-language pathologist.

Dealing with Emotional and Social Issues

Though they might encounter social, psychological, and educational challenges, kids with a cleft just want to be treated like everyone else.

Some kids struggle growing up with a cleft lip or cleft palate and might need help handling certain situations. The psychologists and social workers on the cleft palate team are available to guide you through these difficult times. The good news is that most kids with cleft lip or cleft palate grow up to be healthy, happy adults.

In the meantime, you can support your child with these tips:

- Try not to focus on the cleft and don't allow it to define who your child is.

- Create a warm, supportive, and accepting home environment where each person's individual worth is openly celebrated.

- Encourage your child to develop friendships with people from diverse backgrounds. Lead by example.

- Point out positive attributes in others that do not involve physical appearance.

- Encourage independence by giving your child the freedom to make decisions and take appropriate risks, letting his or her accomplishments lead to a sense of personal value. Having opportunities to make decisions early on—like picking out which clothes to wear—gives kids confidence and the skills to make bigger decisions later.

- Consider encouraging your child to present information about cleft lip and palate to his/her class with a special presentation that you arrange with the teacher. Perhaps your child would like you and/or a member from the cleft palate team to talk to the class. This can be especially effective with young children.

If your child is teased, talk about it and be a patient listener. Provide tools to confront the teasers by asking what your child would like to say and then practicing those statements. And it's important to keep the lines of communication open as your child approaches adolescence so that you can address his or her concerns about appearance.

If your child has difficulty with self-esteem or other psychosocial situations, contact a child psychologist or social worker for support and management. Together with the cleft palate team, you can help your child through tough times.

Chapter 11

Cystic Fibrosis

What Is Cystic Fibrosis?

Cystic fibrosis, or CF, is an inherited disease of your secretory glands, including the glands that make mucus and sweat.

"Inherited" means that the disease is passed through the genes from parents to children. People who have CF inherit two faulty CF genes—one from each parent. The parents likely don't have the disease themselves.

CF mostly affects the lungs, pancreas, liver, intestines, sinuses, and sex organs.

Causes of Cystic Fibrosis

A defect in the CFTR [cystic fibrosis transmembrane conductance regulator] gene causes cystic fibrosis (CF). This gene makes a protein that controls the movement of salt and water in and out of your body's cells. In people who have CF, the gene makes a protein that doesn't work right. This causes thick, sticky mucus and very salty sweat.

Research suggests that the CFTR protein also affects the body in other ways. This may help explain other symptoms and complications of CF.

More than a thousand known defects can affect the CFTR gene. What type of defect you or your child has may influence how severe CF is. Other genes also may play a role in how severe the disease is.

Excerpted from "Cystic Fibrosis," by the National Heart, Lung, and Blood Institute (NHLBI, www.nhlbi.nih.gov), part of the National Institutes of Health, March 2009.

How Is Cystic Fibrosis Inherited?

Every person inherits two CFTR genes—one from each parent. Children who inherit a faulty CFTR gene from each parent will have CF.

Children who inherit a faulty CFTR gene from one parent and a normal CFTR gene from the other parent will be "CF carriers." CF carriers usually have no symptoms of CF and live normal lives. However, carriers can pass the faulty CFTR gene on to their children.

Risk for Cystic Fibrosis

About 30,000 people in the United States have cystic fibrosis (CF). CF is one of the most common inherited diseases among Caucasians. About 1,000 new cases of CF are diagnosed each year.

CF affects both males and females and people from all racial and ethnic groups. However, the disease is most common among Caucasians of Northern European descent.

CF also is common among Latinos and Native Americans, especially the Pueblo and Zuni. The disease is much less common among African Americans and Asian Americans.

About 12 million Americans are carriers of a faulty CF gene. Many of them don't know that they're CF carriers.

Signs and Symptoms of Cystic Fibrosis

The symptoms of CF vary from person to person and over time. Sometimes you will have few symptoms. Other times, your symptoms may become more severe.

One of the first signs of cystic fibrosis (CF) that parents may notice is that their baby's skin tastes salty when kissed or the baby doesn't pass stool when first born.

Most of the other signs and symptoms of CF develop later. They are related to how CF affects the respiratory, digestive, or reproductive systems of the body.

Respiratory System Signs and Symptoms

People who have CF have thick, sticky mucus that builds up in their airways. This buildup of mucus makes it easier for bacteria to grow and cause infections. Infections can block the airways and cause frequent coughing that brings up thick sputum (spit) or mucus that's sometimes bloody.

People who have CF tend to have lung infections caused by unusual germs that don't respond to standard antibiotics. For example, lung infections due to bacteria called mucoid Pseudomonas are much more common in people who have CF. An infection caused by this bacteria may be a sign of CF.

People who have CF have frequent bouts of sinusitis, an infection of the air-filled spaces behind your eyes, nose, and forehead. Frequent bouts of bronchitis and pneumonia also occur. These infections can cause long-term lung damage.

As CF gets worse, you may develop more serious complications, such as pneumothorax, or collapsed lung; or bronchiectasis.

Some people who have CF also develop nasal polyps (growths in the nose) that may require surgery.

Digestive System Signs and Symptoms

Mucus that blocks tubes, or ducts, in your pancreas and prevents enzymes from reaching your intestines causes most digestive system signs and symptoms.

Without these enzymes, your intestines can't fully absorb fats and proteins. This can cause ongoing diarrhea or bulky, foul-smelling, greasy stools. Intestinal blockage also may occur, especially in newborns. Too much gas or severe constipation in the intestines may cause stomach pain and discomfort.

A hallmark of CF in children is poor weight gain and growth. These children are unable to get enough nutrients from their food due to the lack of enzymes to help absorb fats and proteins.

As CF gets worse, other complications may occur, such as the following:

- Pancreatitis (a condition in which the pancreas becomes inflamed, which causes pain)

- Rectal prolapse (frequent coughing or problems passing stools may cause rectal tissue from inside you to move out of your rectum)

- Liver disease due to inflamed or blocked bile ducts

- Diabetes

- Gallstones

Reproductive System Signs and Symptoms

Men who have CF are infertile because they're born without a vas deferens. This is the tube that delivers sperm from the testicle to the penis.

A woman who has CF may have a hard time getting pregnant because of mucus blocking her cervix or other CF complications.

Other Signs, Symptoms, and Complications

Other signs and symptoms of CF are related to an upset of the balance of minerals in your blood.

CF causes your sweat to become very salty. As a result, your body loses large amounts of salt when you sweat. This can cause dehydration (a condition in which your body doesn't have enough fluids), increased heart rate, tiredness, weakness, decreased blood pressure, heat stroke, and, rarely, death.

CF also can cause clubbing and low bone density. Clubbing is the widening and rounding of the tips of your fingers and toes. It develops late in CF because your lungs aren't moving enough oxygen into your bloodstream.

Low bone density also tends to occur late in CF. It can lead to a bone-thinning disorder called osteoporosis.

Treating Cystic Fibrosis

Cystic fibrosis (CF) has no cure. However, treatments have greatly improved in recent years. The goals of CF treatment are to do the following:

- Prevent and control lung infections

- Loosen and remove thick, sticky mucus from the lungs

- Prevent or treat blockages in the intestines

- Provide enough nutrition

- Prevent dehydration (a condition in which the body doesn't have enough fluids)

Depending on how severe the disease is, you or your child may be treated in a hospital.

Chapter 12

Inherited Disorders
of Metabolism

Recent innovations in medical technology have changed newborn screening programs in the United States. The widespread use of tandem mass spectrometry is helping to identify more inborn errors of metabolism. Primary care physicians often are the first to be contacted by state and reference laboratories when neonatal screening detects the possibility of an inborn error of metabolism. Physicians must take immediate steps to evaluate the infant and should be able to access a regional metabolic disorder subspecialty center. Detailed knowledge of biochemical pathways is not necessary to treat patients during the initial evaluation. Nonspecific metabolic abnormalities (e.g., hypoglycemia, metabolic acidosis, hyperammonemia) must be treated urgently even if the specific underlying metabolic disorder is not yet known. Similarly, physicians still must recognize inborn errors of metabolism that are not detected reliably by tandem mass spectrometry and know when to pursue additional diagnostic testing. The early and specific diagnosis of inborn errors of metabolism and prompt initiation of appropriate therapy are still the best determinants of outcome for these patients.

The topic of inborn errors of metabolism is challenging for most physicians. The number of known metabolic disorders is probably as large as the number of presenting symptoms that may indicate metabolic disturbances. Furthermore, physicians know they may not encounter certain rare inborn errors of metabolism during a lifetime of practice. Nonetheless, with a collective incidence of one in 1,500 persons, at least one of these disorders will be encountered by almost all practicing physicians.[1–3]

Improvements in medical technology and greater knowledge of the human genome are resulting in significant changes in the diagnosis, classification, and treatment of inherited metabolic disorders. Many known inborn errors of metabolism will be recognized earlier or treated differently because of these changes. It is important for primary care physicians to recognize the clinical signs of inborn errors of metabolism and to know when to pursue advanced laboratory testing or referral to a children's subspecialty center.

Early Diagnosis and Screening in Asymptomatic Infants

The principles of population screening to identify persons with biologic markers of disease and to apply interventions to prevent disease progression are well established. Screening tests must be timely and effective with a high predictive value. Current approaches to detecting inborn errors of metabolism revolve around laboratory screening for certain disorders in asymptomatic newborns, follow-up and verification of abnormal laboratory results, prompt physician recognition of unscreened disorders in symptomatic persons, and rapid implementation of appropriate therapies.

The increasing application of new technologies such as electrospray ionization–tandem mass spectrometry to newborn screening[4] in asymptomatic persons allows earlier identification of clearly defined inborn errors of metabolism. It also detects some conditions of uncertain clinical significance.[5] The inborn errors of metabolism detected by tandem mass spectrometry generally include aminoacidemias, urea cycle disorders, organic acidurias, and fatty acid oxidation disorders. Earlier recognition of these inborn errors of metabolism has the potential to reduce morbidity and mortality rates in these infants.[6]

Tandem mass spectrometry has been introduced or mandated in many states, with some states testing for up to seven conditions and others screening for up to 40 conditions. Therefore, physicians must be aware of variability in newborn screening among individual hospitals and states. Current state-by-state information on newborn screening programs can be obtained through the internet resource GeNeS-R-US (Genetic and Newborn Screening Resource Center of the United States; http://genes-r-us.uthscsa.edu).[7] Primary care physicians are most likely to be the first to inform parents of an abnormal result from a newborn screening program. In many instances, primary care physicians may need to clarify preliminary laboratory results or explain the possibility of a false-positive result.[6]

Early Diagnosis in Symptomatic Infants

Within a few days or weeks after birth, a previously healthy neonate may begin to show signs of an underlying metabolic disorder. Although the clinical picture may vary, infants with metabolic disorders typically present with lethargy, decreased feeding, vomiting, tachypnea (from acidosis), decreased perfusion, and seizures. As the metabolic illness progresses, there may be increasing stupor or coma associated with progressive abnormalities of tone (hypotonia, hypertonia), posture (fisting, opisthotonos), and movements (tongue-thrusting, lip-smacking, myoclonic jerks), and with sleep apnea.[8] Metabolic screening tests should be initiated. Elevated plasma ammonia levels, hypoglycemia, and metabolic acidosis, if present, are suggestive of inborn errors of metabolism. In addition, the parent or physician may notice an unusual odor in an infant with certain inborn errors of metabolism (e.g., maple syrup urine disease, phenylketonuria [PKU], hepatorenal tyrosinemia type 1, isovaleric acidemia). A disorder similar to Reye's syndrome (i.e., nonspecific hepatic encephalopathy, possibly with hypoglycemia) may be present secondary to abnormalities of gluconeogenesis, fatty acid oxidation, the electron transport chain, or organic acids.

Most metabolic disorders associated with organ system manifestations are not detected by tandem mass spectrometry screening. These highly diverse presentations of inborn errors of metabolism may be associated with dysfunction of the central nervous system (CNS), liver, kidney, eye, bone, blood, muscle, gastrointestinal tract, and integument. Infants with symptoms of acute or chronic encephalopathy usually require a focused but systematic evaluation by a children's neurologist and appropriate testing (e.g., magnetic resonance imaging, additional genetic or metabolic analysis). Subspecialty referral is likewise necessary for infants or children presenting with hepatic, renal, or cardiac syndromes; dysmorphic syndromes; ocular findings; or significant orthopedic abnormalities.

A "pattern recognition" approach helps guide the physician toward a differential diagnosis and targeted biochemical and molecular testing.[9] However, this approach is not to be confused with the identification of congenital malformations, particularly those related to chromosomal disorders. Patients generally have a normal appearance in the early stages of most inborn metabolic disorders. Because most inborn errors of metabolism are single-gene disorders, chromosomal testing usually is not indicated.

Considerations in Older Infants and Children

Older infants with inborn errors of metabolism may demonstrate paroxysmal stupor, lethargy, emesis, failure to thrive, or organomegaly. Neurologic findings of neurometabolic disorders are acquired macrocephaly or microcephaly (CNS storage, dysmyelination, atrophy), hypotonia, hypertonia/spasticity, seizures, or other movement disorders. General non-neurologic manifestations of neurometabolic disorders include skeletal abnormalities and coarse facial features (e.g., with mucopolysaccharidoses), macular or retinal changes (e.g., with leukodystrophies, poliodystrophies, mitochondrial disorders), corneal clouding (e.g., with Hurler's syndrome, galactosemia), skin changes (e.g., angiokeratomas in Fabry's disease), or hepatosplenomegaly (with various storage diseases).

Consistent features of metabolic disorders in toddlers and preschool-age children include stagnation or loss of cognitive milestones; loss of expressive language skills; progressive deficits in attention, focus, and concentration; and other behavioral changes. The physician should attempt to make fundamental distinctions between primary-genetic and secondary-acquired causes of conditions that present as developmental delay or failure to thrive. Clues can be extracted through careful family, social, environmental, and nutritional history-taking. Syndromes with metabolic disturbances may lead to the identification of clinically recognizable genetic disorders. Referral to a geneticist often is indicated to further evaluate physical findings of primary genetic determinants.

Initial laboratory investigations for older children are the same as for infants. Infants and children presenting with acute metabolic decompensation precipitated by periods of prolonged fasting should be evaluated further for those organic acid, fatty acid oxidation, or peroxisomal disorders that are not detected by tandem mass spectrometry or certain regional neonatal screening programs.

Cerebrospinal fluid (CSF) may be helpful in the evaluation of certain metabolic disorders after neuroimaging studies and basic blood and urine analyses have been completed. Common CSF studies include cells (to rule out inflammatory disorders), glucose (plus plasma glucose to evaluate for blood-brain barrier or glucose transporter disorders), lactate (as a marker of energy metabolism or mitochondrial disorders), total protein, and quantitative amino acids. Nuclear magnetic resonance spectroscopy can provide a noninvasive, in vivo evaluation of proton-containing metabolites and can lead to the diagnosis of certain rare, but potentially treatable, neurometabolic disorders.[10] Electron microscopic evaluation of a skin biopsy is a highly sensitive screening tool that provides valuable clues to stored membrane material or ultrastructural organelle changes.[11]

PKU

PKU is an autosomal-recessive disorder most commonly caused by a mutation in the gene coding for phenylalanine hydroxylase, an enzyme responsible for the conversion of phenylalanine to tyrosine. Sustained phenyl-alanine concentrations higher than 20 mg per dL (1,211 micro mol per L) usually correlate with classic symptoms of PKU, such as impaired head circumference growth, poor cognitive function, irritability, and lighter skin pigmentation. Infants diagnosed with PKU are treated with a special low-phenylalanine formula. Tyrosine is given at approximately 25 mg per kg of weight per day; amino acids are given at about 3 g per kg per day in infancy and 2 g per kg per day in childhood. Infants and children must be monitored regularly during the developmental period, and it is recommended that strict dietary therapy be continued for life. Special considerations for pregnant women with PKU include constant monitoring of phenylalanine concentrations to prevent intrauterine fetal malformation.[12]

Ornithine Transcarbamylase Deficiency

Ornithine transcarbamylase deficiency is the most common urea cycle disorder. Signs of ornithine transcarbamylase deficiency in infant boys include severe emesis, hyperammonemia, and progressive encephalopathy. Heterozygous girls, who demonstrate partial expression of the X-linked ornithine transcarbamylase deficiency disorder, may present with symptoms such as mild hyper-ammonemia and notable avoidance of dietary protein. Acute treatment options include sodium benzoate, sodium phenylacetate, and arginine. Certain persons may benefit from liver transplantation.

Methylmalonicaciduria Disorders

The most common genetic causes of methylmalonicaciduria are deficiencies in methylmalonyl-CoA mutase activity and in enzymatic synthesis of cobalamin. Pernicious anemia and dietary cobalamin deficiency also can result in abnormal methylmalonic acid metabolism. Metabolic ketoacidosis is the clinical hallmark of methylmalonicaciduria in infants. Therapy consists of protein restriction, restriction of methylmalonate precursors, and pharmacologic doses of vitamin B12.

MCAD Deficiency

The most common fatty acid oxidation disorder is MCAD [Medium-chain acyl-CoA dehydrogenase] deficiency. The majority of infants diagnosed with MCAD deficiency are homozygous for the A985G missense mutation and have northwestern European ancestry. Infants with MCAD deficiency appear to develop normally but present with rapidly progressive hypoglycemia, lethargy, and seizures, typically secondary to acute vomiting or fasting. Treatment of MCAD deficiency includes frequent cornstarch feeds and avoidance of fasting. Parents must have a basic understanding of the metabolic deficit in their child and should carry a letter from their treating physicians to alert emergency caregivers about the need for urgent attention in a crisis situation.

Galactosemia

There are three known enzymatic errors in galactose metabolism. The most common defect is confirmed by measuring decreased activity of erythrocyte galactose 1-phosphate uridyltransferase (GALT). Clinical manifestations of galactosemia include lethargy, hypotonia, jaundice, hypoglycemia, elevated liver enzymes, and coagulopathy. It is important to distinguish the galactosemia disease genotype (G/G) from asymptomatic variant genotypes (e.g., G/D, G/N, D/D), which can be picked up as "positive" in newborn screening.

The main treatment for infants with the G/G mutation or very low GALT activity is lactose-free formula followed by dietary restriction of all lactose-containing foods later in life. Untreated infants who survive the neonatal period may have severe growth failure, mental retardation, cataracts, ovarian failure, and liver cirrhosis. Despite early and adequate intervention, some children still may develop milder signs of these clinical manifestations.

Gaucher's Disease

Type 1 Gaucher's disease, the most common lysosomal storage disorder, typically presents with hepatosplenomegaly, pancytopenia, and destructive bone disease. Types 2 and 3 Gaucher's disease present with strabismus, bulbar signs, progressive cognitive deterioration, and myoclonic seizures. Treatment options for type 1 Gaucher's disease include regular infusions with recombinant human acid beta-glucosidase.

Importance of Early Treatment

Often, empiric therapeutic measures are needed before a definitive diagnosis is available. In a critically ill infant, aggressive treatment before the definitive confirmation of diagnosis is lifesaving and may reduce neurologic sequelae. Infants with a treatable organic acidemia (e.g., methylmalonic acidemia) may respond to 1 mg of intramuscular vitamin B12. Metabolic acidosis should be treated aggressively with sodium bicarbonate. Seizures in infancy should be treated initially with traditional antiepileptic drugs, but patients with rare inborn errors of metabolism may respond to other treatments (e.g., oral pyridoxine in a dosage of 5 mg per kg per day) if rare disorders such as pyridoxine-dependent epilepsy are clinically suspected by the consulting neurologist.

Long-Term Treatment

Traditional therapies for metabolic diseases include dietary therapy such as protein restriction, avoidance of fasting, or cofactor supplements. Evolving therapies include organ transplantation and enzyme replacement. Efforts to provide treatment through somatic gene therapy are in early stages, but there is hope that this approach will provide additional therapeutic possibilities. Even when no effective therapy exists or when an infant dies from a metabolic disorder, the family still needs an accurate diagnosis for clarification, reassurance, genetic counseling, and potential prenatal screening. Additional resources, including information about regional biochemical genetic consultation services, are available online.[13–15]

References

1. Beaudet AL, Scriver CR, Sly WS, Valle D. Molecular bases of variant human phenotypes. In: Scriver CR, ed. *The Metabolic and Molecular Bases of Inherited Disease.* 8th ed. New York: McGraw-Hill, 2001:3–51.

2. Applegarth DA, Toone JR, Lowry RB. Incidence of inborn errors of metabolism in British Columbia, 1969–1996. *Pediatrics.* 2000;105:e10.

3. Meikle PJ, Hopwood JJ, Clague AE, Carey WF. Prevalence of lysosomal storage disorders. *JAMA.* 1999;281:249–54.

4. Wilcken B, Wiley V, Hammond J, Carpenter K. Screening newborns for inborn errors of metabolism by tandem mass spectrometry. *N Engl J Med.* 2003;348:2304–12.

5. Holtzman NA. Expanding newborn screening: how good is the evidence?. *JAMA.* 2003;290:2606–8.

6. Waisbren SE, Albers S, Amato S, Ampola M, Brewster TG, Demmer L, et al. Effect of expanded newborn screening for biochemical genetic disorders on child outcomes and parental stress. *JAMA.* 2003;290:2564–72.

7. University of Texas Health Science Center at San Antonio. National Newborn Screening and Genetics Resource Center. Accessed online January 10, 2006, at: http://genes-r-us.uthscsa.edu.

8. Clarke JT. *A Clinical Guide to Inherited Metabolic Diseases.* 2nd ed. New York: Cambridge University Press, 2002.

9. Blau N, Duran M, Blaskovics ME, Gibson KM. *Physician's Guide to the Laboratory Diagnosis of Metabolic Diseases.* 2nd ed. New York: Springer, 2003.

10. Novotny E, Ashwal S, Shevell M. Proton magnetic resonance spectroscopy: an emerging technology in pediatric neurology research. *Pediatr Res.* 1998;44:1–10.

11. Prasad A, Kaye EM, Alroy J. Electron microscopic examination of skin biopsy as a cost-effective tool in the diagnosis of lysosomal storage diseases. *J Child Neurol.* 1996;11:301–8.

12. Levy HL, Ghavami M. Maternal phenylketonuria: a metabolic teratogen. *Teratology.* 1996;53:176–84.

13. GeneTests. National Institutes of Health. Accessed online January 10, 2006, at: http://www.genetests.org.

14. National Human Genome Research Institute. National Institutes of Health. Accessed online January 10, 2006, at: http://www.genome.gov.

15. American Society of Human Genetics. Accessed online January 10, 2006, at: http://www.ashg.org.

Chapter 13

Muscular Dystrophy

Muscular dystrophy (MD) refers to a group of more than 30 genetic diseases that cause progressive weakness and degeneration of skeletal muscles used during voluntary movement. The word dystrophy is derived from the Greek dys, which means "difficult" or "faulty," and troph, or "nourish." These disorders vary in age of onset, severity, and pattern of affected muscles. All forms of MD grow worse as muscles progressively degenerate and weaken. Many patients eventually lose the ability to walk.

Some types of MD also affect the heart, gastrointestinal system, endocrine glands, spine, eyes, brain, and other organs. Respiratory and cardiac diseases may occur, and some patients may develop a swallowing disorder. MD is not contagious and cannot be brought on by injury or activity.

What causes MD?

All of the muscular dystrophies are inherited and involve a mutation in one of the thousands of genes that program proteins critical to muscle integrity. The body's cells don't work properly when a protein is altered or produced in insufficient quantity (or sometimes missing completely). Many cases of MD occur from spontaneous mutations

Excerpted from "Muscular Dystrophy: Hope Through Research," by the National Institute of Neurological Disorders and Stroke (NINDS, www.ninds.nih.gov), part of the National Institutes of Health, June 22, 2011.

that are not found in the genes of either parent, and this defect can be passed to the next generation.

Genes are like blueprints: They contain coded messages that determine a person's characteristics or traits. They are arranged along 23 rod-like pairs of chromosomes, with one half of each pair being inherited from each parent. Each half of a chromosome pair is similar to the other, except for one pair, which determines the sex of the individual. Muscular dystrophies can be inherited in three ways:

Autosomal dominant inheritance occurs when a child receives a normal gene from one parent and a defective gene from the other parent. Autosomal means the genetic mutation can occur on any of the 22 non-sex chromosomes in each of the body's cells. Dominant means only one parent needs to pass along the abnormal gene in order to produce the disorder. In families where one parent carries a defective gene, each child has a 50 percent chance of inheriting the gene and therefore the disorder. Males and females are equally at risk and the severity of the disorder can differ from person to person.

Autosomal recessive inheritance means that both parents must carry and pass on the faulty gene. The parents each have one defective gene but are not affected by the disorder. Children in these families have a 25 percent chance of inheriting both copies of the defective gene and a 50 percent chance of inheriting one gene and therefore becoming a carrier, able to pass along the defect to their children. Children of either sex can be affected by this pattern of inheritance.

X-linked (or sex-linked) recessive inheritance occurs when a mother carries the affected gene on one of her two X chromosomes and passes it to her son (males always inherit an X chromosome from their mother and a Y chromosome from their father, while daughters inherit an X chromosome from each parent).

Sons of carrier mothers have a 50 percent chance of inheriting the disorder. Daughters also have a 50 percent chance of inheriting the defective gene but usually are not affected, since the healthy X chromosome they receive from their father can offset the faulty one received from their mother. Affected fathers cannot pass an X-linked disorder to their sons but their daughters will be carriers of that disorder. Carrier females occasionally can exhibit milder symptoms of MD.

How many people have MD?

MD occurs worldwide, affecting all races. Its incidence varies, as some forms are more common than others. Its most common forms in children, Duchenne and Becker muscular dystrophy, alone affect approximately one in every 3,500 to 5,000 boys, or between 400 and 600 live male births each year in the United States.

Some types of MD are more prevalent in certain countries and regions of the world. Most muscular dystrophies are familial, meaning there is some family history of the disease.

There are nine major groups of the muscular dystrophies. The disorders are classified by the extent and distribution of muscle weakness, age of onset, rate of progression, severity of symptoms, and family history (including any pattern of inheritance). Although some forms of MD become apparent in infancy or childhood, others may not appear until middle age or later. Overall, incidence rates and severity vary, but each of the dystrophies causes progressive skeletal muscle deterioration, and some types affect cardiac muscle.

How are the muscular dystrophies treated?

There is no specific treatment that can stop or reverse the progression of any form of MD. All forms of MD are genetic and cannot be prevented. Treatment is aimed at keeping the patient independent for as long as possible and preventing complications that result from weakness, reduced mobility, and cardiac and respiratory difficulties. Treatment may involve a combination of approaches, including physical therapy, drug therapy, and surgery.

What is the prognosis?

The prognosis varies according to the type of MD and the speed of progression. Some types are mild and progress very slowly, allowing normal life expectancy, while others are more severe and result in functional disability and loss of ambulation. Life expectancy may depend on the degree of muscle weakness and any respiratory and/or cardiac complications.

Chapter 14

Spina Bifida

The human nervous system develops from a small, specialized plate of cells along the back of an embryo. Early in development, the edges of this plate begin to curl up toward each other, creating the neural tube—a narrow sheath that closes to form the brain and spinal cord of the embryo. As development progresses, the top of the tube becomes the brain and the remainder becomes the spinal cord.

This process is usually complete by the 28th day of pregnancy. But if problems occur during this process, the result can be brain disorders called neural tube defects, including spina bifida.

What is spina bifida?

Spina bifida, which literally means "cleft spine," is characterized by the incomplete development of the brain, spinal cord, and/or meninges (the protective covering around the brain and spinal cord). It is the most common neural tube defect in the United States—affecting 1,500 to 2,000 of the more than 4 million babies born in the country each year.

What are the different types of spina bifida?

There are four types of spina bifida: occulta, closed neural tube defects, meningocele, and myelomeningocele.

Excerpted from "Spina Bifida Fact Sheet," by the National Institute of Neurological Disorders and Stroke (NINDS, www.ninds.nih.gov), part of the National Institutes of Health, December 18, 2009.

Occulta is the mildest and most common form in which one or more vertebrae are malformed. The name "occulta," which means "hidden," indicates that the malformation, or opening in the spine, is covered by a layer of skin. This form of spina bifida rarely causes disability or symptoms.

Closed neural tube defects make up the second type of spina bifida. This form consists of a diverse group of spinal defects in which the spinal cord is marked by a malformation of fat, bone, or membranes. In some patients there are few or no symptoms; in others the malformation causes incomplete paralysis with urinary and bowel dysfunction.

In the third type, meningocele, the meninges protrude from the spinal opening, and the malformation may or may not be covered by a layer of skin. Some patients with meningocele may have few or no symptoms while others may experience symptoms similar to closed neural tube defects.

Myelomeningocele, the fourth form, is the most severe and occurs when the spinal cord is exposed through the opening in the spine, resulting in partial or complete paralysis of the parts of the body below the spinal opening. The paralysis may be so severe that the affected individual is unable to walk and may have urinary and bowel dysfunction.

What causes spina bifida?

The exact cause of spina bifida remains a mystery. No one knows what disrupts complete closure of the neural tube, causing a malformation to develop. Scientists suspect genetic, nutritional, and environmental factors play a role.

Research studies indicate that insufficient intake of folic acid—a common B vitamin—in the mother's diet is a key factor in causing spina bifida and other neural tube defects. Prenatal vitamins that are prescribed for the pregnant mother typically contain folic acid as well as other vitamins.

What are the signs and symptoms of spina bifida?

The symptoms of spina bifida vary from person to person, depending on the type. Often, individuals with occulta have no outward signs of the disorder. Closed neural tube defects are often recognized early in life due to an abnormal tuft or clump of hair or a small dimple or birthmark on the skin at the site of the spinal malformation.

Meningocele and myelomeningocele generally involve a fluid-filled sac—visible on the back—protruding from the spinal cord. In meningocele, the sac may be covered by a thin layer of skin, whereas in most cases of myelomeningocele, there is no layer of skin covering the sac and a section of spinal cord tissue usually is exposed.

What are the complications of spina bifida?

Complications of spina bifida can range from minor physical problems to severe physical and mental disabilities. It is important to note, however, that most people with spina bifida are of normal intelligence. Severity is determined by the size and location of the malformation, whether or not skin covers it, whether or not spinal nerves protrude from it, and which spinal nerves are involved. Generally all nerves located below the malformation are affected. Therefore, the higher the malformation occurs on the back, the greater the amount of nerve damage and loss of muscle function and sensation.

In addition to loss of sensation and paralysis, another neurological complication associated with spina bifida is Chiari II malformation—a rare condition (but common in children with myelomeningocele) in which the brainstem and the cerebellum, or rear portion of the brain, protrude downward into the spinal canal or neck area. This condition can lead to compression of the spinal cord and cause a variety of symptoms including difficulties with feeding, swallowing, and breathing; choking; and arm stiffness.

Chiari II malformation may also result in a blockage of cerebrospinal fluid, causing a condition called hydrocephalus, which is an abnormal buildup of cerebrospinal fluid in the brain. Cerebrospinal fluid is a clear liquid that surrounds the brain and spinal cord. The buildup of fluid puts damaging pressure on the brain. Hydrocephalus is commonly treated by surgically implanting a shunt—a hollow tube—in the brain to drain the excess fluid into the abdomen.

Some newborns with myelomeningocele may develop meningitis, an infection in the meninges. Meningitis may cause brain injury and can be life-threatening.

Children with both myelomeningocele and hydrocephalus may have learning disabilities, including difficulty paying attention, problems with language and reading comprehension, and trouble learning math.

Additional problems such as latex allergies, skin problems, gastrointestinal conditions, and depression may occur as children with spina bifida get older.

How is spina bifida treated?

There is no cure for spina bifida. The nerve tissue that is damaged or lost cannot be repaired or replaced, nor can function be restored to the damaged nerves. Treatment depends on the type and severity of the disorder. Generally, children with the mild form need no treatment, although some may require surgery as they grow.

What is the prognosis?

Children with spina bifida can lead relatively active lives. Prognosis depends on the number and severity of abnormalities and associated complications. Most children with the disorder have normal intelligence and can walk, usually with assistive devices. If learning problems develop, early educational intervention is helpful.

Chapter 15

Sensory Disabilities

Chapter Contents

Section 15.1—Hearing Loss.. 98

Section 15.2—Vision Loss.. 102

Section 15.3—Deaf-Blindness 111

Section 15.1

Hearing Loss

From "Hearing Loss," by the National Institute on Aging (NIA, www.nia.nih.gov), part of the National Institutes of Health, April 20, 2010.

Hearing loss can affect your life in many ways. It can range from missing certain sounds to total loss of hearing. Hearing loss can be serious. You may not hear the sound of your smoke detector alerting you to a fire. You may miss out on talks with friends or family.

Hearing problems can make you feel anxious, upset, and left out. It's easy to withdraw from people when you can't follow what is being said at the dinner table or in a restaurant. Friends and family may think you're confused, uncaring, or difficult when you're really having trouble hearing.

If you have a problem hearing, there is help. There are many treatments—hearing aids, certain medicines, or surgery.

How Do I Know If I Have a Hearing Loss?

See your doctor if you experience the following:

- Have trouble hearing over the telephone

- Find it hard to follow conversations when two or more people are talking

- Often ask people to repeat what they are saying

- Need to turn up the TV volume so loud that others complain

- Have a problem hearing because of background noise

- Think that others seem to mumble

- Can't understand when women and children speak to you

Types of Hearing Loss

Hearing loss can have many different causes. Here are two kinds of hearing loss common in older people.

Presbycusis is a common type of hearing loss that comes on slowly as a person ages. It seems to run in families and affects hearing in both ears. The degree of hearing loss varies from person to person. A common sign of early hearing loss is not being able to hear a phone ringing.

Tinnitus causes a ringing, roaring, or hissing noise in your ear. Tinnitus can go hand-in-hand with many types of hearing loss. It can also be a sign of other health problems, such as high blood pressure or allergies. Often it is unclear what causes tinnitus, which may be permanent, come and go, or go away quickly.

Other Hearing Loss Problems

Loud noise is one of the most common causes of hearing loss. Noise from lawn mowers, snowblowers, motorcycles, firecrackers, or loud music can damage the inner ear. This can result in permanent hearing loss. You can prevent most noise-related hearing loss. Protect yourself by turning down the sound on your stereo, television, or headphones; move away from loud noise; or use earplugs or other ear protection.

Ear wax or fluid build-up can block sounds that are carried from the eardrum to the inner ear. If wax blockage is a problem, try using mild treatments, such as mineral oil, baby oil, glycerin, or commercial ear drops, to soften ear wax. A punctured eardrum can also cause hearing loss. The eardrum can be damaged by infection, pressure, or putting objects in the ear, including cotton-tipped swabs. See your doctor if you have pain or fluid draining from the ear.

Viruses and bacteria, heart condition, stroke, brain injuries, or tumors may affect your hearing. If you have hearing problems caused by a new medication, check with your doctor to see if another medicine can be used.

Sudden deafness is a medical emergency that may be curable if treated in time. See a doctor right away.

Talk to Your Doctor

Your family doctor may be able to diagnose and treat your hearing problem. Or, your doctor may refer you to other clinicians such as an otolaryngologist, a doctor who specializes in medical problems of the ear, nose, and throat (also called an ENT doctor), or an audiologist, who is trained to measure hearing and provide services to improve hearing. Audiologists can help select the best hearing aid for you and teach you how to use it.

What Devices Can Help?

There are many hearing devices that can help such as the following:

Hearing aids: Hearing aids are electronic, battery-run devices that make sounds louder. There are many types of hearing aids available. Before buying a hearing aid, check to find out if your insurance will cover the cost. Ask if you can have a trial period so that you can make sure the device is right for you. An audiologist will teach you how to use your hearing aid.

Hearing aids should fit comfortably in your ear. You may need several visits with the audiologist to get it right. Hearing aids may need repairs, and batteries will have to be changed on a regular basis. Remember, when you buy a hearing aid, you are buying both a product and a service.

Assistive devices: There are many products that can help you hear better. For example:

- Telephone amplifying devices can make it easier to use the phone. TV and radio listening systems can let you hear the TV or radio without being bothered by background noise or needing to turn up the volume.

- Alert systems can work with doorbells, smoke detectors, and alarm clocks to send you visual signals or vibrations. For example, a flashing light could let you know someone is at the door or the phone is ringing, or a vibrating alarm clock under your pillow could wake you in the morning.

- Cochlear implants. These electronic devices are for people with severe hearing loss. Part of the device is surgically implanted under the skin. Another part is visible. You need special training to adjust to an implant. They don't work for all types of hearing loss.

What Can I Do If I Have Trouble Hearing?

- Let people know that you have trouble hearing.

- Ask people to face you and to speak more slowly and clearly. Also, ask them to speak without shouting.

- Pay attention to what is being said and to facial expressions or gestures.

- Let the person talking know if you do not understand.

- Ask the person speaking to reword a sentence and try again.

How Can I Help a Person with Hearing Loss?

Here are some tips you can use when talking with someone who has a hearing problem:

- Include people with hearing loss in the conversation.
- Find a quiet place to talk to help reduce background noise, especially in restaurants and social gatherings.
- Stand in good lighting and use facial expressions or gestures to give clues.
- Face the person and talk clearly.
- Speak a little more loudly than normal, but don't shout.
- Speak at a reasonable speed; do not hide your mouth, eat, or chew gum.
- Repeat yourself if necessary, using different words.
- Try to make sure only one person talks at a time.
- Be patient. Stay positive and relaxed.
- Ask how you can help.

Many people develop hearing problems as they grow older. Today, there are many ways to improve your hearing. Asking for professional help as soon as you notice a problem is the best way to handle the problem.

Section 15.2

Vision Loss

Nearly 3.5 million Americans over 40 have some degree of vision loss, most commonly from age-related conditions. This number is expected to double in the next few decades as the baby boomers grow older.

Most people with age-related vision loss will not become completely blind; instead they will experience partial or moderate loss of vision. They may need to develop new skills to remain self-reliant. This text discusses age-related vision loss and how you, as caregiver, can help your loved one adjust to the challenges.

What Causes Adult-Onset Vision Loss?

Most people experience some decline in vision as they age. It becomes more difficult to read small print, to get around in dim lighting, or to tell the difference between dark blue and black, for example. Such changes in vision are a normal part of aging. However, more serious changes to eyesight also occur as one ages.

People of any age who have a stroke, traumatic brain injury, or a brain tumor may experience many physical changes, including vision loss. The loss may be temporary or permanent.

Most older adults experiencing low vision, however, will be affected by one of four conditions: Macular degeneration, glaucoma, cataracts, and diabetic retinopathy. Table 15.1 summarizes the most common symptoms or warning signs of these conditions; more detailed information follows.

It is important to remember that a person may have one of these conditions but not have any or all of the symptoms listed in Table 15.1.

Table 15.1. Common Symptoms and Warning Signs of Vision Loss

Conditions	Most Common Symptoms & Warning Signs
Macular Degeneration	Vision loss in center of eye; blurred vision; straight lines look wavy; need for more light; affects one or both eyes
Glaucoma	Gradual loss of peripheral, or side, vision; difficulty driving at night; loss of contrast
Cataracts	Hazy vision; difficulty driving at night; double vision; trouble distinguishing colors; sensitivity to glare
Diabetic Retinopathy	Blurred or changing vision; difficulty reading; floaters; affects central or peripheral vision

Macular Degeneration

What Is It?

Age-related macular degeneration (AMD) is the leading cause of vision loss for people over 50 in the Western world. There are two types of macular degeneration, the wet form and the dry form.

Dry macular degeneration is the more common form of the condition and develops slowly. Vision loss may be mild for years, although it will eventually worsen. It may also lead to wet macular degeneration. With dry macular degeneration, small fatty deposits called drusen gather on the macula, which is a part of the eye that helps us see sharp details.

Wet macular degeneration is more severe and accounts for about 10 percent of cases of macular degeneration. It is caused by the growth of abnormal blood vessels under the macula. These blood vessels leak blood into the tissue at the back of the eye, producing scar tissue and rapid changes to the macula. Wet macular degeneration often develops very quickly and causes sudden loss of vision in the center of the eye.

One unusual effect of rapid vision loss is called Charles Bonnet Syndrome. This condition, which sometimes accompanies macular degeneration, produces hallucinations. These hallucinations do not reflect mental illness or another neurological disorder; they are, in effect, occasional visual "additions" to limited sight, and may even be pleasant—flowers, animals, faces. An estimated 10 to 40 percent of those with AMD experience this syndrome.

Treatment Options

There is no cure for macular degeneration, but early detection means more treatment options may be available and research into the condition is ongoing. While there are currently no direct treatments for dry macular degeneration, there are some recommendations to follow which may help slow the progress of either the wet or dry form. These include stopping smoking, eating lots of vegetables and fruits, especially dark green leafy vegetables (such as spinach, kale, and collards) and taking, with your doctor's approval, supplements with zinc, copper, and antioxidant vitamins (vitamins C, E, and beta carotene). The National Eye Institute is studying other supplements that can affect eye health including omega-3 (fish oil), lutein, and zeaxanthin.

Wet macular degeneration can be treated, and early detection and treatment may prevent severe vision loss. Medications currently available are delivered to the eye by injection. These treatments help reduce the growth of abnormal blood vessels and help preserve, or in some cases improve, the vision that remains. Other options, used less frequently, include photodynamic or laser surgery; additional options are under investigation. For most people, therapies require multiple treatments, and can result in slower loss of vision.

Glaucoma

What Is It?

Glaucoma causes the loss of peripheral, or side, vision caused by optic nerve damage usually associated with high eye pressure. Glaucoma is a leading cause of blindness in the United States and while it can affect people of all ages, it is most common in older adults. It is important that the symptoms of glaucoma are caught early, through screening by an eye care professional, to prevent total blindness.

Treatment Options

The damage caused by glaucoma is permanent, but treatments are available to prevent further vision loss. The most common treatment for glaucoma is eyedrops used daily to lower eye pressure. These medications can preserve vision but may cause side effects. Laser and conventional surgery are also sometimes options to treat glaucoma.

Cataracts

What Is It?

A cataract is the clouding of the normally clear lens of the eye. This clouding causes hazy vision, as if you were looking through a frosted or yellow window. Cataracts typically develop gradually over a period of years and are a common cause of vision loss among older adults.

Treatment Options

Cataracts can be removed through surgery in which the lens of the eye is removed and replaced by a plastic lens. This operation is fairly short and is highly successful. After surgery, patients often have a change in their eyeglass prescription. However, some individuals are not bothered too much by their cataracts and are able to manage by changing eyeglass prescriptions and protecting their eyes from too much sunlight, as exposure to sun speeds up the growth of cataracts.

Diabetic Retinopathy

What Is It?

Diabetic retinopathy can occur in people with diabetes, typically in those with advanced diabetes and high blood sugar levels. Diabetic retinopathy is caused by leaking blood vessels. An estimated 25 percent of people with diabetes have some diabetic retinopathy, but for most no severe vision problems will develop. Because there are often no symptoms in the early stages of diabetic retinopathy, people with advanced diabetes should have regular vision exams to check for this condition.

Treatment Options

Maintaining stable blood sugar levels is the best way for a diabetic to prevent diabetic retinopathy. Once the condition has developed, laser surgery can sometimes prevent further vision loss. Advanced retinopathy can be treated through microsurgery called vitrectomy which removes and replaces eye fluid.

Getting an Accurate Diagnosis

The National Eye Institute and the American Academy of Ophthalmology recommend that everyone over age 60 get a full, dilated eye exam every 2 years, or more often if there is an eye disease involved.

If your loved one experiences the symptoms of low vision, such as blurred vision or sensitivity to glare, he or she should seek the care of a low vision specialist—an optometrist or ophthalmologist with particular expertise in this area. This specialist will do a vision assessment and then make a referral for specific treatment, vision-related training, and/or assistive devices.

It is important that your loved one continues to see the vision specialist every year to catch any changes in vision. The sooner such changes are found and possibly treated, the better the chance that your loved one will still be able to retain his or her vision and live as independently as possible.

Vision-Related Rehabilitation Services and Vision Training

Helping your loved one find vision-related rehabilitation services may be one of the best ways for you as a caregiver to provide practical support. Rehabilitation services include adaptive living, orientation and mobility training (including the possibility of using a cane to move around in public), vision training, and assistive devices.

Because some people with low vision do still retain usable vision, it's helpful to work with a vision rehabilitation specialist to learn how to best use the vision they have. If your loved one has macular degeneration, for example, and has lost vision in the center of his or her eye, the vision rehabilitation specialist will teach how to best use the peripheral vision that remains.

Rehabilitation services are provided by state and private agencies serving blind and visually impaired persons. You can locate these services by checking your local telephone directory, or calling the American Foundation for the Blind for a referral.

Home Alterations (Adaptive Living)

There are many inexpensive and relatively simple changes that you can make in the house to help your loved one remain safe and comfortable.

Improve Lighting and Reduce Glare

Adding more lamps and lighting throughout the house will help your loved one use their remaining vision effectively. Consider adding gooseneck lamps in places where extra light is needed for such tasks as writing checks, cooking, or reading. Illuminate stairs, especially top and bottom steps. Install night lights in key places.

It is useful to find out which types of bulbs provide the best kind of lighting to help your loved one see most clearly. Depending on the type of vision loss, different qualities of light (more white or yellow, for example) might make it easier to see.

Reducing glare is important as well. Installing blinds or shades on windows in the house and wearing anti-glare sunglasses and visors outdoors will be beneficial.

Accentuate Dark and Light Contrasts throughout the Home

Many alterations are simply ways to make things show up more easily. Use paint or tape in contrasting colors to help your loved one find and use items throughout the house. For example, having outlet or switch plate covers in colors that contrast with wall paint makes light switches or thermostats easier to find. Similarly, using plates, cups, and utensils in a color that contrasts with the countertop and table aids in food preparation and dining. Use towels in the bathroom that do not blend with the wall color to make them easy to find. Install handrails along the staircase in colors that contrast with walls to help prevent falls.

Organizing the House

Organize cupboards and specify exact locations for important things. If the cereal is always on the middle shelf of the pantry, for example, your loved one will not need to strain to try to determine if it is cereal or something else. Set up consistent places for mail, keys, and other important items.

Use markers to print large labels for such everyday items as cleaning or cooking supplies (and be sure to keep cleaning supplies separate from food storage areas). Clearly mark stove dials and label all medications.

It's extremely important to keep your living space clear of obstacles and hazards. While large area rugs can be useful to define rooms, remove throw rugs and unnecessary furnishings that clutter walking paths to help eliminate tripping hazards. Any measure you can take to reduce the danger of falls is helpful.

Assistive Devices

Many kinds of assistive devices can be of great help and often can be found at drugstores or specialty shops or through websites that specialize in these products. Some of the most useful are:

- Magnifiers: Very effective for those with low vision and come in many different sizes and styles. Different kinds of magnifiers will help accomplish different tasks.

- Penlights: Useful whenever more concentrated light might help your loved one see or read something. Like magnifiers, you might want to keep several penlights around to help in different situations.

- Electronic: Closed circuit televisions (CCTVs) are very useful for those with low vision. CCTVs look something like a computer but consist of a camera and screen. An object can be placed under the camera which magnifies it, and then displays it much larger on the screen. This makes reading and writing easier.

- Audio products: There are also a large number of audio products to help with everyday tasks or hobbies. These include "talking" clocks, calculators, watches, navigation tools, books, and more.

- Telephones: Telephones come with large dials and buttons in various forms; computers offer large print, large screens, and special keyboards.

Many other ingenious devices have been developed to help.

Traveling outside the Home (Orientation and Mobility Training)

Vision rehabilitation services introduce techniques to make travel as independent as possible. This is called orientation and mobility training, and will include learning how to best use existing vision. Other techniques include using a white cane, and learning how to better use one's hearing while walking. While not everyone is eager to use a cane, if your loved one is receptive, this can be a very useful tool to maintain independence.

To assist someone while walking, use the sighted guide technique: Walk a half step in front of them and have them hold your arm just above the elbow. You can also announce any hazards, like steps or holes in the sidewalk to help them (and you!) avoid falling. Other tips:

- Carry magnifiers and/or penlights when shopping or going to appointments outside the home.

- Fold each denomination of dollar bill a different way to help your loved one shop or use public transportation.

- When needed, let bus drivers, shopkeepers, or others know that your loved one has low vision to make traveling outside the home safe.

Paying for Low-Vision Care and Devices

Medicare covers only certain low-vision care, including some surgery for glaucoma and for intraocular lenses used in cataract surgery. It also pays for treatment for certain patients with age-related macular degeneration in which the central part of the eye deteriorates.

Some nonprofit groups also provide financial assistance to needy patients with low vision.

Emotional Effects of Vision Loss

Anyone diagnosed with a condition causing vision loss may experience many difficult emotions, including grief, shock, anger, and depression. These feelings may last only a short time or could persist for years. Losing the ability to drive may be an emotional blow, and your loved one may worry about whether he or she will still be able to live independently. Vision loss might be one of the first definite signs of aging that people experience, making them feel vulnerable or frail.

Acknowledging these negative emotions is important. As a caregiver, you may also have concerns about how your relationship with your loved one will change. You might be worried about increased dependence. You might be unhappy about being asked to take on tasks that you do not want to do. You will most likely experience emotions about your loved one's vision loss that you will need to address. Being open and honest about these feelings will help you move past them and allow you to continue as a caregiver.

Most people with vision loss do find that their confidence about living with reduced eyesight increases over time. By participating in rehabilitation training and trying the techniques taught there, your loved one will likely begin to trust their new skills and feel better about the future.

How Can You Help Your Loved One Adjust to Low Vision?

To help your loved one deal with the challenges of reduced vision, you'll want to be as informed, supportive, and caring as possible. Learning as much as you can about the condition and best adaptation strategies will help reduce early feelings of despair or fear, and move to acceptance and confidence. Counseling and support groups can be significant sources of help. Finally, by treating the vision loss as a family issue you will help your loved one feel supported as he or she adjusts to life with vision loss.

It might not be obvious where or when your loved one needs assistance. Although it's hard for any of us to ask for help, communicating openly and clearly is important. Encourage your loved one to be specific about the kinds of tasks that she or he finds challenging and exactly what you can do to help.

Remember that you may need to use speech in specific ways to tell your loved one things. For example, upon leaving the room you may need to let them know you are going. Similarly, when greeting people, you may need to announce who someone is, as your loved one might not be able to recognize them. Also, remember that pointing, nodding the head, or using other body language will not be effective communication.

Although your loved one now has a vision impairment, it is very important to encourage self-reliance. By continuing to treat your loved one with respect and care, you can help him or her feel empowered to overcome challenges and remain as independent as possible.

Recommended Reading

Aging and Vision Loss: A Handbook for Families, Alberta L. Orr, MSW and Priscilla A. Rogers, PhD, 2006, AFB Press. Available at: 800-AFB-LINE (800-232-5463) or www.afb.org.

Living Better: A Guide for People with Vision Loss, Lighthouse International, 2008. Available at: 800-829-0500 or www.lighthouse.org.

Fact Sheet on Assistive Technology, Family Caregiver Alliance, 2005. Available at: http://caregiver.org/caregiver/jsp/content_node.jsp?nodeid=1412

Section 15.3

Deaf-Blindness

"Overview on Deaf-Blindness," by Barbara Miles, M.Ed., DB-Link, October 2008, © National Consortium on Deaf-Blindness. Reprinted with permission. The National Consortium on Deaf-Blindness is home to DB-LINK, the largest collection of information related to deaf-blindness worldwide. For additional information, visit http://nationaldb.org.

What Is Deaf-Blindness?

It may seem that deaf-blindness refers to a total inability to see or hear. However, in reality deaf-blindness is a condition in which the combination of hearing and visual losses in children cause "such severe communication and other developmental and educational needs that they cannot be accommodated in special education programs solely for children with deafness or children with blindness" (34 CFR 300.8 (c) (2), 2006) or multiple disabilities. Children who are called deaf-blind are singled out educationally because impairments of sight and hearing require thoughtful and unique educational approaches in order to ensure that children with this disability have the opportunity to reach their full potential.

A person who is deaf-blind has a unique experience of the world. For people who can see and hear, the world extends outward as far as his or her eyes and ears can reach. For the young child who is deaf-blind, the world is initially much narrower. If the child is profoundly deaf and totally blind, his or her experience of the world extends only as far as the fingertips can reach. Such children are effectively alone if no one is touching them. Their concepts of the world depend upon what or whom they have had the opportunity to physically contact.

If a child who is deaf-blind has some usable vision and/or hearing, as many do, her or his world will be enlarged. Many children called deaf-blind have enough vision to be able to move about in their environments, recognize familiar people, see sign language at close distances, and perhaps read large print. Others have sufficient hearing to recognize familiar sounds, understand some speech, or develop speech themselves. The range of sensory impairments included in the term "deaf-blindness" is great.

Who Is Deaf-Blind, and What Are the Causes of Deaf-Blindness?

As far as it has been possible to count them, there are over 10,000 children (ages birth to 22 years) in the United States who have been classified as deaf-blind (NCDB, 2008). It has been estimated that the adult deaf-blind population numbers 35,000–40,000 (Watson, 1993). The causes of deaf-blindness are many. In the following text is a list of many of the possible etiologies of deaf-blindness.

Major Causes of Deaf-Blindness

This list is adapted from Etiologies and Characteristics of Deaf-Blindness, Heller & Kennedy, (1994), p. viii, Table 1.

Syndromes

- Down
- Trisomy 13
- Usher

Multiple Congenital Anomalies

- CHARGE (Coloboma of the eye, heart defects, atresia of the nasal choanae, retardation of growth and/or development, genital and/or urinary abnormalities, and ear abnormalities and deafness) Association
- Fetal alcohol syndrome
- Hydrocephaly
- Maternal drug abuse
- Microcephaly

Congenital Prenatal Dysfunction

- AIDS [acquired immunodeficiency syndrome]
- Herpes
- Rubella
- Syphilis
- Toxoplasmosis

Postnatal Causes

- Asphyxia
- Encephalitis
- Head injury/trauma
- Meningitis
- Stroke

Prematurity is also a major cause of deaf-blindness.

Some people are deaf-blind from birth. Others may be born deaf or hard-of-hearing and become blind or visually impaired later in life; or the reverse may be the case.

Still others may be adventitiously deaf-blind—that is, they are born with both sight and hearing but lose some or all of these senses as a result of accident or illness.

Deaf-blindness is often accompanied by additional disabilities. Causes such as maternal rubella can also affect the heart and the brain. Some genetic syndromes or brain injuries that cause deaf-blindness may also cause cognitive disabilities and/or physical disabilities.

What Are the Challenges Facing a Person Who Is Deaf-Blind?

A person who is deaf-blind must somehow make sense of the world using the limited information available to him or her. If the person's sensory disabilities are great, and if people in the environment have not made an effort to order the world for him or her in a way that makes it easier to understand, this challenge may be overwhelming. Behavioral and emotional difficulties often accompany deaf-blindness and are the natural outcomes of the child's or adult's inability to understand and communicate.

People who can see and hear often take for granted the information that those senses provide. Events such as the approach of another person, an upcoming meal, the decision to go out, a change in routine are all signaled by sights and sounds that allow a person to prepare for them. The child or adult who misses these cues because of limited sight and/or hearing may come to experience the world as an unpredictable, and possibly threatening, place. To a great extent, persons who are deaf-blind must depend upon the goodwill and sensitivity of those around them to make their world safe and understandable.

113

The challenge of learning to communicate is perhaps the greatest one that children who are deaf-blind face. It is also the greatest opportunity, since communication and language hold the power to make their thoughts, needs, and desires known.

The ability to use words can also open up worlds beyond the reach of their fingertips through the use of interpreters, books, and an ever-increasing array of electronic communication devices. In order to learn language, children who are deaf-blind must depend upon others to make language accessible to them. Given that accessibility, children who are deaf-blind face the challenges of engaging in interactions to the best of their abilities and of availing themselves of the language opportunities provided for them.

A person who is deaf-blind also faces, further, the challenge of learning to move about in the world as freely and independently as possible. Adult individuals also must eventually find adult living and work situations that allow them to use their talents and abilities in the best way possible. Many adults who are deaf-blind lead independent or semi-independent lives and have productive work and enjoyable social lives. The achievement of such success depends in large part upon the education they have received since childhood, and particularly upon the communication with others that they have been able to develop.

What Are the Particular Challenges Facing the Family, Teachers, and Caregivers of a Person Who Is Deaf-Blind?

Communication

The disability of deaf-blindness presents unique challenges to families, teachers, and caregivers, who must make sure that the person who is deaf-blind has access to the world beyond the limited reach of his or her eyes, ears, and fingertips. The people in the environment of children or adults who are deaf-blind must seek to include them—moment-by-moment—in the flow of life and in the physical environments that surround them. If they do not, the child will be isolated and will not have the opportunity to grow and to learn. If they do, the child will be afforded the opportunity to develop to his or her fullest potential.

The most important challenge for parents, caregivers, and teachers is to communicate meaningfully with the child who is deaf-blind. Continual good communication will help foster his or her healthy development. Communication involves much more than mere language. Good communication can best be thought of as conversation. Conversations employ body language and gestures, as well as both signed and spoken words. A conversation with a child who is deaf-blind can begin with a partner who simply notices what the child is paying attention to at the moment and finds a way to let the child know that his or her interest is shared. This shared interest, once established, can become a topic around which a conversation can be built.

Mutual conversational topics are typically established between a parent and a sighted or hearing child by making eye contact and by gestures such as pointing or nodding, or by exchanges of sounds and facial expressions. Lacking significant amounts of sight and hearing, children who are deaf-blind will often need touch in order for them to be sure that their partner shares their focus of attention. The parent or teacher may, for example, touch an interesting object along with the child in a nondirective way. Or, the mother may imitate a child's movements, allowing the child tactual access to that imitation, if necessary. (This is the tactual equivalent of the actions of a mother who instinctively imitates her child's babbling sounds.) Establishing a mutual interest like this will open up the possibility for conversational interaction.

Teachers, parents, siblings, and peers can continue conversations with children who are deaf-blind by learning to pause after each turn in the interaction to allow time for response. These children frequently have very slow response times. Respecting the child's own timing is crucial to establishing successful interactions. Pausing long enough to allow the child to take another turn in the interaction, then responding to that turn, pausing again, and so on—this back-and-forth exchange becomes a conversation. Such conversations, repeated consistently, build relationships and become the eventual basis for language learning.

As the child who is deaf-blind becomes comfortable interacting nonverbally with others, she or he becomes ready to receive some form of symbolic communication as part of those interactions. Often it is helpful to accompany the introduction of words (spoken or signed) with the use of simple gestures and/or objects which serve as symbols or representations for activities. Doing so may help a child develop the understanding that one thing can stand for another, and will also enable him or her to anticipate events.

Think of the many thousands of words and sentences that most children hear before they speak their own first words. A child who is deaf-blind needs comparable language stimulation, adjusted to his or her ability to receive and make sense of it. Parents, caregivers, and teachers face the challenge of providing an environment rich in language that is meaningful and accessible to the child who is deaf-blind. Only with such a rich language environment will the child have the opportunity to acquire language herself or himself. Those around the child can create a rich language environment by continually commenting on the child's own experience using sign language, speech, or whatever symbol system is accessible to the child. These comments are best made during conversational interactions. A teacher or a parent may, for example, use gesture or sign language to name the object that he or she and the child are both touching, or name the movement that they share. This naming of objects and actions, done many, many times, may begin to give the child who is deaf-blind a similar opportunity afforded to the hearing child—that of making meaningful connections between words and the things for which they stand.

Principal communication systems for persons who are deaf-blind are these:

- Touch cues

- Gestures

- Object symbols

- Picture symbols

- Sign language

- Finger spelling

- Signed English

- Pidgin Signed English

- Braille writing and reading

- Tadoma method of speech reading

- American Sign Language

- Large print writing and reading

- Lip-reading speech

Along with nonverbal and verbal conversations, a child who is deaf-blind needs a reliable routine of meaningful activities, and some way or ways that this routine can be communicated to her or him.

Touch cues, gestures, and use of object symbols are some typical ways in which to let a child who is deaf-blind know what is about to happen to her or him. Each time before the child is picked up, for example, the caregiver may gently lift his or her arms a bit, and then pause, giving the child time to ready herself or himself for being handled. Such consistency will help the child to feel secure and to begin to make the world predictable, thus allowing the child to develop expectations. Children and adults who are deaf-blind and are able to use symbolic communication may also be more reliant on predictable routine than people who are sighted and hearing. Predictable routine may help to ease the anxiety which is often caused by the lack of sensory information.

Orientation and Mobility

In addition, the child who is deaf-blind will need help learning to move about in the world. Without vision, or with reduced vision, he or she will not only have difficulty navigating, but may also lack the motivation to move outward in the first place.

Helping a young child who is deaf-blind learn to move may begin with thoughtful attention to the physical space around him or her (crib or other space) so that whatever movements the child instinctively makes are rewarded with interesting stimulation that motivates further movement.

Orientation and mobility specialists can help parents and teachers to construct safe and motivating spaces for the young child who is deaf-blind. In many instances children who are deaf-blind may also have additional physical and health problems that limit their ability to move about. Parents and teachers may need to include physical and occupational therapists, vision teachers, health professionals, and orientation and mobility specialists on the team to plan accessible and motivating spaces for these children. Older children or adults who have lost vision can also use help from trained specialists in order to achieve as much confidence and independence as possible in moving about in their world.

Individualized Education

Education for a child or youth with deaf-blindness needs to be highly individualized; the limited channels available for learning necessitate organizing a program for each child that will address the child's unique ways of learning and his or her own way. Sensory deficits can easily mislead even experienced educators into underestimating (or occasionally overestimating) intelligence and constructing inappropriate programs.

Helen Keller said, "Blindness separates a person from things, but deafness separates him from people." This potential isolation is one important reason why it is necessary to engage the services of persons familiar with the combination of both blindness and deafness when planning an educational program for a child who is deaf-blind. Doing so will help a child or youth with these disabilities receive an education which maximizes her or his potential for learning and for meaningful contact with her or his environment. The earlier these services can be obtained, the better for the child.

Transition

When a person who is deaf-blind nears the end of his or her school-based education, transition and rehabilitation help will be required to assist in planning so that as an adult the individual can find suitable work and living situations. Because of the diversity of needs, such services for a person who is deaf-blind can rarely be provided by a single person or agency; careful and respectful team work is required among specialists and agencies concerned with such things as housing, vocational and rehabilitation needs, deafness, blindness, orientation and mobility, medical needs, and mental health.

The adult who is deaf-blind must be central to the transition planning. The individual's own goals, directions, interests, and abilities must guide the planning at every step of the way. Skilled interpreters, family members, and friends who know the person well can help the adult who is deaf-blind have the most important voice in planning his or her own future.

Inclusion in Family

Clearly, the challenges for parents, teachers, and caregivers of children who are deaf-blind are many. Not least among them is the challenge of including the child in the flow of family and community life. Since such a child does not necessarily respond to care in the ways we might expect, parents will be particularly challenged in their efforts to include her or him. The mother or father of an infant who can see is usually rewarded with smiles and lively eye contact from the child. The parent of a child who is deaf-blind must look for more subtle rewards: Small hand or body movements, for instance, may be the child's way of expressing pleasure or connection. Parents may also need to change their perceptions regarding typical developmental milestones. They can learn, as many have, to rejoice as fully in the ability of their child who is deaf-blind to sign a new word, or to feed herself, or to return a greeting as they do over another child's college scholarship or success in basketball or election to class office.

Parents, then, may need to shift expectations and perceptions in significant ways. They also need to do the natural grieving that

118

accompanies the birth of a child who is disabled. Teachers and care-givers must also make these perceptual shifts. Parents' groups and resources for teachers can provide much-needed support for those who live and work with children and adults who are deaf-blind. Such supports will help foster the mutually rewarding inclusion of children who are deaf-blind into their families and communities.

Summary

Though deaf-blindness presents many unique challenges to both those who have visual and hearing impairments and to their caregivers and friends, these challenges are by no means insurmountable. Many persons who are deaf-blind have achieved a quality of life that is excellent. The persons who are deaf-blind who have high quality lives have several things in common.

First, they have each, in their own way, come to accept themselves as individuals who have unique experiences of the world, and valuable gifts to share. This fundamental acceptance of self can occur regardless of the severity of the particular sensory losses or other challenges that a person has.

Second, they have had educational experiences which have helped them maximize their abilities to communicate and to function productively.

Finally, these happy, involved persons who are deaf-blind live in families, communities, or social groups that have an attitude of welcoming acceptance. They have friends, relatives, and co-workers who value their presence as individuals with significant contributions to make to the world around them. For these persons with limited sight and hearing, and for those near them, deaf-blindness fosters opportunities for learning and mutual enrichment.

References

The National Consortium on Deaf-Blindness (2008). 2007 National child count of children and youth who are deaf-blind. Monmouth: Teaching Research Division.

Wolff Heller, K. & Kennedy, C. (1994). Etiologies and characteristics of deaf-blindness. Monmouth: Teaching Research Publications.

Watson, D., & Taff-Watson, M. (Eds.), (1993). Second edition. A model service delivery system for persons who are deaf-blind. Arkansas: University of Arkansas.

Chapter 16

Speech Disorders

Chapter Contents

Section 16.1—Aphasia 122

Section 16.2—Apraxia 124

Section 16.1

Aphasia

Excerpted from "Aphasia," by the National Institute on Deafness and Other Communication Disorders (NIDCD, www.nidcd.nih.gov), part of the National Institutes of Health, October 2008.

What is aphasia?

Aphasia is a disorder that results from damage to portions of the brain that are responsible for language. For most people, these are areas on the left side (hemisphere) of the brain. Aphasia usually occurs suddenly, often as the result of a stroke or head injury, but it may also develop slowly, as in the case of a brain tumor, an infection, or dementia. The disorder impairs the expression and understanding of language as well as reading and writing. Aphasia may co-occur with speech disorders such as dysarthria or apraxia of speech, which also result from brain damage.

What types of aphasia are there?

There are two broad categories of aphasia—fluent and non-fluent. Damage to the temporal lobe (the side portion) of the brain may result in a fluent aphasia called Wernicke aphasia. In most people, the damage occurs in the left temporal lobe, although it can result from damage to the right lobe as well. People with Wernicke aphasia may speak in long sentences that have no meaning, add unnecessary words, and even create made-up words. For example, someone with Wernicke aphasia may say, "You know that smoodle pinkered and that I want to get him round and take care of him like you want before." As a result, it is often difficult to follow what the person is trying to say. People with Wernicke aphasia usually have great difficulty understanding speech, and they are often unaware of their mistakes. These individuals usually have no body weakness because their brain injury is not near the parts of the brain that control movement.

A type of non-fluent aphasia is Broca aphasia. People with Broca aphasia have damage to the frontal lobe of the brain. They frequently speak in short phrases that make sense but are produced with great effort. They often omit small words such as "is," "and," and "the." For example, a person with Broca aphasia may say, "Walk dog," meaning, "I will take the dog for a walk," or "book book two table," for "There are two books on the table." People with Broca aphasia typically understand the speech of others fairly well. Because of this, they are often aware of their difficulties and can become easily frustrated.

People with Broca aphasia often have right-sided weakness or paralysis of the arm and leg because the frontal lobe is also important for motor movements.

Another type of non-fluent aphasia, global aphasia, results from damage to extensive portions of the language areas of the brain. Individuals with global aphasia have severe communication difficulties and may be extremely limited in their ability to speak or comprehend language.

There are other types of aphasia, each of which results from damage to different language areas in the brain. Some people may have difficulty repeating words and sentences even though they can speak and they understand the meaning of the word or sentence. Others may have difficulty naming objects even though they know what the object is and what it may be used for.

How is aphasia treated?

In some cases, a person will completely recover from aphasia without treatment. This type of spontaneous recovery usually occurs following a type of stroke in which blood flow to the brain is temporarily interrupted but quickly restored, called a transient ischemic attack. In these circumstances, language abilities may return in a few hours or a few days.

For most cases, however, language recovery is not as quick or as complete. While many people with aphasia experience partial spontaneous recovery, in which some language abilities return a few days to a month after the brain injury, some amount of aphasia typically remains. In these instances, speech-language therapy is often helpful. Recovery usually continues over a 2-year period. Many health professionals believe that the most effective treatment begins early in the recovery process. Some of the factors that influence the amount of improvement include the cause of the brain damage, the area of the brain that was damaged, the extent of the brain injury, and the age and health of the individual.

Section 16.2

Apraxia

Excerpted from "Apraxia of Speech," by the National Institute on Deafness and Other Communication Disorders (NIDCD, www.nidcd.nih.gov), part of the National Institutes of Health, November 2002. Reviewed by David A. Cooke, MD, FACP, May 5, 2011.

What is apraxia of speech?

Apraxia of speech, also known as verbal apraxia or dyspraxia, is a speech disorder in which a person has trouble saying what he or she wants to say correctly and consistently. It is not due to weakness or paralysis of the speech muscles (the muscles of the face, tongue, and lips). The severity of apraxia of speech can range from mild to severe.

What are the types and causes of apraxia?

There are two main types of speech apraxia—acquired apraxia of speech and developmental apraxia of speech. Acquired apraxia of speech can affect a person at any age, although it most typically occurs in adults. It is caused by damage to the parts of the brain that are involved in speaking, and involves the loss or impairment of existing speech abilities. The disorder may result from a stroke, head injury, tumor, or other illness affecting the brain. Acquired apraxia of speech may occur together with muscle weakness affecting speech production (dysarthria) or language difficulties caused by damage to the nervous system (aphasia).

Developmental apraxia of speech (DAS) occurs in children and is present from birth. It appears to affect more boys than girls. This speech disorder goes by several other names, including developmental verbal apraxia, developmental verbal dyspraxia, articulatory apraxia, and childhood apraxia of speech. DAS is different from what is known as a developmental delay of speech, in which a child follows the typical path of speech development but does so more slowly than normal.

The cause or causes of DAS are not yet known. Some scientists believe that DAS is a disorder related to a child's overall language development. Others believe it is a neurological disorder that affects the brain's ability to send the proper signals to move the muscles involved in speech. However, brain imaging and other studies have not found evidence of specific brain lesions or differences in brain structure in children with DAS. Children with DAS often have family members who have a history of communication disorders or learning disabilities. This observation and recent research findings suggest that genetic factors may play a role in the disorder.

How is it treated?

In some cases, people with acquired apraxia of speech recover some or all of their speech abilities on their own. This is called spontaneous recovery.

Children with developmental apraxia of speech will not outgrow the problem on their own. Speech-language therapy is often helpful for these children and for people with acquired apraxia who do not spontaneously recover all of their speech abilities.

Speech-language pathologists use different approaches to treat apraxia of speech, and no single approach has been proven to be the most effective. Therapy is tailored to the individual and is designed to treat other speech or language problems that may occur together with apraxia. Each person responds differently to therapy, and some people will make more progress than others. People with apraxia of speech usually need frequent and intensive one-on-one therapy.

Support and encouragement from family members and friends are also important. In severe cases, people with acquired or developmental apraxia of speech may need to use other ways to express themselves. These might include formal or informal sign language, a language notebook with pictures or written words that the person can show to other people, or an electronic communication device such as a portable computer that writes and produces speech.

Chapter 17

Intellectual and Cognitive Disabilities

Chapter Contents

Section 17.1—Down Syndrome 128

Section 17.2—Fetal Alcohol Spectrum Disorders 130

Section 17.3—Head Trauma in Infants
(Shaken Baby Syndrome) 132

Section 17.1

Down Syndrome

From "Facts about Down Syndrome," by the National Institute of
Child Health and Human Development (NICHD, www.nichd.nih.gov),
part of the National Institutes of Health, March 24, 2010.

Down syndrome is set of mental and physical symptoms that result
from having an extra copy of Chromosome 21.

Normally, a fertilized egg has 23 pairs of chromosomes. In most
people with Down syndrome, there is an extra copy of Chromosome
21 (also called trisomy 21 because there are three copies of this chromosome
instead of two), which changes the body's and brain's normal
development.

Signs and Symptoms of Down Syndrome

Even though people with Down syndrome may have some physical
and mental features in common, symptoms of Down syndrome can
range from mild to severe. Usually, mental development and physical
development are slower in people with Down syndrome than in those
without the condition.

Intellectual and Developmental Disabilities (IDDs) is a disability
that causes limits on intellectual abilities and adaptive behaviors
(conceptual, social, and practical skills people use to function in everyday
lives). Most people with Down syndrome have IQs that fall in
the mild to moderate range of IDDs. They may have delayed language
development and slow motor development.

Some common physical signs of Down syndrome include the following:

- Flat face with an upward slant to the eye, short neck, and abnormally
  shaped ears
- Deep crease in the palm of the hand
- White spots on the iris of the eye
- Poor muscle tone, loose ligaments
- Small hands and feet

There are a variety of other health conditions that are often seen in people who have Down syndrome, including the following:

- Congenital heart disease

- Hearing problems

- Intestinal problems, such as blocked small bowel or esophagus

- Celiac disease

- Eye problems, such as cataracts

- Thyroid dysfunctions

- Skeletal problems

- Dementia—similar to Alzheimer disease

Treatment for Down Syndrome

Down syndrome is not a condition that can be cured. However, early intervention can help many people with Down syndrome live productive lives well into adulthood.

Children with Down syndrome can often benefit from speech therapy, occupational therapy, and exercises for gross and fine motor skills. They might also be helped by special education and attention at school. Many children can integrate well into regular classes at school. For more information about treatments for Down syndrome, ask your health care provider.

Section 17.2

Fetal Alcohol Spectrum Disorders

Excerpted from "Fetal Alcohol Spectrum Disorders (FASDs)," by the National Center on Birth Defects and Developmental Disabilities (NCBDDD, www.cdc.gov/ncbddd), Centers for Disease Control and Prevention (CDC), October 6, 2010.

Fetal alcohol spectrum disorders (FASDs) are a group of conditions that can occur in a person whose mother drank alcohol during pregnancy. These effects can include physical problems and problems with behavior and learning. Often, a person with an FASD has a mix of these problems.

Signs and Symptoms

FASDs refer to the whole range of effects that can happen to a person whose mother drank alcohol during pregnancy. These conditions can affect each person in different ways, and can range from mild to severe.

A person with an FASD might have the following:

- Abnormal facial features, such as a smooth ridge between the nose and upper lip (this ridge is called the philtrum)
- Small head size
- Shorter-than-average height
- Low body weight
- Poor coordination
- Hyperactive behavior
- Difficulty paying attention
- Poor memory
- Difficulty in school (especially with math)
- Learning disabilities
- Speech and language delays
- Intellectual disability or low IQ

- Poor reasoning and judgment skills
- Sleep and sucking problems as a baby
- Vision or hearing problems
- Problems with the heart, kidneys, or bones

Types of FASDs

Different terms are used to describe FASDs, depending on the type of symptoms.

- **Fetal Alcohol Syndrome (FAS):** FAS represents the severe end of the FASD spectrum. Fetal death is the most extreme outcome from drinking alcohol during pregnancy. People with FAS might have abnormal facial features, growth problems, and central nervous system (CNS) problems. People with FAS can have problems with learning, memory, attention span, communication, vision, or hearing. They might have a mix of these problems. People with FAS often have a hard time in school and trouble getting along with others.

- **Alcohol-Related Neurodevelopmental Disorder (ARND):** People with ARND might have intellectual disabilities and problems with behavior and learning. They might do poorly in school and have difficulties with math, memory, attention, judgment, and poor impulse control.

- **Alcohol-Related Birth Defects (ARBD):** People with ARBD might have problems with the heart, kidneys, or bones or with hearing. They might have a mix of these.

The term fetal alcohol effects (FAE) was previously used to describe intellectual disabilities and problems with behavior and learning in a person whose mother drank alcohol during pregnancy. In 1996, the Institute of Medicine (IOM) replaced FAE with the terms alcohol-related neurodevelopmental disorder (ARND) and alcohol-related birth defects (ARBD).

Treatment

FASDs last a lifetime. There is no cure for FASDs, but research shows that early intervention treatment services can improve a child's development.

Section 17.3

Head Trauma in Infants (Shaken Baby Syndrome)

Excerpted from "A Journalist's Guide to Shaken Baby Syndrome:
A Preventable Tragedy," by the Centers for Disease Control and
Prevention (CDC, www.cdc.gov), 2010.

Shaken baby syndrome (SBS) is a preventable, severe form of physical child abuse resulting from violently shaking an infant by the shoulders, arms, or legs. SBS may result from both shaking alone or from shaking with impact.

SBS is not just a crime—it is a public health issue. SBS resulting in head injury is a leading cause of child abuse death in the United States. Nearly all victims of SBS suffer serious health consequences and at least one of every four babies who are violently shaken dies from this form of child maltreatment.

The bottom line is that vigorously shaking a baby can be fatal or result in a permanent disability. Shaking most often occurs in response to a baby crying or other factors that can lead the person caring for a baby to become frustrated or angry. All babies cry and do things that can frustrate caregivers; however, not all caregivers are prepared to care for a baby.

Babies, newborn to 1 year (especially babies ages 2 to 4 months), are at greatest risk of injury from shaking. Shaking them violently can trigger a "whiplash" effect that can lead to internal injuries—including bleeding in the brain or in the eyes. Often there are no obvious external physical signs, such as bruising or bleeding, to indicate an injury.

In more severe cases of SBS, babies may exhibit the following— unresponsiveness, loss of consciousness, breathing problems (irregular breathing or not breathing), and no pulse.

Chapter 18

Learning Disabilities

Chapter Contents

Section 18.1—Dyscalculia.. 134

Section 18.2—Dyslexia 138

Section 18.3—Dysgraphia 142

Section 18.4—Dyspraxia... 147

Section 18.5—Executive Functioning Problems...................... 149

Section 18.6—Information Processing Disorders..................... 155

Section 18.1

Dyscalculia

What Is Dyscalculia?

Dyscalculia refers to a wide range of lifelong learning disabilities involving math. There is no single type of math disability. Dyscalculia can vary from person to person. And, it can affect people differently at different stages of life.

Two major areas of weakness can contribute to math learning disabilities:

- Visual-spatial difficulties, which result in a person having trouble processing what the eye sees

- Language processing difficulties, which result in a person having trouble processing and making sense of what the ear hears

Using alternate learning methods, people with dyscalculia can achieve success.

What Are the Effects of Dyscalculia?

Disabilities involving math vary greatly. So, the effects they have on a person's development can vary just as much. For instance, a person who has trouble processing language will face different challenges in math than a person who has trouble with visual-spatial relationships. Another person may have trouble remembering facts and keeping a sequence of steps in order. This person will have yet a different set of math-related challenges to overcome.

For individuals with visual-spatial troubles, it may be hard to visualize patterns or different parts of a math problem. Language processing problems can make it hard for a person to get a grasp of the vocabulary of math. Without the proper vocabulary and a clear understanding of what the words represent, it is difficult to build on math knowledge. When basic math facts are not mastered earlier, teens and adults with dyscalculia may have trouble moving on to more advanced math applications. These require that a person be able to follow multi-step procedures and be able to identify critical information needed to solve equations and more complex problems.

What Are the Warning Signs of Dyscalculia?

Having trouble learning math skills does not necessarily mean a person has a learning disability. All students learn at different paces. It can take young people time and practice for formal math procedures to make practical sense. So how can you tell if someone has dyscalculia? If a person continues to display trouble with the areas listed in the following text, consider testing for dyscalculia. Extra help may be beneficial.

Warning signs for young children:

- Difficulty learning to count

- Trouble recognizing printed numbers

- Difficulty tying together the idea of a number (4) and how it exists in the world (4 horses, 4 cars, 4 children)

- Poor memory for numbers

- Trouble organizing things in a logical way—putting round objects in one place and square ones in another

Warning signs for school-age children:

- Trouble learning math facts (addition, subtraction, multiplication, division)

- Difficulty developing math problem-solving skills

- Poor long-term memory for math functions

- Not familiar with math vocabulary

- Difficulty measuring things

- Avoiding games that require strategy

Warning signs for teenagers and adults:

- Difficulty estimating costs like groceries, bills

- Difficulty learning math concepts beyond the basic math facts

- Poor ability to budget or balance a checkbook

- Trouble with concepts of time, such as sticking to a schedule or approximating time

- Trouble with mental math

- Difficulty finding different approaches to one problem

How Is Dyscalculia Identified?

When a teacher or trained professional evaluates a student for learning disabilities in math, the student is interviewed about a full range of math-related skills and behaviors.

Pencil and paper math tests are often used, but an evaluation needs to accomplish more. It is meant to reveal how a person understands and uses numbers and math concepts to solve advanced-level, as well as every day, problems. The evaluation compares a person's expected and actual levels of skill and understanding while noting the person's specific strengths and weaknesses. In the following text are some of the areas that may be addressed:

- Ability with basic math skills like counting, adding, subtracting, multiplying, and dividing

- Ability to predict appropriate procedures based on understanding patterns—knowing when to add, subtract, multiply, divide, or do more advanced computations

- Ability to organize objects in a logical way

- Ability to measure—telling time, using money

- Ability to estimate number quantities

- Ability to self-check work and find alternate ways to solve problems

How Is Dyscalculia Treated?

Helping a student identify his/her strengths and weaknesses is the first step to getting help. Following identification, parents, teachers, and other educators can work together to establish strategies that will help the student learn math more effectively. Help outside the classroom lets a student and tutor focus specifically on the difficulties that student is having, taking pressure off moving to new topics too quickly. Repeated reinforcement and specific practice of straightforward ideas can make understanding easier. Other strategies for inside and outside the classroom include [the following]:

- Use graph paper for students who have difficulty organizing ideas on paper.

- Work on finding different ways to approach math facts; i.e., instead of just memorizing the multiplication tables, explain that 8 x 2 = 16, so if 16 is doubled, 8 x 4 must = 32.

- Practice estimating as a way to begin solving math problems.

- Introduce new skills beginning with concrete examples and later moving to more abstract applications.

- For language difficulties, explain ideas and problems clearly and encourage students to ask questions as they work.

- Provide a place to work with few distractions and have pencils, erasers, and other tools on hand as needed.

- Help students become aware of their strengths and weaknesses.

Understanding how a person learns best is a big step in achieving academic success and confidence.

Section 18.2

Dyslexia

"Dyslexia Basics," a fact sheet published by the International
Dyslexia Association © 2008 International Dyslexia Association.
Reprinted with permission.

What Is Dyslexia?

Dyslexia is a language-based learning disability. Dyslexia refers
to a cluster of symptoms, which result in people having difficulties
with specific language skills, particularly reading. Students with dyslexia usually experience difficulties with other language skills such as
spelling, writing, and pronouncing words. Dyslexia affects individuals
throughout their lives; however, its impact can change at different
stages in a person's life. It is referred to as a learning disability because
dyslexia can make it very difficult for a student to succeed academically
in the typical instructional environment, and in its more severe forms,
will qualify a student for special education, special accommodations,
or extra support services.

What Causes Dyslexia?

The exact causes of dyslexia are still not completely clear, but anatomical and brain imagery studies show differences in the way the
brain of a dyslexic person develops and functions.

Moreover, most people with dyslexia have been found to have problems with identifying the separate speech sounds within a word and/
or learning how letters represent those sounds, a key factor in their
reading difficulties. Dyslexia is not due to either lack of intelligence
or desire to learn; with appropriate teaching methods, dyslexics can
learn successfully.

How Widespread Is Dyslexia?

About 13–14% of the school population nationwide has a handicapping condition that qualifies them for special education. Current
studies indicate that one-half of all the students who qualify for

special education are classified as having a learning disability (LD) (6–7%). About 85% of those LD students have a primary learning disability in reading and language processing. Nevertheless, many more people—perhaps as many as 15–20% of the population as a whole—have some of the symptoms of dyslexia, including slow or inaccurate reading, poor spelling, poor writing, or mixing up similar words. Not all of these will qualify for special education, but they are likely to struggle with many aspects of academic learning and are likely to benefit from systematic, explicit, instruction in reading, writing, and language.

Dyslexia occurs in people of all backgrounds and intellectual levels. People who are very bright can be dyslexic. They are often capable or even gifted in areas that do not require strong language skills, such as art, computer science, design, drama, electronics, math, mechanics, music, physics, sales, and sports.

In addition, dyslexia runs in families; dyslexic parents are very likely to have children who are dyslexic. Some people are identified as dyslexic early in their lives, but for others, their dyslexia goes unidentified until they get older.

What Are the Effects of Dyslexia?

The impact that dyslexia has is different for each person and depends on the severity of the condition and the effectiveness of instruction or remediation. The core difficulty is with word recognition and reading fluency, spelling, and writing. Some dyslexics manage to learn early reading and spelling tasks, especially with excellent instruction, but later experience their most debilitating problems when more complex language skills are required, such as grammar, understanding textbook material, and writing essays.

People with dyslexia can also have problems with spoken language, even after they have been exposed to good language models in their homes and good language instruction in school. They may find it difficult to express themselves clearly, or to fully comprehend what others mean when they speak. Such language problems are often difficult to recognize, but they can lead to major problems in school, in the workplace, and in relating to other people. The effects of dyslexia reach well beyond the classroom.

Dyslexia can also affect a person's self-image. Students with dyslexia often end up feeling "dumb" and less capable than they actually are. After experiencing a great deal of stress due to academic problems, a student may become discouraged about continuing in school.

How Is Dyslexia Diagnosed?

Schools may use a new process called Response to Intervention (RTI) to identify children with learning disabilities. Under an RTI model, schools provide those children not readily progressing with the acquisition of critical early literacy skills with intensive and individualized supplemental reading instruction. If a student's learning does not accelerate enough with supplemental instruction to reach the established grade-level benchmarks, and other kinds of developmental disorders are ruled out, he or she may be identified as learning disabled in reading.

The majority of students thus identified are likely dyslexic and they will probably qualify for special education services. Schools are encouraged to begin screening children in kindergarten to identify any child who exhibits the early signs of potential reading difficulties.

For children and adults who do not go through this RTI process, an evaluation to formally diagnose dyslexia is needed. Such an evaluation traditionally has included intellectual and academic achievement testing, as well as an assessment of the critical underlying language skills that are closely linked to dyslexia. These include receptive (listening) and expressive language skills, phonological skills including phonemic awareness, and also a student's ability to rapidly name letters and names. A student's ability to read lists of words in isolation, as well as words in context, should also be assessed. If a profile emerges that is characteristic of dyslexic readers, an individualized intervention plan should be developed, which should include appropriate accommodations, such as extended time. The testing can be conducted by trained school or outside specialists.

What Are the Signs of Dyslexia?

The problems displayed by individuals with dyslexia involve difficulties in acquiring and using written language. It is a myth that dyslexic individuals "read backwards," although spelling can look quite jumbled at times because students have trouble remembering letter symbols for sounds and forming memories for words. Other problems experienced by dyslexics include the following:

- Learning to speak
- Learning letters and their sounds
- Organizing written and spoken language
- Memorizing number facts

- Reading quickly enough to comprehend

- Persisting with and comprehending longer reading assignments

- Spelling

- Learning a foreign language

- Correctly doing math operations

Not all students who have difficulties with these skills are dyslexic. Formal testing of reading, language, and writing skills is the only way to confirm a diagnosis of suspected dyslexia.

How Is Dyslexia Treated?

Dyslexia is a life-long condition. With proper help, many people with dyslexia can learn to read and write well. Early identification and treatment is the key to helping dyslexics achieve in school and in life. Most people with dyslexia need help from a teacher, tutor, or therapist specially trained in using a multisensory, structured language approach. It is important for these individuals to be taught by a systematic and explicit method that involves several senses (hearing, seeing, touching) at the same time. Many individuals with dyslexia need one-on-one help so that they can move forward at their own pace. In addition, students with dyslexia often need a great deal of structured practice and immediate, corrective feedback to develop automatic word recognition skills. When students with dyslexia receive academic therapy outside of school, the therapist should work closely with classroom teachers, special education providers, and other school personnel.

Schools can implement academic accommodations and modifications to help dyslexic students succeed. For example, a student with dyslexia can be given extra time to complete tasks, help with taking notes, and work assignments that are modified appropriately. Teachers can give taped tests or allow dyslexic students to use alternative means of assessment. Students can benefit from listening to books on tape and using the computer for text reading programs and for writing.

Students may also need help with emotional issues that sometimes arise as a consequence of difficulties in school. Mental health specialists can help students cope with their struggles.

What Are the Rights of a Dyslexic Person?

The Individuals with Disabilities Education Act 2004 (IDEA), Section 504 of the Rehabilitation Act of 1973, and the Americans with

Disabilities Act (ADA) define the rights of students with dyslexia and other specific learning disabilities.

These individuals are legally entitled to special services to help them overcome and accommodate their learning problems. Such services include education programs designed to meet the needs of these students. The Acts also protect people with dyslexia against unfair and illegal discrimination.

Section 18.3

Dysgraphia

Dysgraphia is a learning disability that affects writing, which requires a complex set of motor and information processing skills. Dysgraphia makes the act of writing difficult. It can lead to problems with spelling, poor handwriting, and putting thoughts on paper. People with dysgraphia can have trouble organizing letters, numbers, and words on a line or page. This can result partly from [the following]:

• Visual-spatial difficulties: Trouble processing what the eye sees

• Language processing difficulty: Trouble processing and making sense of what the ear hears

As with all learning disabilities (LD), dysgraphia is a lifelong challenge, although how it manifests may change over time. A student with this disorder can benefit from specific accommodations in the learning environment. Extra practice learning the skills required to be an accomplished writer can also help.

What Are the Warning Signs of Dysgraphia?

Just having bad handwriting doesn't mean a person has dysgraphia. Since dysgraphia is a processing disorder, difficulties can change throughout a lifetime. However since writing is a developmental process—children learn the motor skills needed to write, while learning the thinking skills needed to communicate on paper—difficulties can also overlap.

In Early Writers

- Tight, awkward pencil grip and body position
- Avoiding writing or drawing tasks
- Trouble forming letter shapes
- Inconsistent spacing between letters or words
- Poor understanding of uppercase and lowercase letters
- Inability to write or draw in a line or within margins
- Tiring quickly while writing

In Young Students

- Illegible handwriting
- Mixture of cursive and print writing
- Saying words out loud while writing
- Concentrating so hard on writing that comprehension of what's written is missed
- Trouble thinking of words to write
- Omitting or not finishing words in sentences

In Teenagers and Adults

- Trouble organizing thoughts on paper
- Trouble keeping track of thoughts already written down
- Difficulty with syntax structure and grammar
- Large gap between written ideas and understanding demonstrated through speech

What Strategies Can Help?

There are many ways to help a person with dysgraphia achieve success. Generally strategies fall into three main categories:

- Accommodations: Providing alternatives to written expression

- Modifications: Changing expectations or tasks to minimize or avoid the area of weakness

- Remediation: Providing instruction for improving handwriting and writing skills

Each type of strategy should be considered when planning instruction and support. A person with dysgraphia will benefit from help from both specialists and those who are closest to the person. Finding the most beneficial type of support is a process of trying different ideas and openly exchanging thoughts on what works best.

Although teachers and employers are required by law to make "reasonable accommodations" for individuals with learning disabilities, they may not be aware of how to help. Speak to them about dysgraphia and explain the challenges faced as a result of this learning disability.

Here are examples of how to teach individuals with dysgraphia to overcome some of their difficulties with written expression.

Early Writers

Be patient and positive, encourage practice, and praise effort. Becoming a good writer takes time and practice.

- Use paper with raised lines for a sensory guide to staying within the lines.

- Try different pens and pencils to find one that's most comfortable.

- Practice writing letters and numbers in the air with big arm movements to improve motor memory of these important shapes. Also practice letters and numbers with smaller hand or finger motions.

- Encourage proper grip, posture, and paper positioning for writing. It's important to reinforce this early as it's difficult for students to unlearn bad habits later on.

- Use multi-sensory techniques for learning letters, shapes, and numbers. For example, speaking through motor sequences, such as "b" is "big stick down, circle away from my body."

- Introduce a word processor on a computer early; however do not eliminate handwriting for the child. While typing can make it easier to write by alleviating the frustration of forming letters, handwriting is a vital part of a person's ability to function in the world.

Young Students

Encourage practice through low-stress opportunities for writing. This might include writing letters or in a diary, making household lists, or keeping track of sports teams.

- Allow use of print or cursive—whichever is more comfortable.

- Use large graph paper for math calculation to keep columns and rows organized.

- Allow extra time for writing assignments.

- Begin writing assignments creatively with drawing, or speaking ideas into a tape recorder.

- Alternate focus of writing assignments—put the emphasis on some for neatness and spelling, others for grammar or organization of ideas.

- Explicitly teach different types of writing—expository and personal essays, short stories, poems, etc.

- Do not judge timed assignments on neatness and spelling.

- Have students proofread work after a delay—it's easier to see mistakes after a break.

- Help students create a checklist for editing work—spelling, neatness, grammar, syntax, clear progression of ideas, etc.

- Encourage use of a spell checker—speaking spell checkers are available for handwritten work.

- Reduce amount of copying; instead, focus on writing original answers and ideas.

- Have student complete tasks in small steps instead of all at once.

- Find alternative means of assessing knowledge, such as oral reports or visual projects.

Teenagers and Adults

Many of these tips can be used by all age groups. It is never too early or too late to reinforce the skills needed to be a good writer.

- Provide tape recorders to supplement note taking and to prepare for writing assignments.

- Create a step-by-step plan that breaks writing assignments into small tasks.

- When organizing writing projects, create a list of keywords that will be useful.

- Provide clear, constructive feedback on the quality of work, explaining both the strengths and weaknesses of the project, commenting on the structure as well as the information that is included.

- Use assistive technology such as voice-activated software if the mechanical aspects of writing remain a major hurdle.

How to Approach Writing Assignments

- Plan your paper (pull together your ideas and consider how you want them in your writing).

- Organize your thoughts and ideas.

- Create an outline or graphic organizer to be sure you've included all your ideas.

- Make a list of key thoughts and words you will want to use in your paper.

1. Write a Draft

This first draft should focus on getting your ideas on paper—don't worry about making spelling or grammar errors. Using a computer is helpful because it will be easier to edit later on.

2. Edit Your Work

- Check your work for proper spelling, grammar, and syntax; use a spell checker if necessary.

- Edit your paper to elaborate and enhance content—a thesaurus is helpful for finding different ways to make your point.

3. Revise Your Work, Producing a Final Draft

- Rewrite your work into a final draft.

- Be sure to read it one last time before submitting it.

Section 18.4

Dyspraxia

Dyspraxia is a disorder that affects motor skill development. People with dyspraxia have trouble planning and completing fine motor tasks. This can vary from simple motor tasks such as waving goodbye to more complex tasks like brushing teeth. [See Table 18.1.]

It is estimated that dyspraxia affects at least two percent of the general population, and 70% of those affected are male. As many as six percent of all children show some signs of dyspraxia.

A person with dyspraxia can learn to function independently. Special learning methods and repeated practice of basic tasks can help. Sometimes occupational, physical, or speech therapy is also needed.

Dyspraxia often exists along with other learning disabilities and other conditions that impact learning, such as attention deficit hyperactivity disorder (ADHD). Coexisting learning disabilities might include dyslexia (trouble reading, writing, and spelling) or dyscalculia (trouble with mathematics). Some symptoms of all these learning disabilities and ADHD are similar.

Weaknesses in comprehension, information processing, and listening can contribute to the troubles experienced by people with dyspraxia. They may also have low self-esteem, depression, and other emotional and behavioral troubles.

What Are the Warning Signs of Dyspraxia?

Babies with dyspraxia may avoid crawling and rolling over and other tasks involving motor skills. As they become older, children with dyspraxia are prone to problems such as those listed in the following text. Having these problems does not necessarily mean a person has dyspraxia. But if they continue over time, consider testing by trained professionals. You or your child may benefit from special help.

Table 18.1. Dyspraxia by Category

Category	May cause trouble with:
Ideomotor dyspraxia	Inability to complete single-step motor tasks such as combing hair and waving goodbye
Ideational dyspraxia	Difficulty with multi-step tasks like brushing teeth, making a bed, putting clothes on in order, as well as buttoning and buckling
Oromotor dyspraxia	Difficulties coordinating the muscle movements needed to pronounce words
Constructional dyspraxia	Problems with establishing spatial relationships—for instance being able to accurately position or move objects from one place to another

Dyspraxia at Different Ages

- Difficulty learning to walk, jump, and skip
- Trouble pronouncing words and being understood
- Slow to establish left- or right-handedness
- Frequently bumps into things
- Easily irritated by touch—clothing on skin, hair brushing, etc.

School-Age Children

- Trouble with activities that require fine motor skills, like holding a pencil, buttoning, cutting with scissors
- Poor coordination—trouble with sports activities
- Slow or difficult-to-understand speech
- Speech difficulties can cause severe social awkwardness and unwillingness to attempt social interactions

Teenagers and Adults

- Trouble with speech control—volume, pitch, articulation
- Difficulty writing
- Extreme sensitivity to light, touch, space, taste, smells
- Difficulty with personal grooming
- Difficulty driving
- Very clumsy

How Is Dyspraxia Identified and Treated?

There is no cure for dyspraxia. However, early identification and intervention can greatly help. Depending upon the severity of the disability, work with occupational, speech, and physical therapists can improve a person's ability to function and succeed independently.

It can be very frustrating to have trouble communicating or moving. Beginning at an early age, it is vital that parents offer patience, encouragement, help, and support.

All people with dyspraxia need help practicing simple tasks. They can benefit from step-by-step progress into more complex activities. Start with easy physical activities that develop coordination. This can increase confidence. Encourage friendships to broaden experience and understanding of social relationships.

Section 18.5

Executive Functioning Problems

I have often written about learning strategies, and how important it is to help students become "strategic" in their approach to learning, and I discussed some ways that teachers can promote student learning by both teaching and reinforcing the use of effective strategies to their students and by imbedding effective teaching strategies into their classroom instruction. What was missing from that discussion was any real focus on the kinds of "thinking" students need to do when they are confronted with different types of learning challenges and opportunities. These "thinking ingredients" fall under the umbrella term "executive functioning."

A Working Definition of "Executive Functioning"

"Executive functioning" is a term used to describe the many different cognitive processes that individuals use to control their behavior and to get ready to respond to different situations. Whether the task at hand is to read a newspaper article, write an e-mail to a friend, have a telephone conversation with a relative, or join in a soccer game at the park, executive functioning is at work behind the scenes, helping to accomplish the desired goal. In other words, executive functioning:

- is conscious, purposeful, and thoughtful;

- involves activating, orchestrating, monitoring, evaluating, and adapting different strategies to accomplish different tasks;

- includes an understanding of how people tap their knowledge and skills and how they stay motivated to accomplish their goals;

- requires the ability to analyze situations, plan, and take action, focus and maintain attention, and adjust actions as needed to get the job done.

We All Have It and We All Do It

Sometimes these processes seem to happen in a seamless and automatic way, and at other times they seem to not happen quickly enough (or not at all), resulting in what some people refer to as "getting stuck," not knowing what went wrong and having a hard time discerning what to do next. At its best, executive functioning allows us to be mentally and behaviorally flexible to all sorts of task demands, to adjust our thinking to accomplish our goal (even when there are changing conditions along the way), and to adapt our reflexes and responses in ways that result in coherence and smoothness of responses.

How does someone know if their executive functioning abilities are well tuned and ready for action? A few indicators might be if you:

- make good use of past knowledge and experience (both before you start an activity and while it is ongoing);

- take notice of the current situation for cues about what is expected of you and how you might best proceed doing the task at hand;

- think about what you are doing (or are about to start doing), imagine what if any implications it has for you in the future, and allow yourself to feel whether this activity has any personal values or relevance to you (taking your emotional temperature really does matter because it often has a very real impact on how you think!);

- feel you are ready and can be flexible in changing your thinking along the way if need be;

- can delay gratification (not jump to conclusions too quickly) and inhibit any impulsive responses that might take you off track or distract you from your goal;

- are able to adjust the way you think and respond when the rules change unexpectedly.

Learning Disabilities and Executive Functioning

In school, at home, or in the workplace, we're called on all day, every day, to self-regulate behavior. Normally, features of executive functioning are seen in our ability to:

- make plans;

- keep track of time;

- keep track of more than one thing at once;

- meaningfully include past knowledge in discussions;

- engage in group dynamics;

- evaluate ideas;

- reflect on our work;

- change our minds and make mid-course corrections while thinking, reading, and writing;

- finish work on time;

- ask for help;

- wait to speak until we're called on;

- seek more information when we need it.

Problems with executive functioning may be manifested when a person:

- has difficulty planning a project;

- has trouble comprehending how much time a project will take to complete;

- struggles to tell a story (verbally or in writing);

151

- has trouble communicating details in an organized, sequential manner;

- has difficulty with the mental strategies involved in memorization and retrieving information from memory;

- has trouble initiating activities or tasks, or generating ideas independently;

- has difficulty retaining information while doing something with it; e.g., remembering a phone number while dialing.

These problem behaviors are often the descriptors we hear about students with learning disabilities (LD) as well as those with ADHD (attention deficit hyperactivity disorder) and language processing disorders. Parents and teachers complain that they:

- "forget to look ahead," and have trouble planning and setting goals;

- have difficulty sorting, organizing, and prioritizing information;

- focus either on details or the big picture at the expense of the other;

- have difficulty shifting from one activity to another (especially when rules/task demand change);

- have a hard time juggling multiple details in working memory;

- struggle shifting between information that is literal vs. figurative, past vs. current, etc.;

- are often overwhelmed by the increased and varied work load in the middle and upper grades;

- "get it" (e.g., the information being taught, the work tasks assigned) but often "don't know what to do with it" (e.g., how to complete the task in a way that demonstrates their knowledge).

For individuals with LD, problems with executive functioning are often complicated by performance anxiety. Feeling anxious about what to do and how well you're doing (especially when, as is the case with LD, you are "winging it" without a strategy or plan of attack) can easily lead to feeling overloaded and overwhelmed. This in turn leads to exhaustion, inattentiveness, and a cycle of insecurity and feeling out of control. Not a great scenario for learning!

An Excellent Resource

A fine summary of executive function difficulties and learning disabilities can be found in the fifth chapter of a book titled *Executive Function in Education: From Theory to Practice,* edited by Dr. Lynn Meltzer (2007, Guilford Press). The chapter discusses some of the core executive function processes that affect academic performance:

- Selecting appropriate goals
- Initiating work
- Organizing
- Prioritizing
- Memorizing
- Shifting strategies and being flexible in thinking
- Self-monitoring/checking

The chapter also includes an explanation of the inter-relationships between strategy use, effort, self-concept, and academic performance.

Useful sections can also be found on reading comprehension, written language, independent study, homework, and long-term projects and test taking. This chapter also addresses the challenge of identifying difficulties in executive function because of "diagnostic fuzziness," a term that means exactly what it sounds like. There is much overlap between the shared behaviors we typically attribute to executive function LD, and ADHD. There is also considerable controversy around how motivation, effort, and persistence affect the types of behaviors that fall under the executive function umbrella.

And the part of this chapter that I like the best talks about "intervention approaches" on two different levels: The environment and the person. It offers (as simplified and paraphrased below) a set of principles that are important for teaching all students, and are especially critical for students who show weakness in executive function processes:

- Executive function strategies should be taught explicitly and systematically.
- Teach students how when and why specific strategies should be used.
- Embed strategy instruction into the curriculum.
- Students should be encouraged to modify and personalize strategies to match their own learning preferences.

- Practice using strategies with different tasks across content areas.

- Keep motivation high (as being a strategic learner can be very hard work!).

- Help students set realistic goals and use self-monitoring and self-management strategies to identify areas of weakness and self-correct behaviors and performance.

- Make sure that students experience success in using strategies and encourage their consistent use over time.

- Count "strategy use" as part of a student's grade (focus on the "how" of learning, not just the "what").

- Help students understand the limitations of hard work without a strategic plan for learning; effective executive function tools and strategies can greatly improve learning efficiency.

Additional Resources

Denckla, M.B. (1994). Measurement of executive functioning. In G.R. Lyon (Ed.), *Frames of Reference for the Assessment of Learning Disabilities: New Views on Measurement Issues* (pp117–142). Baltimore: Paul H. Brookes Publishing Company.

What Are Executive Functions and Self-Regulation and What Do They Have to Do With Language-Learning Disorders? A paper by Bonnie D. Singer and Anthony S. Bashir printed in *Language, Speech, and Hearing Services in Schools*, Vol. 30, 265–273 July 1999 © American Speech-Language-Hearing Association 265.

Section 18.6

Information Processing Disorders

What Is Information Processing?

Sight, smell, hearing, taste, and touch are all ways the body collects information. But the act of using those senses is only the first step toward being able to use the data they've collected. The information the body collects is sent to the brain which recognizes it, understands it, responds to it, and stores it; repeating this pattern hundreds and even thousands of times each day. Information processing makes it possible for a person to complete all the tasks that are required in a given day, from brushing teeth to grocery shopping to watching TV.

While there are several different and often overlapping types of information processing, two important groups are:

Visual processing:

- Visual discrimination

- Visual sequencing

- Visual memory

- Visual motor processing

- Visual closure

- Spatial relationships

Auditory processing:

- Auditory discrimination

- Auditory memory

- Auditory sequencing

What Is an Information Processing Disorder?

An information processing disorder is a deficiency in a person's ability to effectively use the information the senses have gathered. It is not the result of hearing loss, impaired vision, an attention deficit disorder, or any kind of intellectual or cognitive deficit.

Though information processing disorders are often not named as specific types of learning disabilities, they are seen in many individuals with learning disabilities and can often help explain why a person is having trouble with learning and performance. The inability to process information efficiently can lead to frustration, low self-esteem, and social withdrawal, especially with speech/language impairments.

Many people experience problems with learning and behavior occasionally, but if a person consistently displays difficulties with these tasks over time, testing for information processing disorders by trained professionals should be considered.

Chapter 19

Autism Spectrum Disorders

The autism spectrum disorders (ASDs) are more common in the pediatric population than are some better known disorders such as diabetes, spina bifida, or Down syndrome. The earlier the disorder is diagnosed, the sooner the child can be helped through treatment interventions. Pediatricians, family physicians, daycare providers, teachers, and parents may initially dismiss signs of ASD, optimistically thinking the child is just a little slow and will catch up.

All children with ASD demonstrate deficits in 1) social interaction, 2) verbal and nonverbal communication, and 3) repetitive behaviors or interests. In addition, they will often have unusual responses to sensory experiences, such as certain sounds or the way objects look. Each of these symptoms runs the gamut from mild to severe. They will present in each individual child differently. For instance, a child may have little trouble learning to read but exhibit extremely poor social interaction. Each child will display communication, social, and behavioral patterns that are individual but fit into the overall diagnosis of ASD.

Children with ASD do not follow the typical patterns of child development. In some children, hints of future problems may be apparent from birth. In most cases, the problems in communication and social skills become more noticeable as the child lags further behind other

Excerpted from "Autism Spectrum Disorders (Pervasive Developmental Disorders)," by the National Institute of Mental Health (NIMH, www.nimh.nih.gov), part of the National Institutes of Health, December 8, 2010.

children the same age. Some other children start off well enough. Oftentimes between 12 and 36 months old, the differences in the way they react to people and other unusual behaviors become apparent. Some parents report the change as being sudden, and that their children start to reject people, act strangely, and lose language and social skills they had previously acquired. In other cases, there is a plateau, or leveling, of progress so that the difference between the child with autism and other children the same age becomes more noticeable.

ASD is defined by a certain set of behaviors that can range from the very mild to the severe.

Possible Indicators of Autism Spectrum Disorders

- Does not babble, point, or make meaningful gestures by 1 year of age
- Does not speak one word by 16 months
- Does not combine two words by 2 years
- Does not respond to name
- Loses language or social skills

  Some other indicators include the following:
- Poor eye contact
- Doesn't seem to know how to play with toys
- Excessively lines up toys or other objects
- Is attached to one particular toy or object
- Doesn't smile
- At times seems to be hearing impaired

Problems That May Accompany ASD

Sensory problems: When children's perceptions are accurate, they can learn from what they see, feel, or hear. On the other hand, if sensory information is faulty, the child's experiences of the world can be confusing. Many ASD children are highly attuned or even painfully sensitive to certain sounds, textures, tastes, and smells. Some children find the feel of clothes touching their skin almost unbearable. Some sounds—a vacuum cleaner, a ringing telephone, a sudden storm, even the sound of waves lapping the shoreline—will cause these children to cover their ears and scream.

In ASD, the brain seems unable to balance the senses appropriately. Some ASD children are oblivious to extreme cold or pain. An ASD child may fall and break an arm, yet never cry. Another may bash his head against a wall and not wince, but a light touch may make the child scream with alarm.

Mental retardation: Many children with ASD have some degree of mental impairment. When tested, some areas of ability may be normal, while others may be especially weak. For example, a child with ASD may do well on the parts of the test that measure visual skills but earn low scores on the language subtests.

Seizures: One in four children with ASD develops seizures, often starting either in early childhood or adolescence. Seizures, caused by abnormal electrical activity in the brain, can produce a temporary loss of consciousness (a blackout), a body convulsion, unusual movements, or staring spells. Sometimes a contributing factor is a lack of sleep or a high fever. An EEG (electroencephalogram—recording of the electric currents developed in the brain by means of electrodes applied to the scalp) can help confirm the seizure's presence.

In most cases, seizures can be controlled by a number of medicines called anticonvulsants. The dosage of the medication is adjusted carefully so that the least possible amount of medication will be used to be effective.

Fragile X syndrome: This disorder is the most common inherited form of mental retardation. It was so named because one part of the X chromosome has a defective piece that appears pinched and fragile when under a microscope. Fragile X syndrome affects about two to five percent of people with ASD. It is important to have a child with ASD checked for Fragile X, especially if the parents are considering having another child. For an unknown reason, if a child with ASD also has Fragile X, there is a one-in-two chance that boys born to the same parents will have the syndrome. Other members of the family who may be contemplating having a child may also wish to be checked for the syndrome.

A distinction can be made between a father's and mother's ability to pass along to a daughter or son the altered gene on the X chromosome that is linked to Fragile X syndrome. Because both males (XY) and females (XX) have at least one X chromosome, both can pass on the mutated gene to their children.

A father with the altered gene for Fragile X on his X chromosome will only pass that gene on to his daughters. He passes a Y chromosome on to his sons, which doesn't transmit the condition. Therefore, if the father has the altered gene on his X chromosome, but the mother's X chromosomes are normal, all of the couple's daughters would have the altered gene for Fragile X, while none of their sons would have the mutated gene. Because mothers pass on only X chromosomes to their children, if the mother has the altered gene for Fragile X, she can pass that gene to either her sons or her daughters. If the mother has the mutated gene on one X chromosome and has one normal X chromosome, and the father has no genetic mutations, all the children have a 50-50 chance of inheriting the mutated gene.

The odds noted here apply to each child the parents have; in terms of prevalence, the latest statistics are consistent in showing that 5% of people with autism are affected by Fragile X and 10% to 15% of those with Fragile X show autistic traits.

Tuberous sclerosis: Tuberous sclerosis is a rare genetic disorder that causes benign tumors to grow in the brain as well as in other vital organs. It has a consistently strong association with ASD. One to 4 percent of people with ASD also have tuberous sclerosis.

Treatment Options

There is no single best treatment package for all children with ASD. One point that most professionals agree on is that early intervention is important; another is that most individuals with ASD respond well to highly structured, specialized programs.

Before you make decisions on your child's treatment, you will want to gather information about the various options available. Learn as much as you can, look at all the options, and make your decision on your child's treatment based on your child's needs. You may want to visit public schools in your area to see the type of program they offer to special needs children.

Guidelines used by the Autism Society of America include the following questions parents can ask about potential treatments:

- Will the treatment result in harm to my child?

- How will failure of the treatment affect my child and family?

- Has the treatment been validated scientifically?

- Are there assessment procedures specified?

- How will the treatment be integrated into my child's current program? Do not become so infatuated with a given treatment that functional curriculum, vocational life, and social skills are ignored.

Chapter 20

Attention Deficit Hyperactivity Disorder

What is attention deficit hyperactivity disorder?

Attention deficit hyperactivity disorder (ADHD) is one of the most common childhood disorders and can continue through adolescence and adulthood. Symptoms include difficulty staying focused and paying attention, difficulty controlling behavior, and hyperactivity (overactivity). ADHD has three subtypes.

Predominantly hyperactive-impulsive is one subtype:

- Most symptoms (six or more) are in the hyperactivity-impulsivity categories.

- Fewer than six symptoms of inattention are present, although inattention may still be present to some degree.

Predominantly inattentive is another subtype:

- The majority of symptoms (six or more) are in the inattention category and fewer than six symptoms of hyperactivity-impulsivity are present, although hyperactivity-impulsivity may still be present to some degree.

- Children with this subtype are less likely to act out or have difficulties getting along with other children. They may sit quietly,

Excerpted from "Attention Deficit Hyperactivity Disorder (ADHD)," by the National Institute of Mental Health (NIMH, www.nimh.nih.gov), part of the National Institutes of Health, 2008.

but they are not paying attention to what they are doing. Therefore, the child may be overlooked, and parents and teachers may not notice that he or she has ADHD.

Combined hyperactive-impulsive and inattentive is the third subtype:

- Six or more symptoms of inattention and six or more symptoms of hyperactivity-impulsivity are present.

- Most children have the combined type of ADHD.

Treatments can relieve many of the disorder's symptoms, but there is no cure. With treatment, most people with ADHD can be successful in school and lead productive lives. Researchers are developing more effective treatments and interventions, and using new tools such as brain imaging, to better understand ADHD and to find more effective ways to treat and prevent it.

What are the symptoms of ADHD in children?

Inattention, hyperactivity, and impulsivity are the key behaviors of ADHD. It is normal for all children to be inattentive, hyperactive, or impulsive sometimes, but for children with ADHD, these behaviors are more severe and occur more often. To be diagnosed with the disorder, a child must have symptoms for 6 or more months and to a degree that is greater than other children of the same age.

Children who have symptoms of inattention may do the following:

- Be easily distracted, miss details, forget things, and frequently switch from one activity to another

- Have difficulty focusing on one thing

- Become bored with a task after only a few minutes, unless they are doing something enjoyable

- Have difficulty focusing attention on organizing and completing a task or learning something new

- Have trouble completing or turning in homework assignments, often losing things (e.g., pencils, toys, assignments) needed to complete tasks or activities

- Not seem to listen when spoken to

- Daydream, become easily confused, and move slowly

- Have difficulty processing information as quickly and accurately as others

- Struggle to follow instructions

Children who have symptoms of hyperactivity may do the following:

- Fidget and squirm in their seats
- Talk nonstop
- Dash around, touching or playing with anything and everything in sight
- Have trouble sitting still during dinner, school, and story time
- Be constantly in motion
- Have difficulty doing quiet tasks or activities

Children who have symptoms of impulsivity may do the following:

- Be very impatient
- Blurt out inappropriate comments, show their emotions without restraint, and act without regard for consequences
- Have difficulty waiting for things they want or waiting their turns in games
- Often interrupt conversations or others' activities

Parents and teachers can miss the fact that children with symptoms of inattention have the disorder because they are often quiet and less likely to act out. They may sit quietly, seeming to work, but they are often not paying attention to what they are doing. They may get along well with other children, compared with those with the other subtypes, who tend to have social problems.

But children with the inattentive kind of ADHD are not the only ones whose disorders can be missed. For example, adults may think that children with the hyperactive and impulsive subtypes just have emotional or disciplinary problems.

How is ADHD treated?

Currently available treatments focus on reducing the symptoms of ADHD and improving functioning. Treatments include medication, various types of psychotherapy, education or training, or a combination of treatments.

Medications: The most common type of medication used for treating ADHD is called a stimulant. Although it may seem unusual to

163

treat ADHD with a medication considered a stimulant, it actually has a calming effect on children with ADHD.

Many types of stimulant medications are available. A few other ADHD medications are non-stimulants and work differently than stimulants. For many children, ADHD medications reduce hyperactivity and impulsivity and improve their ability to focus, work, and learn. Medication also may improve physical coordination.

However, a one-size-fits-all approach does not apply for all children with ADHD. What works for one child might not work for another. One child might have side effects with a certain medication, while another child may not. Sometimes several different medications or dosages must be tried before finding one that works for a particular child. Any child taking medications must be monitored closely and carefully by caregivers and doctors.

Stimulant medications come in different forms, such as a pill, capsule, liquid, or skin patch. Some medications also come in short-acting, long-acting, or extended release varieties. In each of these varieties, the active ingredient is the same, but it is released differently in the body. Long-acting or extended release forms often allow a child to take the medication just once a day before school, so they don't have to make a daily trip to the school nurse for another dose. Parents and doctors should decide together which medication is best for the child and whether the child needs medication only for school hours or for evenings and weekends, too.

ADHD can be diagnosed and medications prescribed by MDs (usually a psychiatrist) and in some states also by clinical psychologists, psychiatric nurse practitioners, and advanced psychiatric nurse specialists. Check with your state's licensing agency for specifics.

Psychotherapy: Different types of psychotherapy are used for ADHD. Behavioral therapy aims to help a child change his or her behavior. It might involve practical assistance, such as help organizing tasks or completing schoolwork, or working through emotionally difficult events. Behavioral therapy also teaches a child how to monitor his or her own behavior. Learning to give oneself praise or rewards for acting in a desired way, such as controlling anger or thinking before acting, is another goal of behavioral therapy. Parents and teachers also can give positive or negative feedback for certain behaviors. In addition, clear rules, chore lists, and other structured routines can help a child control his or her behavior.

Therapists may teach children social skills, such as how to wait their turn, share toys, ask for help, or respond to teasing. Learning to read facial expressions and the tone of voice in others, and how to respond appropriately can also be part of social skills training.

Chapter 21

Psychiatric Disability and Mental Disorders

The evaluation of disability on the basis of mental disorders requires documentation of a medically determinable impairment(s), consideration of the degree of limitation such impairment(s) may impose on the individual's ability to work, and consideration of whether these limitations have lasted or are expected to last for a continuous period of at least 12 months. The listings for mental disorders are arranged in nine diagnostic categories: Organic mental disorders; schizophrenic, paranoid, and other psychotic disorders; affective disorders; mental retardation; anxiety-related disorders; somatoform disorders; personality disorders; substance addiction disorders; and autistic disorder and other pervasive developmental disorders.

For a person to be classified with a disabling psychiatric condition, there must be evidence from an acceptable medical source showing that you have a medically determinable mental impairment. The SSA will make every reasonable effort to obtain all relevant and available medical evidence about your mental impairment(s), including its history, and any records of mental status examination, psychological testing, and hospitalizations and treatment. Whenever possible, and appropriate, medical source evidence should reflect the medical source's considerations of information from you and other concerned persons who are aware of your activities of daily living; social functioning; concentration, persistence, or pace; or episodes of decompensation.

Excerpted from "Mental Disorders—Adult," Disability Evaluation Under Social Security, by the Social Security Administration (SSA, www.socialsecurity.gov), September 2008. Updated March 24, 2011.

Also, in accordance with standard clinical practice, any medical source assessment of your mental functioning should take into account any sensory, motor, or communication abnormalities, as well as your cultural and ethnic background.

Individuals with mental impairments can often provide accurate descriptions of their limitations. The presence of a mental impairment does not automatically rule you out as a reliable source of information about your own functional limitations. When you have a mental impairment and are willing and able to describe your limitations, the SSA will try to obtain such information from you. However, you may not be willing or able to fully or accurately describe the limitations resulting from your impairment(s). Thus, the SSA will carefully examine the statements you provide to determine if they are consistent with the information about, or general pattern of, the impairment as described by the medical and other evidence, and to determine whether additional information about your functioning is needed from you or other sources.

Other professional health care providers (e.g., psychiatric nurse, psychiatric social worker) can normally provide valuable functional information, which should be obtained when available and needed. If necessary, information should also be obtained from nonmedical sources, such as family members and others who know you, to supplement the record of your functioning in order to establish the consistency of the medical evidence and longitudinality of impairment severity. Other sources of information about functioning include, but are not limited to, records from work evaluations and rehabilitation progress notes.

Your level of functioning may vary considerably over time. The level of your functioning at a specific time may seem relatively adequate or, conversely, rather poor. Proper evaluation of your impairment(s) must take into account any variations in the level of your functioning in arriving at a determination of severity over time. Thus, it is vital to obtain evidence from relevant sources over a sufficiently long period prior to the date of adjudication to establish your impairment severity.

You may have attempted to work or may actually have worked during the period of time pertinent to the determination of disability. This may have been an independent attempt at work or it may have been in conjunction with a community mental health or sheltered program, and it may have been of either short or long duration. Information concerning your behavior during any attempt to work and the circumstances surrounding termination of your work effort are particularly useful in determining your ability or inability to function in a work setting. In addition, the SSA should also examine the degree to which you require special supports (such as those provided through supported employment or transitional employment programs) in order to work.

The mental status examination is performed in the course of a clinical interview and is often partly assessed while the history is being obtained. A comprehensive mental status examination generally includes a narrative description of your appearance, behavior, and speech; thought process (e.g., loosening of associations); thought content (e.g., delusions); perceptual abnormalities (e.g., hallucinations); mood and affect (e.g., depression, mania); sensorium and cognition (e.g., orientation, recall, memory, concentration, fund of information, and intelligence); and judgment and insight. The individual case facts determine the specific areas of mental status that need to be emphasized during the examination.

Psychological tests, intelligence tests, and other factors may play a role in the decision of whether your psychiatric condition causes disability.

Types of Mental Impairment

Organic Mental Disorders

These disorders are psychological or behavioral abnormalities associated with a dysfunction of the brain. History and physical examination or laboratory tests demonstrate the presence of a specific organic factor judged to be etiologically related to the abnormal mental state and loss of previously acquired functional abilities.

Schizophrenic, Paranoid, and Other Psychotic Disorders

These disorders are characterized by the onset of psychotic features with deterioration from a previous level of functioning.

Affective Disorders

These disorders are characterized by a disturbance of mood, accompanied by a full or partial manic or depressive syndrome. Mood refers to a prolonged emotion that colors the whole psychic life; it generally involves either depression or elation.

Mental Retardation

Mental retardation refers to significantly subaverage general intellectual functioning with deficits in adaptive functioning initially manifested during the developmental period; i.e., the evidence demonstrates or supports onset of the impairment before age 22.

Anxiety-Related Disorders

In these disorders anxiety is either the predominant disturbance or it is experienced if the individual attempts to master symptoms; for example, confronting the dreaded object or situation in a phobic disorder or resisting the obsessions or compulsions in obsessive compulsive disorders.

Somatoform Disorders

Physical symptoms for which there are no demonstrable organic findings or known physiological mechanisms.

Personality Disorders

A personality disorder exists when personality traits are inflexible and maladaptive and cause either significant impairment in social or occupational functioning or subjective distress. Characteristic features are typical of the individual's long-term functioning and are not limited to discrete episodes of illness.

Substance Addiction Disorders

These disorders include behavioral changes or physical changes associated with the regular use of substances that affect the central nervous system.

Autistic Disorder and Other Pervasive Developmental Disorders

These disorders are characterized by qualitative deficits in the development of reciprocal social interaction, in the development of verbal and nonverbal communication skills, and in imaginative activity. Often, there is a markedly restricted repertoire of activities and interests, which frequently are stereotyped and repetitive.

Chapter 22

Degenerative Diseases That Cause Disability

Chapter Contents

Section 22.1—Alzheimer Disease 170

Section 22.2—Amyotrophic Lateral Sclerosis 172

Section 22.3—Arthritis 175

Section 22.4—Multiple Sclerosis 179

Section 22.5—Parkinson Disease 183

Section 22.1

Alzheimer Disease

From "Alzheimer's Disease Fact Sheet," by the National Institute on Aging (NIA, www.nia.nih.gov), part of the National Institutes of Health, February 2010.

Alzheimer disease is an irreversible, progressive brain disease that slowly destroys memory and thinking skills, and eventually even the ability to carry out the simplest tasks. In most people with Alzheimer disease, symptoms first appear after age 60.

Alzheimer disease is the most common cause of dementia among older people. Dementia is the loss of cognitive functioning—thinking, remembering, and reasoning—to such an extent that it interferes with a person's daily life and activities. Estimates vary, but experts suggest that as many as 5.1 million Americans may have Alzheimer disease.

Alzheimer disease is named after Dr. Alois Alzheimer. In 1906, Dr. Alzheimer noticed changes in the brain tissue of a woman who had died of an unusual mental illness. Her symptoms included memory loss, language problems, and unpredictable behavior. After she died, he examined her brain and found many abnormal clumps (now called amyloid plaques) and tangled bundles of fibers (now called neurofibrillary tangles). Plaques and tangles in the brain are two of the main features of Alzheimer disease. The third is the loss of connections between nerve cells (neurons) in the brain.

What changes in the brain occur in Alzheimer disease?

Although we still don't know what starts the Alzheimer disease process, we do know that damage to the brain begins as many as 10 to 20 years before any problems are evident. Tangles begin to develop deep in the brain, in an area called the entorhinal cortex, and plaques form in other areas. As more and more plaques and tangles form in particular brain areas, healthy neurons begin to work less efficiently. Then, they lose their ability to function and communicate with each other, and eventually they die. This damaging process spreads to a nearby structure, called the hippocampus, which is essential in forming memories. As the death of neurons increases, affected brain regions begin to shrink. By the final stage of Alzheimer disease, damage is widespread and brain tissue has shrunk significantly.

Very early signs and symptoms: Memory problems are one of the first signs of Alzheimer disease. Some people with memory problems have a condition called amnestic mild cognitive impairment (MCI). People with this condition have more memory problems than normal for people their age, but their symptoms are not as severe as those with Alzheimer disease. More people with MCI, compared with those without MCI, go on to develop Alzheimer disease.

Other changes may also signal the very early stages of Alzheimer disease. For example, brain imaging and biomarker studies of people with MCI and those with a family history of Alzheimer disease are beginning to detect early changes in the brain like those seen in Alzheimer disease. These findings will need to be confirmed by other studies but appear promising. Other recent research has found links between some movement difficulties and MCI. Researchers also have seen links between some problems with the sense of smell and cognitive problems. Such findings offer hope that someday we may have tools that could help detect Alzheimer disease early, track the course of the disease, and monitor response to treatments.

Mild Alzheimer disease: As Alzheimer disease progresses, memory loss continues and changes in other cognitive abilities appear. Problems can include getting lost, trouble handling money and paying bills, repeating questions, taking longer to complete normal daily tasks, poor judgment, and small mood and personality changes. People often are diagnosed in this stage.

Moderate Alzheimer disease: In this stage, damage occurs in areas of the brain that control language, reasoning, sensory processing, and conscious thought. Memory loss and confusion increase, and people begin to have problems recognizing family and friends. They may be unable to learn new things, carry out tasks that involve multiple steps (such as getting dressed), or cope with new situations. They may have hallucinations, delusions, and paranoia, and may behave impulsively.

Severe Alzheimer disease: By the final stage, plaques and tangles have spread throughout the brain and brain tissue has shrunk significantly. People with severe Alzheimer disease cannot communicate and are completely dependent on others for their care. Near the end, the person may be in bed most or all of the time as the body shuts down.

Section 22.2

Amyotrophic Lateral Sclerosis

Excerpted from "Amyotrophic Lateral Sclerosis Fact Sheet," by the National Institute of Neurological Disorders and Stroke (NINDS, www .ninds.nih.gov), part of the National Institutes of Health, June 6, 2011.

What is amyotrophic lateral sclerosis?

Amyotrophic lateral sclerosis (ALS), sometimes called Lou Gehrig disease, is a rapidly progressive, invariably fatal neurological disease that attacks the nerve cells (neurons) responsible for controlling voluntary muscles. The disease belongs to a group of disorders known as motor neuron diseases, which are characterized by the gradual degeneration and death of motor neurons.

Motor neurons are nerve cells located in the brain, brainstem, and spinal cord that serve as controlling units and vital communication links between the nervous system and the voluntary muscles of the body. Messages from motor neurons in the brain (called upper motor neurons) are transmitted to motor neurons in the spinal cord (called lower motor neurons) and from them to particular muscles. In ALS, both the upper motor neurons and the lower motor neurons degenerate or die, ceasing to send messages to muscles. Unable to function, the muscles gradually weaken, waste away (atrophy), and twitch (fasciculations). Eventually, the ability of the brain to start and control voluntary movement is lost.

ALS causes weakness with a wide range of disabilities. Eventually, all muscles under voluntary control are affected, and patients lose their strength and the ability to move their arms, legs, and body. When muscles in the diaphragm and chest wall fail, patients lose the ability to breathe without ventilatory support. Most people with ALS die from respiratory failure, usually within 3 to 5 years from the onset of symptoms. However, about 10 percent of ALS patients survive for 10 or more years.

Although the disease usually does not impair a person's mind or intelligence, several recent studies suggest that some ALS patients may have alterations in cognitive functions such as depression and problems with decision-making and memory.

ALS does not affect a person's ability to see, smell, taste, hear, or recognize touch. Patients usually maintain control of eye muscles and bladder and bowel functions, although in the late stages of the disease most patients will need help getting to and from the bathroom.

Who gets ALS?

As many as 20,000–30,000 people in the United States have ALS, and an estimated 5,000 people in the United States are diagnosed with the disease each year. ALS is one of the most common neuromuscular diseases worldwide, and people of all races and ethnic backgrounds are affected. ALS most commonly strikes people between 40 and 60 years of age, but younger and older people also can develop the disease. Men are affected more often than women.

In 90 to 95 percent of all ALS cases, the disease occurs apparently at random with no clearly associated risk factors. Patients do not have a family history of the disease, and their family members are not considered to be at increased risk for developing ALS.

About 5 to 10 percent of all ALS cases are inherited. The familial form of ALS usually results from a pattern of inheritance that requires only one parent to carry the gene responsible for the disease. About 20 percent of all familial cases result from a specific genetic defect that leads to mutation of the enzyme known as superoxide dismutase 1 (SOD1). Research on this mutation is providing clues about the possible causes of motor neuron death in ALS. Not all familial ALS cases are due to the SOD1 mutation, therefore other unidentified genetic causes clearly exist.

What are the symptoms?

The onset of ALS may be so subtle that the symptoms are frequently overlooked. The earliest symptoms may include twitching, cramping, or stiffness of muscles; muscle weakness affecting an arm or a leg; slurred and nasal speech; or difficulty chewing or swallowing. These general complaints then develop into more obvious weakness or atrophy that may cause a physician to suspect ALS.

The parts of the body affected by early symptoms of ALS depend on which muscles in the body are damaged first. In some cases, symptoms initially affect one of the legs, and patients experience awkwardness when walking or running or they notice that they are tripping or stumbling more often. Some patients first see the effects of the disease on a hand or arm as they experience difficulty with simple tasks requiring manual dexterity such as buttoning a shirt, writing, or turning a key in a lock. Other patients notice speech problems.

Regardless of the part of the body first affected by the disease, muscle weakness and atrophy spread to other parts of the body as the disease progresses. Patients have increasing problems with moving, swallowing (dysphagia), and speaking or forming words (dysarthria). Symptoms of upper motor neuron involvement include tight and stiff muscles (spasticity) and exaggerated reflexes (hyperreflexia) including an overactive gag reflex. An abnormal reflex commonly called Babinski sign (the large toe extends upward as the sole of the foot is stimulated in a certain way) also indicates upper motor neuron damage. Symptoms of lower motor neuron degeneration include muscle weakness and atrophy, muscle cramps, and fleeting twitches of muscles that can be seen under the skin (fasciculations).

To be diagnosed with ALS, patients must have signs and symptoms of both upper and lower motor neuron damage that cannot be attributed to other causes.

Although the sequence of emerging symptoms and the rate of disease progression vary from person to person, eventually patients will not be able to stand or walk, get in or out of bed on their own, or use their hands and arms. Difficulty swallowing and chewing impair the patient's ability to eat normally and increase the risk of choking. Maintaining weight will then become a problem. Because the disease usually does not affect cognitive abilities, patients are aware of their progressive loss of function and may become anxious and depressed. A small percentage of patients may experience problems with memory or decision-making, and there is growing evidence that some may even develop a form of dementia. Health care professionals need to explain the course of the disease and describe available treatment options so that patients can make informed decisions in advance. In later stages of the disease, patients have difficulty breathing as the muscles of the respiratory system weaken. Patients eventually lose the ability to breathe on their own and must depend on ventilatory support for survival. Patients also face an increased risk of pneumonia during later stages of ALS.

Section 22.3

Arthritis

Excerpted from "Questions and Answers about Arthritis and Degenerative Diseases," by the National Institute of Arthritis and Musculoskeletal and Skin Diseases (NIAMS, www .niams.nih.gov), part of the National Institutes of Health, October 2008.

Arthritis literally means joint inflammation. Although joint inflammation describes a symptom or sign rather than a specific diagnosis, the term "arthritis" is often used to refer to any disorder that affects the joints. These disorders fall within the broader category of rheumatic diseases. These are diseases characterized by inflammation (signs include redness or heat, swelling, and symptoms such as pain) and loss of function of one or more connecting or supporting structures of the body. These diseases especially affect joints, tendons, ligaments, bones, and muscles. Common signs and symptoms are pain, swelling, and stiffness. Some rheumatic diseases also can involve internal organs.

There are more than 100 rheumatic diseases. Some are described as connective tissue diseases because they affect the supporting framework of the body and its internal organs. Others are known as autoimmune diseases because they occur when the immune system, which normally protects the body from infection and disease, harms the body's own healthy tissues. Throughout this text, the terms "arthritis" and "rheumatic diseases" are used interchangeably.

The burden of arthritis in the United States is enormous. More than 46 million people in the United States have arthritis or other rheumatic conditions. Adults with arthritis and other rheumatic conditions incurred mean medical care expenditures of $6,978 in 2003, of which $1,635 was for prescriptions. Expenditures for adults with arthritis and other rheumatic conditions totaled $321.8 billion in 2003. Persons age 18 to 64 with arthritis and other rheumatic conditions earned $3,613 less than other persons. Of this amount, $1,590 in lost wages was attributable to arthritis and other rheumatic conditions.

What are some examples of rheumatic diseases?

Osteoarthritis: This is the most common type of arthritis, affecting an estimated 27 million adults in the United States. Osteoarthritis affects both the cartilage, which is the tissue that cushions the ends of bones within the joint, as well as the underlying bone. In osteoarthritis, there is damage to the cartilage, which begins to fray and may wear away entirely. There is also damage to the bond stock of the joint. Osteoarthritis can cause joint pain and stiffness. Disability results most often when the disease affects the spine and the weight-bearing joints (the knees and hips).

Rheumatoid arthritis: This inflammatory disease of the immune system targets first the synovium, or lining of the joint, resulting in pain, stiffness, swelling, joint damage, and loss of function of the joints. Inflammation most often affects joints of the hands and feet and tends to be symmetrical (occurring equally on both sides of the body). This symmetry helps distinguish rheumatoid arthritis from other forms of the disease. About 0.6 percent of the U.S. population (about 1.3 million people) has rheumatoid arthritis.

Juvenile idiopathic arthritis: This disease is the most common form of arthritis in childhood, causing pain, stiffness, swelling, and loss of function of the joints. This condition may be associated with rashes or fevers and may affect various parts of the body.

Fibromyalgia: Fibromyalgia is a chronic disorder that causes pain throughout the tissues that support and move the bones and joints. Pain, stiffness, and localized tender points occur in the muscles and tendons, particularly those of the neck, spine, shoulders, and hips. Patients also may experience fatigue and sleep disturbances. Fibromyalgia affects millions of adults in the United States.

Systemic lupus erythematosus: Systemic lupus erythematosus (also known as lupus or SLE) is an autoimmune disease in which the immune system harms the body's own healthy cells and tissues. This can result in inflammation of and damage to the joints, skin, kidneys, heart, lungs, blood vessels, and brain. By conservative estimates, lupus affects about 150,000 people.

Scleroderma: Also known as systemic sclerosis, scleroderma means literally "hard skin." The disease affects the skin, blood vessels, and joints. It may also affect internal organs, such as the lungs and kidneys. In scleroderma, there is an abnormal and excessive production of collagen (a fiber-like protein) in the skin and internal organs.

Spondyloarthropathies: This group of rheumatic diseases principally affects the spine. One common form—ankylosing spondylitis—also may affect the hips, shoulders, and knees. The tendons and ligaments around the bones and joints become inflamed, resulting in pain and stiffness. Ankylosing spondylitis tends to affect people in late adolescence or early adulthood. Reactive arthritis, sometimes called Reiter syndrome, is another spondyloarthropathy. It develops after an infection involving the lower urinary tract, bowel, or other organ. It is commonly associated with eye problems, skin rashes, and mouth sores.

Infectious arthritis: This is a general term used to describe forms of arthritis that are caused by infectious agents, such as bacteria or viruses. Parvovirus arthritis and gonococcal arthritis are examples of infectious arthritis. Arthritis symptoms also may occur in Lyme disease, which is caused by a bacterial infection following the bite of certain ticks. In those cases of arthritis caused by bacteria, early diagnosis and treatment with antibiotics are crucial to removing the infection and minimizing damage to the joints.

Gout: This type of arthritis results from deposits of needle-like crystals of uric acid in the joints. The crystals cause episodic inflammation, swelling, and pain in the affected joint, which is often the big toe. An estimated 2.1 million Americans have gout.

Polymyalgia rheumatica: Because this disease involves tendons, muscles, ligaments, and tissues around the joint, symptoms often include pain, aching, and morning stiffness in the shoulders, hips, neck, and lower back. It is sometimes the first sign of giant cell arteritis, a disease of the arteries characterized by headaches, inflammation, weakness, weight loss, and fever.

Polymyositis: This rheumatic disease causes inflammation and weakness in the muscles. The disease may affect the whole body and cause disability.

Psoriatic arthritis: This form of arthritis occurs in some patients with psoriasis, a scaling skin disorder. Psoriatic arthritis often affects the joints at the ends of the fingers and toes and is accompanied by changes in the fingernails and toenails. Back pain may occur if the spine is involved.

Bursitis:: This condition involves inflammation of the bursae, small, fluid-filled sacs that help reduce friction between bones and other moving structures in the joints. The inflammation may result from arthritis in the joint or injury or infection of the bursae. Bursitis produces pain and tenderness and may limit the movement of nearby joints.

177

Tendonitis: This condition refers to inflammation of tendons (tough cords of tissue that connect muscle to bone) caused by overuse, injury, or a rheumatic condition. Tendonitis produces pain and tenderness and may restrict movement of nearby joints.

Who is affected by rheumatic diseases?

An estimated 46 million people in the United States have arthritis or other rheumatic conditions. By the year 2020, this number is expected to reach 60 million. Rheumatic diseases are a more frequent cause of activity limitation than heart disease, cancer, or diabetes.

Rheumatic diseases affect people of all races and ages. Some rheumatic conditions are more common among certain populations. For example, consider the following:

- Rheumatoid arthritis occurs two to three times more often in women than in men.

- Scleroderma is more common in women than in men.

- Nine out of 10 people who have lupus are women.

- Nine out of 10 people who have fibromyalgia are women.

- Gout is more common in men than in women. After menopause, the incidence of gout for women begins to rise.

- Systemic lupus erythematosus is more common in women than in men, and it occurs more often in African Americans and Hispanics than in Caucasians.

Section 22.4

Multiple Sclerosis

Excerpted from "Multiple Sclerosis: Hope Through Research," by the National Institute of Neurological Disorders and Stroke (NINDS, www .ninds.nih.gov), part of the National Institutes of Health, June 28, 2011.

An unpredictable disease of the central nervous system, multiple sclerosis (MS) can range from relatively benign to somewhat disabling to devastating as communication between the brain and other parts of the body is disrupted.

The majority of patients are mildly affected, but in the worst cases MS can render a person unable to write, speak, or walk. A physician can diagnose MS in some patients soon after the onset of the illness. In others, however, physicians may not be able to readily identify the cause of the symptoms, leading to years of uncertainty and multiple diagnoses punctuated by baffling symptoms that mysteriously wax and wane.

During an MS attack, inflammation occurs in areas of the white matter of the central nervous system in random patches called plaques. This process is followed by destruction of myelin, the fatty covering that insulates nerve cell fibers in the brain and spinal cord. Myelin facilitates the smooth, high-speed transmission of electrochemical messages between the brain, the spinal cord, and the rest of the body; when it is damaged, neurological transmission of messages may be slowed or blocked completely, leading to diminished or lost function. The name "multiple sclerosis" signifies both the number (multiple) and condition (sclerosis, from the Greek term for scarring or hardening) of the demyelinated areas in the central nervous system.

How many people have MS?

No one knows exactly how many people have MS. It is believed that, currently, there are approximately 250,000 to 350,000 people in the United States with MS diagnosed by a physician. This estimate suggests that approximately 200 new cases are diagnosed each week.

What are the symptoms of MS?

Symptoms of MS may be mild or severe, of long duration or short, and may appear in various combinations, depending on the area of the nervous system affected.

Complete or partial remission of symptoms, especially in the early stages of the disease, occurs in approximately 70 percent of MS patients.

The initial symptom of MS is often blurred or double vision, red-green color distortion, or even blindness in one eye. Inexplicably, visual problems tend to clear up in the later stages of MS. Inflammatory problems of the optic nerve may be diagnosed as retrobulbar or optic neuritis. Fifty-five percent of MS patients will have an attack of optic neuritis at some time or other and it will be the first symptom of MS in approximately 15 percent. This has led to general recognition of optic neuritis as an early sign of MS, especially if tests also reveal abnormalities in the patient's spinal fluid.

Most MS patients experience muscle weakness in their extremities and difficulty with coordination and balance at some time during the course of the disease. These symptoms may be severe enough to impair walking or even standing. In the worst cases, MS can produce partial or complete paralysis. Spasticity—the involuntary increased tone of muscles leading to stiffness and spasms—is common, as is fatigue. Fatigue may be triggered by physical exertion and improve with rest, or it may take the form of a constant and persistent tiredness.

Most people with MS also exhibit paresthesias, transitory abnormal sensory feelings such as numbness, prickling, or "pins and needles" sensations; uncommonly, some may also experience pain. Loss of sensation sometimes occurs.

Speech impediments, tremors, and dizziness are other frequent complaints. Occasionally, people with MS have hearing loss.

Approximately half of all people with MS experience cognitive impairments such as difficulties with concentration, attention, memory, and poor judgment, but such symptoms are usually mild and are frequently overlooked. In fact, they are often detectable only through comprehensive testing. Patients themselves may be unaware of their cognitive loss; it is often a family member or friend who first notices a deficit. Such impairments are usually mild, rarely disabling, and intellectual and language abilities are generally spared.

Cognitive symptoms occur when lesions develop in brain areas responsible for information processing. These deficits tend to become more apparent as the information to be processed becomes more complex. Fatigue may also add to processing difficulties. Scientists do not yet know whether altered cognition in MS reflects problems with information acquisition, retrieval, or a combination of both. Types of memory problems may differ depending on the individual's disease course (relapsing-remitting, primary-progressive, etc.), but there does not appear to be any direct correlation between duration of illness and severity of cognitive dysfunction.

Depression, which is unrelated to cognitive problems, is another common feature of MS. In addition, about 10 percent of patients suffer from more severe psychotic disorders such as manic-depression and paranoia. Five percent may experience episodes of inappropriate euphoria and despair—unrelated to the patient's actual emotional state—known as "laughing/weeping syndrome." This syndrome is thought to be due to demyelination in the brainstem, the area of the brain that controls facial expression and emotions, and is usually seen only in severe cases.

As the disease progresses, sexual dysfunction may become a problem. Bowel and bladder control may also be lost.

In about 60 percent of MS patients, heat—whether generated by temperatures outside the body or by exercise—may cause temporary worsening of many MS symptoms. In these cases, eradicating the heat eliminates the problem. Some temperature-sensitive patients find that a cold bath may temporarily relieve their symptoms. For the same reason, swimming is often a good exercise choice for people with MS.

The erratic symptoms of MS can affect the entire family as patients may become unable to work at the same time they are facing high medical bills and additional expenses for housekeeping assistance and modifications to homes and vehicles. The emotional drain on both patient and family is immeasurable.

Support groups and counseling may help MS patients, their families, and friends find ways to cope with the many problems the disease can cause.

Can MS be treated?

There is as yet no cure for MS. Many patients do well with no therapy at all, especially since many medications have serious side effects and some carry significant risks. Naturally occurring or spontaneous remissions make it difficult to determine therapeutic effects of experimental treatments; however, the emerging evidence that MRIs can chart the development of lesions is already helping scientists evaluate new therapies.

In the past, the principal medications physicians used to treat MS were steroids possessing anti-inflammatory properties; these include adrenocorticotropic hormone (better known as ACTH), prednisone, prednisolone, methylprednisolone, betamethasone, and dexamethasone. Studies suggest that intravenous methylprednisolone may be superior to the more traditional intravenous ACTH for patients experiencing acute relapses; no strong evidence exists to support the use of these drugs to treat progressive forms of MS. Also, there is some indication that steroids may be more appropriate for people with movement, rather than sensory, symptoms.

While steroids do not affect the course of MS over time, they can reduce the duration and severity of attacks in some patients. The mechanism behind this effect is not known; one study suggests the medications work by restoring the effectiveness of the blood/brain barrier. Because steroids can produce numerous adverse side effects (acne, weight gain, seizures, psychosis), they are not recommended for long-term use.

One of the most promising MS research areas involves naturally occurring antiviral proteins known as interferons. Three forms of beta interferon (Avonex, Betaseron, and Rebif) have now been approved by the Food and Drug Administration for treatment of relapsing-remitting MS. Beta interferon has been shown to reduce the number of exacerbations and may slow the progression of physical disability. When attacks do occur, they tend to be shorter and less severe. In addition, MRI scans suggest that beta interferon can decrease myelin destruction.

Investigators speculate that the effects of beta interferon may be due to the drug's ability to correct an MS-related deficiency of certain white blood cells that suppress the immune system and/or its ability to inhibit gamma interferon, a substance believed to be involved in MS attacks. Alpha interferon is also being studied as a possible treatment for MS. Common side effects of interferons include fever, chills, sweating, muscle aches, fatigue, depression, and injection site reactions.

Scientists continue their extensive efforts to create new and better therapies for MS. Goals of therapy are threefold—to improve recovery from attacks, to prevent or lessen the number of relapses, and to halt disease progression.

Section 22.5

Parkinson Disease

Excerpted from "Parkinson's Disease: Hope Through Research," by the
National Institute of Neurological Disorders and Stroke (NINDS, www
.ninds.nih.gov), part of the National Institutes of Health, August 2011.

Parkinson disease (PD) is a degenerative disorder of the central nervous system.

Researchers believe that at least 500,000 people in the United States currently have PD, although some estimates are much higher. Society pays an enormous price for PD. The total cost to the nation is estimated to exceed $6 billion annually.

What is Parkinson disease?

Parkinson disease belongs to a group of conditions called movement disorders. The four main symptoms are tremor, or trembling in hands, arms, legs, jaw, or head; rigidity, or stiffness of the limbs and trunk; bradykinesia, or slowness of movement; and postural instability, or impaired balance. These symptoms usually begin gradually and worsen with time. As they become more pronounced, patients may have difficulty walking, talking, or completing other simple tasks.

Not everyone with one or more of these symptoms has PD, as the symptoms sometimes appear in other diseases as well.

PD is both chronic, meaning it persists over a long period of time, and progressive, meaning its symptoms grow worse over time. It is not contagious.

Although some PD cases appear to be hereditary, and a few can be traced to specific genetic mutations, most cases are sporadic—that is, the disease does not seem to run in families. Many researchers now believe that PD results from a combination of genetic susceptibility and exposure to one or more environmental factors that trigger the disease.

PD is the most common form of parkinsonism, the name for a group of disorders with similar features and symptoms. PD is also called primary parkinsonism or idiopathic PD. The term idiopathic means a disorder for which no cause has yet been found. Although most forms of parkinsonism are idiopathic, there are some cases where the cause is known or suspected or where the symptoms result from another disorder. For example, parkinsonism may result from changes in the brain's blood vessels.

What causes the disease?

Parkinson disease occurs when nerve cells, or neurons, in an area of the brain known as the substantia nigra die or become impaired. Normally, these neurons produce an important brain chemical known as dopamine. Dopamine is a chemical messenger responsible for transmitting signals between the substantia nigra and the next "relay station" of the brain, the corpus striatum, to produce smooth, purposeful movement. Loss of dopamine results in abnormal nerve firing patterns within the brain that cause impaired movement. Studies have shown that most Parkinson patients have lost 60 to 80 percent or more of the dopamine-producing cells in the substantia nigra by the time symptoms appear.

Recent studies have shown that people with PD also have loss of the nerve endings that produce the neurotransmitter norepinephrine. Norepinephrine, which is closely related to dopamine, is the main chemical messenger of the sympathetic nervous system, the part of the nervous system that controls many automatic functions of the body, such as pulse and blood pressure. The loss of norepinephrine might help explain several of the non-motor features seen in PD, including fatigue and abnormalities of blood pressure regulation.

Many brain cells of people with PD contain Lewy bodies—unusual deposits or clumps of the protein alpha-synuclein, along with other proteins. Researchers do not yet know why Lewy bodies form or what role they play in development of the disease. The clumps may prevent the cell from functioning normally, or they may actually be helpful, perhaps by keeping harmful proteins "locked up" so that the cells can function.

Scientists have identified several genetic mutations associated with PD, and many more genes have been tentatively linked to the disorder. Studying the genes responsible for inherited cases of PD can help researchers understand both inherited and sporadic cases. The same genes and proteins that are altered in inherited cases may also be altered in sporadic cases by environmental toxins or other factors. Researchers also hope that discovering genes will help identify new ways of treating PD.

Although the importance of genetics in PD is increasingly recognized, most researchers believe environmental exposures increase a person's risk of developing the disease. Even in familial cases, exposure to toxins or other environmental factors may influence when symptoms of the disease appear or how the disease progresses. There are a number of toxins, such as 1-methyl-4-phenyl-1,2,3,6-tetrahydropyridine, or MPTP (found in some kinds of synthetic heroin), that can cause parkinsonian symptoms in humans. Other, still-unidentified environmental factors also may cause PD in genetically susceptible individuals.

Viruses are another possible environmental trigger for PD. People who developed encephalopathy after a 1918 influenza epidemic were later stricken with severe, progressive Parkinson-like symptoms. A group of Taiwanese women developed similar symptoms after contracting herpes virus infections. In these women, the symptoms, which later disappeared, were linked to a temporary inflammation of the substantia nigra.

Several lines of research suggest that mitochondria may play a role in the development of PD. Mitochondria are the energy-producing components of the cell and are major sources of free radicals—molecules that damage membranes, proteins, DNA, and other parts of the cell. This damage is often referred to as oxidative stress. Oxidative stress-related changes, including free radical damage to DNA, proteins, and fats, have been detected in brains of PD patients.

Other research suggests that the cell's protein disposal system may fail in people with PD, causing proteins to build up to harmful levels and trigger cell death. Additional studies have found evidence that clumps of protein that develop inside brain cells of people with PD may contribute to the death of neurons, and that inflammation or overstimulation of cells (because of toxins or other factors) may play a role in the disease. However, the precise role of the protein deposits remains unknown. Some researchers even speculate that the protein buildup is part of an unsuccessful attempt to protect the cell. While mitochondrial dysfunction, oxidative stress, inflammation, and many other cellular processes may contribute to PD, the actual cause of the dopamine cell death is still undetermined.

What are the symptoms of the disease?

Early symptoms of PD are subtle and occur gradually. Affected people may feel mild tremors or have difficulty getting out of a chair. They may notice that they speak too softly or that their handwriting is slow and looks cramped or small. They may lose track of a word or thought, or they may feel tired, irritable, or depressed for no apparent reason. This very early period may last a long time before the more classic and obvious symptoms appear.

Friends or family members may be the first to notice changes in someone with early PD. They may see that the person's face lacks expression and animation (known as "masked face") or that the person does not move an arm or leg normally. They also may notice that the person seems stiff, unsteady, or unusually slow.

As the disease progresses, the shaking or tremor that affects the majority of Parkinson patients may begin to interfere with daily activities. Patients may not be able to hold utensils steady or they may find that the shaking makes reading a newspaper difficult. Tremor is usually the symptom that causes people to seek medical help.

People with PD often develop a so-called parkinsonian gait that includes a tendency to lean forward, small quick steps as if hurrying forward (called festination), and reduced swinging of the arms. They also may have trouble initiating movement (start hesitation), and they may stop suddenly as they walk (freezing).

PD does not affect everyone the same way, and the rate of progression differs among patients. Tremor is the major symptom for some patients, while for others, tremor is nonexistent or very minor.

PD symptoms often begin on one side of the body. However, as it progresses, the disease eventually affects both sides. Even after the disease involves both sides of the body, the symptoms are often less severe on one side than on the other. The four primary symptoms of PD are:

Tremor: The tremor associated with PD has a characteristic appearance. Typically, the tremor takes the form of a rhythmic back-and-forth motion at a rate of 4–6 beats per second. It may involve the thumb and forefinger and appear as a "pill rolling" tremor. Tremor often begins in a hand, although sometimes a foot or the jaw is affected first. It is most obvious when the hand is at rest or when a person is under stress. For example, the shaking may become more pronounced a few seconds after the hands are rested on a table. Tremor usually disappears during sleep or improves with intentional movement.

Rigidity: Rigidity, or a resistance to movement, affects most people with PD. A major principle of body movement is that all muscles have an opposing muscle. Movement is possible not just because one muscle becomes more active, but because the opposing muscle relaxes. In PD, rigidity comes about when, in response to signals from the brain, the delicate balance of opposing muscles is disturbed. The muscles remain constantly tensed and contracted so that the person aches or feels stiff or weak. The rigidity becomes obvious when another person tries to move the patient's arm, which will move only in ratchet-like or short, jerky movements known as "cogwheel" rigidity.

Bradykinesia: Bradykinesia, or the slowing down and loss of spontaneous and automatic movement, is particularly frustrating because it may make simple tasks somewhat difficult. The person cannot rapidly perform routine movements. Activities once performed quickly and easily—such as washing or dressing—may take several hours.

Postural instability: Postural instability, or impaired balance, causes patients to fall easily. Affected people also may develop a stooped posture in which the head is bowed and the shoulders are drooped.

How is the disease treated?

At present, there is no cure for PD. But medications or surgery can sometimes provide dramatic relief from the symptoms.

Drug treatments: Medications for PD fall into three categories. The first category includes drugs that work directly or indirectly to increase the level of dopamine in the brain. The most common drugs for PD are dopamine precursors—substances such as levodopa that cross the blood-brain barrier and are then changed into dopamine.

Other drugs mimic dopamine or prevent or slow its breakdown. The second category of PD drugs affects other neurotransmitters in the body in order to ease some of the symptoms of the disease. For example, anticholinergic drugs interfere with production or uptake of the neurotransmitter acetylcholine. These drugs help to reduce tremors and muscle stiffness, which can result from having more acetylcholine than dopamine.

The third category of drugs prescribed for PD includes medications that help control the non-motor symptoms of the disease, that is, the symptoms that don't affect movement. For example, people with PD-related depression may be prescribed antidepressants.

Surgery: Treating PD with surgery was once a common practice. But after the discovery of levodopa, surgery was restricted to only a few cases. Studies in the past few decades have led to great improvements in surgical techniques, and surgery is again being used in people with advanced PD for whom drug therapy is no longer sufficient.

Complementary and supportive therapies: A wide variety of complementary and supportive therapies may be used for PD. Among these therapies are standard physical, occupational, and speech therapy techniques, which can help with such problems as gait and voice disorders, tremors and rigidity, and cognitive decline.

Chapter 23

Disability Caused
by Injury and Trauma

Chapter Contents

Section 23.1—Amputation and Limb Loss 190

Section 23.2—Back Pain 193

Section 23.3—Spinal Cord Injury: Understanding
                Paralysis, Paraplegia, and Quadriplegia 196

Section 23.4—Traumatic Brain Injury 200

189

Section 23.1

Amputation and Limb Loss

What are limb loss and limb differences?

Limb loss generally refers to the absence of any part of a limb (arm or leg) due to surgical or traumatic amputation. The term "limb differences" is used in reference to the congenital absence or malformation of limbs.

How frequently does it occur in the population?

- There are nearly 2 million people living with limb loss in the United States.

- The main causes of limb loss are dysvascular disease—including diabetes (54 percent), trauma (45 percent), and cancer (less than 2 percent).

- Approximately, 185,000 amputations occur in the United States each year.

- Every day 507 people lose a limb in the United States.

- Hospital costs associated with having a limb amputated totaled more than $6.5 billion in 2007.

- African Americans are up to four times more likely to undergo an amputation than white Americans.

- Survival rates after an amputation vary based on a variety of factors. Those who have amputations from trauma tend to have good long-term survival, but those from vascular disease (including peripheral arterial disease and diabetes) face a 30-day mortality rate reported to be between 9–15 percent and a long-term survival rate of 60 percent at 1 year, 42 percent at 3 years, and 35–45 percent at 5 years.

- Nearly half of the people who lose a limb to dysvascular disease will die within 5 years. This is higher than the 5-year mortality rate experienced by people with colorectal, breast, and prostate cancer.

- Of people with diabetes who have a lower-limb amputation, up to 55 percent will require amputation of the second leg within 2 to 3 years.

What causes limb loss and limb differences?

Limb loss can occur due to trauma, infection, diabetes, vascular disease, cancer, and other diseases. The causes of congenital limb differences are often unknown. In the past, many cases of limb difference were attributed to the use of drugs, such as thalidomide, by the mother during pregnancy.

How can I reduce the risk of amputation?

Practice good foot hygiene and care, especially if you have diabetes. Stop smoking, or don't start. Practice good safety habits when operating machinery (lawn mowers, power tools, farming equipment, etc.). Reduce the risk of limb difference in your unborn child by taking medications only when absolutely necessary and under your doctor's supervision.

Are there increased risks for other health problems?

Limb loss is more often the result, rather than the cause, of other health problems. Since the loss of a limb can result in decreased activity, the risk of health problems associated with a sedentary lifestyle may be increased. Residual limb and phantom pain, as well as skin problems associated with prosthesis use, are also common.

What is involved in caring for people with limb loss and limb differences?

Care for a person who has undergone amputation will depend greatly upon his or her overall health and strength. People who are candidates for prosthesis use will make several visits to their prosthetic facility to obtain a correctly fitting device. Physical/occupational therapy or gait training may be needed to facilitate successful use of prostheses and other assistive devices to regain independence. Some new amputees may also need professional assistance with emotional adjustment to limb loss. Amputees whose health does not permit prosthesis use may require more assistance with mobility and transfers.

Who can I contact for more information?

Amputee Coalition's National Limb Loss Information Center: Toll-Free: 888-267-5669; Online: Ask the NLLIC Form (www.amputee -coalition.org/forms/nllicask)

Where can I find managed care, Medicare, and other funding information?

Your patient advocate or the social services department at your hospital can assist you with finding appropriate funding resources. For further information, you may contact:

- Amputee Coalition's National Limb Loss Information Center: 888-267-5669

- Medicare Consumer Information: 800-MEDICARE (800-633-4227)

Suggested reading:

- *inMotion* Magazine (www.amputee-coalition.org/inmotion_about .html)

- Amputee Coalition's NLLIC Library Catalog (see Information Center at www.amputee-coalition.org/nllic_library.html)

- Amputee Coalition's Print Resources (store.amputee-coalition.org)

Section 23.2

Back Pain

Excerpted from "Low Back Pain Fact Sheet," by the National Institute of Neurological Disorders and Stroke (NINDS, www.ninds.nih.gov), part of the National Institutes of Health, June 15, 2011.

If you have lower back pain, you are not alone. Nearly everyone at some point has back pain that interferes with work, routine daily activities, or recreation. Americans spend at least $50 billion each year on low back pain, the most common cause of job-related disability and a leading contributor to missed work. Back pain is the second most common neurological ailment in the United States—only headache is more common. Fortunately, most occurrences of low back pain go away within a few days. Others take much longer to resolve or lead to more serious conditions.

Acute or short-term low back pain generally lasts from a few days to a few weeks. Most acute back pain is mechanical in nature—the result of trauma to the lower back or a disorder such as arthritis. Pain from trauma may be caused by a sports injury, work around the house or in the garden, or a sudden jolt such as a car accident or other stress on spinal bones and tissues. Symptoms may range from muscle ache to shooting or stabbing pain, limited flexibility and/or range of motion, or an inability to stand straight. Occasionally, pain felt in one part of the body may "radiate" from a disorder or injury elsewhere in the body. Some acute pain syndromes can become more serious if left untreated.

Chronic back pain is measured by duration—pain that persists for more than 3 months is considered chronic. It is often progressive and the cause can be difficult to determine.

What conditions are associated with low back pain?

Conditions that may cause low back pain and require treatment by a physician or other health specialist include the following:

Bulging disk (also called protruding, herniated, or ruptured disk): The intervertebral disks are under constant pressure. As disks degenerate and weaken, cartilage can bulge or be pushed into the space containing the spinal cord or a nerve root, causing pain. Studies have shown that most herniated disks occur in the lower, lumbar portion of the spinal column. A much more serious complication of a ruptured disk is cauda equina syndrome, which occurs when disk material is pushed into the spinal canal and compresses the bundle of lumbar and sacral nerve roots. Permanent neurological damage may result if this syndrome is left untreated.

Sciatica is a condition in which a herniated or ruptured disk presses on the sciatic nerve, the large nerve that extends down the spinal column to its exit point in the pelvis and carries nerve fibers to the leg. This compression causes shock-like or burning low back pain combined with pain through the buttocks and down one leg to below the knee, occasionally reaching the foot. In the most extreme cases, when the nerve is pinched between the disk and an adjacent bone, the symptoms involve not pain but numbness and some loss of motor control over the leg due to interruption of nerve signaling. The condition may also be caused by a tumor, cyst, metastatic disease, or degeneration of the sciatic nerve root.

Spinal degeneration from disk wear and tear can lead to a narrowing of the spinal canal. A person with spinal degeneration may experience stiffness in the back upon awakening or may feel pain after walking or standing for a long time.

Spinal stenosis related to congenital narrowing of the bony canal predisposes some people to pain related to disk disease.

Osteoporosis is a metabolic bone disease marked by progressive decrease in bone density and strength. Fracture of brittle, porous bones in the spine and hips results when the body fails to produce new bone and/or absorbs too much existing bone. Women are four times more likely than men to develop osteoporosis. Caucasian women of northern European heritage are at the highest risk of developing the condition.

Skeletal irregularities produce strain on the vertebrae and supporting muscles, tendons, ligaments, and tissues supported by spinal column. These irregularities include scoliosis, a curving of the spine to the side; kyphosis, in which the normal curve of the upper back is severely rounded; lordosis, an abnormally accentuated arch in the lower back; back extension, a bending backward of the spine; and back flexion, in which the spine bends forward.

Fibromyalgia is a chronic disorder characterized by widespread musculoskeletal pain, fatigue, and multiple "tender points," particularly in the neck, spine, shoulders, and hips. Additional symptoms may include sleep disturbances, morning stiffness, and anxiety.

Spondylitis refers to chronic back pain and stiffness caused by a severe infection to or inflammation of the spinal joints. Other painful inflammations in the lower back include osteomyelitis (infection in the bones of the spine) and sacroiliitis (inflammation in the sacroiliac joints).

How is back pain treated?

Most low back pain can be treated without surgery. Treatment involves using analgesics, reducing inflammation, restoring proper function and strength to the back, and preventing recurrence of the injury. Most patients with back pain recover without residual functional loss. Patients should contact a doctor if there is not a noticeable reduction in pain and inflammation after 72 hours of self-care.

Medications are often used to treat acute and chronic low back pain. Effective pain relief may involve a combination of prescription drugs and over-the-counter remedies. Patients should always check with a doctor before taking drugs for pain relief. Certain medicines, even those sold over the counter, are unsafe during pregnancy, may conflict with other medications, may cause side effects including drowsiness, or may lead to liver damage.

Section 23.3

Spinal Cord Injury: Understanding Paralysis, Paraplegia, and Quadriplegia

Excerpted from "Spinal Cord Injury: Hope Through Research," by the National Institute of Neurological Disorders and Stroke (NINDS, www.ninds.nih.gov), part of the National Institutes of Health, June 22, 2011.

What is a spinal cord injury?

Although the hard bones of the spinal column protect the soft tissues of the spinal cord, vertebrae can still be broken or dislocated in a variety of ways and cause traumatic injury to the spinal cord. Injuries can occur at any level of the spinal cord. The segment of the cord that is injured, and the severity of the injury, will determine which body functions are compromised or lost. Because the spinal cord acts as the main information pathway between the brain and the rest of the body, a spinal cord injury can have significant physiological consequences.

Catastrophic falls, being thrown from a horse or through a windshield, or any kind of physical trauma that crushes and compresses the vertebrae in the neck can cause irreversible damage at the cervical level of the spinal cord and below. Paralysis of most of the body including the arms and legs, called quadriplegia, is the likely result. Automobile accidents are often responsible for spinal cord damage in the middle back (the thoracic or lumbar area), which can cause paralysis of the lower trunk and lower extremities, called paraplegia.

Other kinds of injuries that directly penetrate the spinal cord, such as gunshot or knife wounds, can either completely or partially sever the spinal cord and create lifelong disabilities.

Most injuries to the spinal cord don't completely sever it. Instead, an injury is more likely to cause fractures and compression of the vertebrae, which then crush and destroy the axons, extensions of nerve cells that carry signals up and down the spinal cord between the brain and the rest of the body. An injury to the spinal cord can damage a few, many, or almost all of these axons. Some injuries will allow almost complete recovery. Others will result in complete paralysis.

Until World War II, a serious spinal cord injury usually meant certain death, or at best a lifetime confined to a wheelchair and an ongoing struggle to survive secondary complications such as breathing problems or blood clots. But today, improved emergency care for people with spinal cord injuries and aggressive treatment and rehabilitation can minimize damage to the nervous system and even restore limited abilities.

Advances in research are giving doctors and patients hope that all spinal cord injuries will eventually be repairable. With new surgical techniques and exciting developments in spinal nerve regeneration, the future for spinal cord injury survivors looks brighter every day.

How does a spinal cord injury affect the rest of the body?

People who survive a spinal cord injury will most likely have medical complications such as chronic pain and bladder and bowel dysfunction, along with an increased susceptibility to respiratory and heart problems. Successful recovery depends upon how well these chronic conditions are handled day to day.

Breathing: Any injury to the spinal cord at or above the C3, C4, and C5 segments, which supply the phrenic nerves leading to the diaphragm, can stop breathing. People with these injuries need immediate ventilatory support. When injuries are at the C5 level and below, diaphragm function is preserved, but breathing tends to be rapid and shallow and people have trouble coughing and clearing secretions from their lungs because of weak thoracic muscles. Once pulmonary function improves, a large percentage of those with C4 injuries can be weaned from mechanical ventilation in the weeks following the injury.

Pneumonia: Respiratory complications, primarily as a result of pneumonia, are a leading cause of death in people with spinal cord injury. In fact, intubation increases the risk of developing ventilator-associated pneumonia (VAP) by 1 to 3 percent per day of intubation. More than a quarter of the deaths caused by spinal cord injury are the result of VAP. Spinal cord injury patients who are intubated have to be carefully monitored for VAP and treated with antibiotics if symptoms appear.

Irregular heart beat and low blood pressure: Spinal cord injuries in the cervical region are often accompanied by blood pressure instability and heart arrhythmias. Because of interruptions to the cardiac accelerator nerves, the heart can beat at a dangerously slow pace, or it can pound rapidly and irregularly. Arrhythmias usually appear in the first 2 weeks after injury and are more common and severe in the most serious injuries. Low blood pressure also often occurs due to loss of tone in blood vessels, which widen and cause blood to pool in the small arteries far away from the heart. This is usually treated with an intravenous infusion to build up blood volume.

Blood clots: People with spinal cord injuries are at triple the usual risk for blood clots. The risk for clots is low in the first 72 hours, but afterward anticoagulation drug therapy can be used as a preventive measure.

Spasm: Many of our reflex movements are controlled by the spinal cord but regulated by the brain. When the spinal cord is damaged, information from the brain can no longer regulate reflex activity. Reflexes may become exaggerated over time, causing spasticity. If spasms become severe enough, they may require medical treatment. For some, spasms can be as much of a help as they are a hindrance, since spasms can tone muscles that would otherwise waste away. Some people can even learn to use the increased tone in their legs to help them turn over in bed, propel them into and out of a wheelchair, or stand.

Autonomic dysreflexia: Autonomic dysreflexia is a life-threatening reflex action that primarily affects those with injuries to the neck or upper back. It happens when there is an irritation, pain, or stimulus to the nervous system below the level of injury. The irritated area tries to send a signal to the brain, but since the signal isn't able to get through, a reflex action occurs without the brain's regulation. Unlike spasms that affect muscles, autonomic dysreflexia affects vascular and organ systems controlled by the sympathetic nervous system.

Anything that causes pain or irritation can set off autonomic dysreflexia—the urge to urinate or defecate, pressure sores, cuts, burns, bruises, sunburn, pressure of any kind on the body, ingrown toenails, or tight clothing. For example, the impulse to urinate can set off high blood pressure or rapid heartbeat that, if uncontrolled, can cause stroke, seizures, or death. Symptoms such as flushing or sweating, a pounding headache, anxiety, sudden high blood pressure, vision changes, or goosebumps on the arms and legs can signal the onset of autonomic dysreflexia. Treatment should be swift. Changing position, emptying the bladder or bowels, and removing or loosening tight clothing are just a few of the possibilities that should be tried to relieve whatever is causing the irritation.

Pressure sores (or pressure ulcers): Pressure sores are areas of skin tissue that have broken down because of continuous pressure on the skin. People with paraplegia and quadriplegia are susceptible to pressure sores because they can't move easily on their own. Places that support weight when someone is seated or recumbent are vulner-able areas. When these areas press against a surface for a long period of time, the skin compresses and reduces the flow of blood to the area. When the blood supply is blocked for too long, the skin will begin to break down. Since spinal cord injury reduces or eliminates sensation below the level of injury, people may not be aware of the normal signals to change position, and must be shifted periodically by a caregiver. Good nutrition and hygiene can also help prevent pressure sores by encouraging healthy skin.

Pain: People who are paralyzed often have what is called neuro-genic pain resulting from damage to nerves in the spinal cord. For some survivors of spinal cord injury, pain or an intense burning or stinging sensation is unremitting due to hypersensitivity in some parts of the body. Others are prone to normal musculoskeletal pain as well, such as shoulder pain due to overuse of the shoulder joint from pushing a wheelchair and using the arms for transfers. Treatments for chronic pain include medications, acupuncture, spinal or brain electrical stimu-lation, and surgery.

Bladder and bowel problems: Most spinal cord injuries affect bladder and bowel functions because the nerves that control the in-volved organs originate in the segments near the lower termination of the spinal cord and are cut off from brain input. Without coordination from the brain, the muscles of the bladder and urethra can't work to-gether effectively, and urination becomes abnormal. The bladder can empty suddenly without warning, or become overfull without releas-ing. In some cases the bladder releases, but urine backs up into the kidneys because it isn't able to get past the urethral sphincter. Most people with spinal cord injuries use either intermittent catheterization or an indwelling catheter to empty their bladders.

Bowel function is similarly affected. The anal sphincter muscle can remain tight, so that bowel movements happen on a reflex basis whenever the bowel is full. Or the muscle can be permanently relaxed, which is called a flaccid bowel, and result in an inability to have a bowel movement. This requires more frequent attempts to empty the bowel and manual removal of stool to prevent fecal impaction. People with spinal cord injuries are usually put on a regularly scheduled bowel program to prevent accidents.

Reproductive and sexual function: Spinal cord injury has a greater impact on sexual and reproductive function in men than it does in women. Most spinal cord injured women remain fertile and can conceive and bear children. Even those with severe injury may well retain orgasmic function, although many lose some if not all of their ability to reach satisfaction. Depending on the level of injury, men may have problems with erections and ejaculation, and most will have compromised fertility due to decreased motility of their sperm. Treatments for men include vibratory or electrical stimulation and drugs such as sildenafil (Viagra). Many couples may also need assisted fertility treatments to allow a spinal cord injured man to father children.

Once someone has survived the injury and begun to psychologically and emotionally cope with the nature of his or her situation, the next concern will be how to live with disabilities. Doctors are now able to predict with reasonable accuracy the likely long-term outcome of spinal cord injuries. This helps patients set achievable goals for themselves, and gives families and loved ones a realistic set of expectations for the future.

Section 23.4

Traumatic Brain Injury

Excerpted from "Traumatic Brain Injury: Hope Through Research," by the National Institute of Neurological Disorders and Stroke (NINDS, www .ninds.nih.gov), part of the National Institutes of Health, April 15, 2011.

Traumatic brain injury (TBI) is a major public health problem, especially among male adolescents and young adults ages 15 to 24, and among elderly people of both sexes 75 years and older. Children aged 5 and younger are also at high risk for TBI.

TBI costs the country more than $56 billion a year, and more than 5 million Americans alive today have had a TBI resulting in a permanent need for help in performing daily activities. Survivors of TBI are often left with significant cognitive, behavioral, and communicative disabilities, and some patients develop long-term medical complications, such as epilepsy.

Other statistics dramatically tell the story of head injury in the United States. Each year:

- approximately 1.4 million people experience a TBI;

- approximately 50,000 people die from head injury;

- approximately 1 million head-injured people are treated in hospital emergency rooms; and

- approximately 230,000 people are hospitalized for TBI and survive.

What is a traumatic brain injury?

TBI, a form of acquired brain injury, occurs when a sudden trauma causes damage to the brain. The damage can be focal—confined to one area of the brain—or diffuse—involving more than one area of the brain. TBI can result from a closed head injury or a penetrating head injury. A closed injury occurs when the head suddenly and violently hits an object but the object does not break through the skull. A penetrating injury occurs when an object pierces the skull and enters brain tissue.

What disabilities can result from a TBI?

Disabilities resulting from a TBI depend upon the severity of the injury, the location of the injury, and the age and general health of the patient. Some common disabilities include problems with cognition (thinking, memory, and reasoning), sensory processing (sight, hearing, touch, taste, and smell), communication (expression and understanding), and behavior or mental health (depression, anxiety, personality changes, aggression, acting out, and social inappropriateness).

Within days to weeks of the head injury approximately 40 percent of TBI patients develop a host of troubling symptoms collectively called postconcussion syndrome (PCS). A patient need not have suffered a concussion or loss of consciousness to develop the syndrome and many patients with mild TBI suffer from PCS. Symptoms include headache, dizziness, vertigo (a sensation of spinning around or of objects spinning around the patient), memory problems, trouble concentrating, sleeping problems, restlessness, irritability, apathy, depression, and anxiety.

These symptoms may last for a few weeks after the head injury. The syndrome is more prevalent in patients who had psychiatric symptoms, such as depression or anxiety, before the injury. Treatment for PCS may include medicines for pain and psychiatric conditions, and psychotherapy and occupational therapy to develop coping skills.

Cognition is a term used to describe the processes of thinking, reasoning, problem solving, information processing, and memory. Most patients with severe TBI, if they recover consciousness, suffer from cognitive disabilities, including the loss of many higher level mental skills. The most common cognitive impairment among severely head-injured patients is memory loss, characterized by some loss of specific memories and the partial inability to form or store new ones. Some of these patients may experience posttraumatic amnesia (PTA), either anterograde or retrograde. Anterograde PTA is impaired memory of events that happened after the TBI, while retrograde PTA is impaired memory of events that happened before the TBI.

Many patients with mild to moderate head injuries who experience cognitive deficits become easily confused or distracted and have problems with concentration and attention. They also have problems with higher level, so-called executive functions, such as planning, organizing, abstract reasoning, problem solving, and making judgments, which may make it difficult to resume preinjury work-related activities. Recovery from cognitive deficits is greatest within the first 6 months after the injury and more gradual after that.

Patients with moderate to severe TBI have more problems with cognitive deficits than patients with mild TBI, but a history of several mild TBIs may have an additive effect, causing cognitive deficits equal to a moderate or severe injury.

Many TBI patients have sensory problems, especially problems with vision. Patients may not be able to register what they are seeing or may be slow to recognize objects. Also, TBI patients often have difficulty with hand-eye coordination. Because of this, TBI patients may be prone to bumping into or dropping objects, or may seem generally unsteady. TBI patients may have difficulty driving a car, working complex machinery, or playing sports. Other sensory deficits may include problems with hearing, smell, taste, or touch. Some TBI patients develop tinnitus, a ringing or roaring in the ears. A person with damage to the part of the brain that processes taste or smell may develop a persistent bitter taste in the mouth or perceive a persistent noxious smell. Damage to the part of the brain that controls the sense of touch may cause a TBI patient to develop persistent skin tingling, itching, or pain. Although rare, these conditions are hard to treat.

Language and communication problems are common disabilities in TBI patients. Some may experience aphasia, defined as difficulty with understanding and producing spoken and written language; others may have difficulty with the more subtle aspects of communication, such as body language and emotional, nonverbal signals. In nonfluent aphasia, also called Broca aphasia or motor aphasia, TBI patients often have trouble recalling words and speaking in complete sentences. They may speak in broken phrases and pause frequently. Most patients are aware of these deficits and may become extremely frustrated. Patients with fluent aphasia, also called Wernicke aphasia or sensory aphasia, display little meaning in their speech, even though they speak in complete sentences and use correct grammar. Instead, they speak in flowing gibberish, drawing out their sentences with nonessential and invented words. Many patients with fluent aphasia are unaware that they make little sense and become angry with others for not understanding them. Patients with global aphasia have extensive damage to the portions of the brain responsible for language and often suffer severe communication disabilities.

TBI patients may have problems with spoken language if the part of the brain that controls speech muscles is damaged. In this disorder, called dysarthria, the patient can think of the appropriate language, but cannot easily speak the words because they are unable to use the muscles needed to form the words and produce the sounds. Speech is often slow, slurred, and garbled. Some may have problems with intonation or inflection, called prosodic dysfunction. An important aspect of speech, inflection conveys emotional meaning and is necessary for certain aspects of language, such as irony.

Communication disabilities such as language and speech problems are common among TBI patients. These language deficits can lead to miscommunication, confusion, and frustration for the patient as well as those interacting with him or her.

Most TBI patients have emotional or behavioral problems that fit under the broad category of psychiatric health. Family members of TBI patients often find that personality changes and behavioral problems are the most difficult disabilities to handle. Psychiatric problems that may surface include depression, apathy, anxiety, irritability, anger, paranoia, confusion, frustration, agitation, insomnia or other sleep problems, and mood swings. Problem behaviors may include aggression and violence, impulsivity, disinhibition, acting out, noncompliance, social inappropriateness, emotional outbursts, childish behavior, impaired self-control, impaired self-awareness, inability to take responsibility or accept criticism, egocentrism, inappropriate sexual activity, and alcohol or drug abuse/addiction. Some patients' personality problems may be so severe that they are diagnosed with borderline personality disorder, a psychiatric condition characterized by many of the problems mentioned above. Sometimes TBI patients suffer from developmental stagnation, meaning that they fail to mature emotionally, socially, or psychologically after the trauma. This is a serious problem for children and young adults who suffer from a TBI. Attitudes and behaviors that are appropriate for a child or teenager become inappropriate in adulthood. Many TBI patients who show psychiatric or behavioral problems can be helped with medication and psychotherapy.

Part Three

Technologies and Services That Help People with Disabilities and Their Families

Chapter 24

What Is Assistive Technology?

Assistive technology is any service or tool that helps the elderly or disabled do the activities they have always done but must now do differently. These tools are also sometimes called adaptive devices.

For many seniors, assistive technology makes the difference between being able to live independently and having to get long-term nursing or home-health care. For others, assistive technology is critical to the ability to perform simple activities of daily living, such as bathing and going to the bathroom.

Such technology may be something as simple as a walker to make moving around easier or an amplification device to make sounds easier to hear (for talking on the telephone or watching television, for instance). It could also include a magnifying glass that helps someone who has poor vision read the newspaper or a small motor scooter that makes it possible to travel over distances that are too far to walk. In short, anything that helps the elderly continue to participate in daily activities is considered assistive technology.

Just as older people may have many different types of disabilities, many different categories of assistive devices and services are available to help overcome those disabilities. These include the following:

- **Adaptive switches:** Modified switches that seniors can use to adjust air conditioners, computers, telephone answering machines, power wheelchairs, and other types of equipment. These switches might be activated by the tongue or the voice.

Excerpted from "Assistive Technology," by the Administration on Aging (AOA, www.aoa.gov), part of the U.S. Department of Health and Human Services, 2010.

- **Communication equipment:** Anything that enables a person to send and receive messages, such as a telephone amplifier.

- **Computer access:** Special software that helps a senior access the internet, for example, or basic hardware, such as a modified keyboard or mouse, that makes the computer more user friendly.

- **Home modifications:** Construction or remodeling work, such as building a ramp for wheelchair access, that allows a senior to overcome physical barriers and live more comfortably with a disability or recover from an accident or injury.

- **Tools for independent living:** Anything that empowers the elderly to enjoy the normal activities of daily living without assistance from others, such as a handicapped-accessible bathroom with grab bars in the bathtub.

- **Mobility aids:** Any piece of equipment that helps a senior get around more easily, such as a power wheelchair, wheelchair lift, or stair elevator.

- **Orthotic or prosthetic equipment:** A device that compensates for a missing or disabled body part. This could range from orthopedic shoe inserts for someone who has fallen arches to an artificial arm for someone whose limb has been amputated.

- **Sensory enhancements:** Anything that makes it easier for those who are partially or fully blind or deaf to better appreciate the world around them. For instance, a telecaption decoder for a TV set would be an assistive device for a senior who is hard of hearing.

- **Therapy:** Equipment or processes that help someone recover as much as possible from an illness or injury. Therapy might involve a combination of services and technology, such as having a physical therapist use a special massage unit to restore a wider range of motion to stiff muscles.

Seniors must carefully evaluate their needs before deciding to purchase assistive technology. Using assistive technology may change the mix of services that a senior requires or may affect the way that those services are provided. For this reason, the process of needs assessment and planning is important.

Usually, needs assessment has the most value when it is done by a team working with the senior in the place where the assistive technology will be used. For example, an elderly person who has trouble communicating or is hard of hearing should consult with his or her doctor, an audiology specialist, a speech-language therapist, and family and friends. Together, these people can identify the problem precisely and determine a course of action to solve the problem.

By performing the needs assessment, defining goals, and determining what would help the senior communicate more easily in the home, the team can decide what assistive technology tools are appropriate. After that, the team can help select the most effective devices available at the lowest cost. A professional member of the team, such as the audiology specialist, can also arrange for any training that the senior and his or her family may require to use the equipment needed.

When considering all the options of assistive technology, it is often useful to look at the issue in terms of high-tech and low-tech solutions. Seniors must also remember to plan ahead and think about how their needs might change over time. High-tech devices tend to be more expensive but may be able to assist with many different needs. Low-tech equipment is usually cheaper but less adaptable for multiple purposes. Before buying any expensive piece of assistive technology, such as a computer, be sure to find out if it can be upgraded as improvements are introduced.

Whether you are conducting a needs assessment or trying to make a decision after such an assessment, it is always a good idea to ask the following questions about assistive technology:

- Does a more advanced device meet more than one of my needs?

- Does the manufacturer of the assistive technology have a preview policy that will let me try out a device and return it for credit if it does not work as expected?

- How are my needs likely to change over the next 6 months? How about over the next 6 years or longer?

- How up-to-date is this piece of assistive equipment? Is it likely to become obsolete in the immediate future?

- What are the tasks that I need help with, and how often do I need help with these tasks?

- What types of assistive technology are available to meet my needs?

- What, if any, types of assistive technology have I used before, and how did that equipment work?

- What type of assistive technology will give me the greatest personal independence?

- Will I always need help with this task? If so, can I adjust this device and continue to use it as my condition changes?

Chapter 25

Mobility Aids:
From Canes to Wheelchairs

How you get around has a big impact on what you can do and where you can go. Simply being able to take a few steps can be a huge advantage for getting around your home. Some people are able to use the narrow confines of the bathroom to their advantage, holding on to the sink, walls, or grab bars. Counters may offer some support when standing or walking in the kitchen. But once you venture past the front door, there are no walls for support and your lifestyle will likely require long distance mobility to do what you need to do, be it shopping, visiting family or friends, attending school, or going to work.

Many people who have lived with a disability for a long time have found that careful consideration of their mobility needs has been a key to their independence. For some, the solution has included multiple devices—different environments, different devices—a manual wheelchair in the home, a scooter for work, and even a handcycle for exercise. Mobility assistance equipment comes in many forms, shapes, and sizes. The options include:

- **Assistive devices for ambulation:** These are simple devices to help you walk—a cane, crutches, and walkers.

- **Manual wheelchair:** Essentially, a chair with wheels designed to allow you to self-propel or be pushed along by a companion or an attendant.

Excerpted from "Mobility Alternatives: From Canes to Wheelchairs," © 2009 United Spinal Association. Reprinted with permission. Additional information, including the complete text of this document, is available at www.unitedspinal.org.

- **Power assist devices:** These are mechanical devices installed on manual wheelchairs to make it easier for the user to self-propel.

- **Scooters:** Most are three-wheel designs, although some four-wheel models are available, usually with an electric motor, and a tiller for steering. A scooter is an effective mobility device that does not look like a wheelchair.

- **Power wheelchairs:** Front-wheel, mid-wheel, and rear-wheel drive options are available. These chairs operate by an electric motor and are controlled by using a joystick, or an alternate control device. Many offer multiple seating options, including power seating.

Be an Informed Consumer

Ask other users about their experiences. Ask lots of questions. Mobility assistance equipment is often purchased through a third party, such as medical insurance, Medicare/Medicaid, the Department of Veterans Affairs, or vocational rehabilitation programs. Each payer has their own set of coverage criteria and a system for purchasing. As you explore the options, keep in mind that all of these products can also be purchased directly. If you have the resources, a private purchase can offer greater selection at less than the manufacturer's suggested retail price and there is no need to wait for an authorization.

You may also find it helpful to consult an experienced health care provider. Many occupational and physical therapists also specialize in assistive technology and there are rehab technology suppliers who specialize in individualized fittings and repairs Ask other users; they're often a great source of information for locating people in your area who may be able to help you.

"My physical functioning was unchanged, but my mind and my world had finally opened up. With the scooter, I could get around again. And I loved the freedom." In her recent article, "When Walking Fails," Dr. Lisa Lezzonni eloquently articulates the challenges facing people who need mobility assistance. Speaking from personal experience as a woman with multiple sclerosis, Lezzoni explains that, after many years of assisted ambulation, first with one cane and then with two canes, she decided to try a scooter.

Adding a wheeled mobility device to your options is a lot like looking for a new car. There are so many options and choices. How can you begin to make an informed decision? To be truly happy with your choice over time requires some homework up front. There is no one best chair. The best chair is the one that allows you to go where you want to go, when you want to go. To find it, you need to consider the environments you'll be in and what you'll be doing. Some users have no choice about using a chair—it is the only form of mobility available to them. For others, a wheelchair may be augmented mobility, allowing for longer distance travel without fatigue or fear of falling.

Options to Think About—Do Your Homework

Mobility needs: Careful consideration of what you want to be able to do will help focus your choices. As noted earlier, the process is similar to buying a car: You must prioritize your functions to identify the features you'll need. You may come to the conclusion that more than one device is, ultimately, what you need. Many users have come to this conclusion and they add different devices over time. Meet your top priority needs first; later you can purchase additional gear to accommodate different environments.

An important first consideration is: Where will you have the most trouble getting around? If ambulation, even with an assistive device like a cane or a walker, is not an option, then you will be a full-time wheelchair rider. If walking around your home or other small spaces is not a problem, then you may be only looking for equipment to increase your community mobility or allow you access to recreational and leisure activities.

You need to review your requirements in each environment—home, community, and work/school/volunteering activities.

- **Home:** Critical features of the wheelchair will affect your ability to transfer (getting in and out of the chair). What is the height of the seat from the floor? How does that height compare to your bed, for example? How do the armrests or foot supports move to make your transfer easier? What is the overall width of the chair? Will it fit through your doorways?

- **Community:** How do you want to travel in the community? Do you need to fold the walker when riding in the car? If you are using your arms or your legs to propel a manual wheelchair, will you get too tired just getting to the store or to visit friends? Would a power option (power assist wheels, power chair or scooter) provide a more efficient method of getting around? Are there sidewalks and curb cuts or are you sharing the road with cars and trucks? Do you want to be in the great outdoors—trails, grass, gravel? Or are you a mall walker—preferring smooth finished floors and wide open doorways? Your choice of tires, wheels, and type of base can make a world of difference getting around the store versus hitting the trail.

- **Transportation:** Where you live and what your transportation options are will have a major impact on your choices. Public transportation—buses or trains—are increasingly accessible for wheelchair users, providing you want to go where the bus is going. Private transportation, (i.e., owning your own vehicle), gives you the most flexibility and freedom, but fitting your mobility device into the car will present a series of questions. Can the chair or scooter fold? Can you store it in the trunk or within the car? Can you get it in the trunk and then walk to the car door? Many wheelchair and scooter users find that a van or a minivan—especially one adapted with a ramp or lift—is the real key to independent mobility. But modified vans are expensive. For many people, they are just not an option.

Options for Ambulation Aids

- **Cane or walking stick:** The key here is getting the cane fitted to the right height. Ideally, when you hang your arm by your side, your hand should hang just over the top of the cane, your wrist lining up with the very top of the cane. An adjustable cane is easiest for ensuring the correct height, but if you are a long-time user, you may choose a custom cane, cut to your specific height, or even a walking stick to add a little style. When you grasp the top of the cane, your elbow should bend at about 30 degrees. If you are using a cane because of weakness on one side of your body, place the cane in the hand of your stronger side.

- **Crutches:** There are basically two types of crutch styles—under the arm (auxiliary) or cuffed to the forearm (Lofstrand or Canadian crutches). A proper fit and some instruction on safe use is important. Seek the assistance of a health care provider when first using crutches. Long-time crutch users have found the style tip (the rubber tip on the bottom of the crutch) and the grip style for your hand can add to overall comfort for long-term use.

- **Walkers:** Walkers are currently available in many styles—pick-up walkers, which have no wheels; sliders, which have small skis or tennis balls on the rear legs; or rollator walkers, which employ four wheels. Some walkers use three wheels, are triangular in shape, and offer somewhat less support, but are not as bulky;

four-wheel walkers are primarily designed for indoor use. More robust walkers that employ four larger wheels and a full basket are also available and may even include a fold-down seat.

Styles of Wheelchairs and Scooters

Broadly speaking, there are three categories of products that are referred to as wheeled mobility devices—manual wheelchairs, scooters, and power wheelchairs. (See Table 25.1.) As mentioned previously, many long-time wheelchair–users have several of types of chairs, with each chair functioning differently in different environments.

Manual Wheelchairs

Manual wheelchairs are designed for two very different purposes: To allow the user to propel himself or herself, or allow a companion or an attendant to push the chair.

Dependent/transport mobility bases, which are not designed for self-propulsion, often have small rear wheels and may look and function much like a stroller. For transport purposes, these chairs often fold compactly to store in the trunk of a car and provide light duty

Table 25.1. Wheelchair Type Advantages and Disadvantages

	Advantages	Disadvantages
Manual wheelchairs	Lightweight; greater reliability; easier to transport; less expensive; provides exercise; easier to overcome accessibility problems	Self-propulsion: Possible secondary complications after long-term use such as sore shoulders, wrists, and elbows; requires physical effort to be mobile
Scooters	Aesthetics—does not look like a wheelchair; increases mobility range without increased exertion; swivel seat may allow for easier transfers in and out of the seat	More complicated to transport in a car than a manual chair; needs charging; less flexible modifications to meet changing physical conditions than a power chair
Power wheelchairs	Greatest mobility range with least exertion; easier to modify over time, if needed; available power seating options (i.e., tilt and/or recline)	More expensive; more difficult to transport; less reliable than manual wheelchairs

mobility. You may find a transport chair is a convenient back-up to your primary chair, easily folded when not needed, but readily available if your chair breaks down.

Specialty positioning bases are mobility devices that allow for changes in positioning by tilting the seating system, reclining the backrest, or both. These devices are not easy to transport, but they are designed to provide comfortable, full-day seating for users who may be unable to propel themselves or operate a power wheelchair.

Self-propelling manual wheelchairs are equipped with a large wheel and riders self-propel using either both arms, both legs, or one arm/one leg. If you are using your leg(s) for propulsion, then the seat-to-floor height is a critical parameter to ensure maximum mobility.

The most active manual wheelchair–users are able to balance the chair on the back wheels alone—a maneuver known as a wheelie. This can significantly improve access for the user. By "popping a wheelie" you can negotiate a high threshold, get over a two-inch curb and, if you are able to ride in a wheelie position, you may be able to cross soft terrain like grass and gravel without the front casters getting stuck. Manual chairs with adjustable rear wheels (i.e., wheels that can move forward and backward on the frame) need to be fitted to the user to get the best combination of "tippiness," or ease of popping a wheelie, and stability, which is not tipping over when just pushing on the wheels. If you have good balance and want to learn to do a wheelie, ask for training from your physical or occupational therapist.

Power Assist

One of the newest technologies offer hybrid or cross-over products—equipment that falls between traditional manual chairs and power wheelchairs.

The power-assist systems are equipped with new wheels (the larger rear wheel for a manual wheelchair) that are battery operated and designed to increase the number of revolutions the wheel makes per push. The goal is to increase the efficiency of manual propulsion while reducing the effort that the rider must exert on the wheels. Add-on power systems are designed to give power chair operation while mounted on a manual wheelchair base. With a quick release system, these add-on power systems are more easily transportable than traditional power chairs, but do not have the long-term performance or durability of traditional power chairs.

The internet provides a great opportunity to explore product options before ever going to a wheelchair clinic or a medical store showroom.

Each manufacturer has a website describing their product line. Major manufacturers include Invacare, Permobile, Pride Mobility, and Sunrise Medical. Other valuable resources include:

- www.usatechguide.org: Large database of available products by category and wheelchair user reviews;

- www.wheelchairjunkie.com: Consumer direct information regarding commercial products and a wheelchair users forum;

- www.resna.org: Provides a directory of therapists, assistive technology practitioners (ATP), and suppliers (ATS) who specialize in rehab products;

- www.nrrts.org: List of suppliers, by state, that specialize in rehabilitation products.

Conclusion

Purchasing a wheeled mobility device is not a simple matter. Much like a car, there are also aesthetic considerations. What is the image you want to project? Also, as in buying a car, you need to be practical. Many a soccer mom would love the two-seater, convertible roadster. Too bad there's no room for the kids. Function often trumps fantasy.

Both our self-image and the functions we need to perform in our everyday lives change over time. Eventually, you may have different priorities and thus move from one type of mobility device to another. But always do your homework. Ask others about function, reliability, and personal experiences.

With routine maintenance, and a little tender loving care, you can stay mobile for years to come.

Chapter 26

Home Use Devices
and Modifications

Chapter Contents

Section 26.1—What Are Home Use Medical Devices? 220

Section 26.2—Adapting Your Living Space to
            Accommodate Your Disability............................ 225

Section 26.1

What Are Home Use Medical Devices?

This section contains text excerpted from "Home Use Devices," January 2011, "Frequently Asked Questions About Home Use Devices," September 3, 2010, and "Unique Considerations in the Home," March 17, 2010, all by the U.S. Food and Drug Administration (FDA, www.fda.gov).

Home Use Devices

What is a home use device?

A home use medical device is intended for users in any environment, apart from the professional healthcare facility or the emergency medical services, requires adequate instructions for use, and may also require training for the user by a qualified healthcare professional to assure safe and effective use.

- A user is a patient (care recipient), caregiver, or family member that directly uses the device or provides assistance in using the device.

- A qualified healthcare professional is a licensed or non-licensed healthcare professional with proficient skill and experience with the use of the device so that they can aid or train care recipients and caregivers to use and maintain the device.

Changes in health care have moved care from the hospital environment to the home environment. In fact, according to results of the 2000 National Home and Hospice Care Survey "approximately 1,355,300 patients were receiving home health care services from 7,200 agencies." In 2004, the National Association for Home Care & Hospice reported that more than 7 million people in the United States receive home health care annually.

As patients move to the use of home health care services for recuperation or long-term care, the medical devices necessary for their care have followed them. As a result, complex medical devices are used more frequently in the home, many times under unsuitable conditions. This in turn has implications for the safe and effective operation of these devices, especially those with sophisticated requirements for proper operation or maintenance.

Frequently Asked Questions about Home Use Devices

What devices does FDA recommend for home use?

FDA is responsible for regulating companies that manufacture, re-package, relabel, and import medical devices sold in the United States. This is accomplished through scientific review of premarket data submitted by a medical device manufacturer to establish a device's safety and efficacy and then once on the market, monitoring medical device adverse event reports to detect and correct device-related problems in a timely manner.

It is important to note because the FDA's scope of work is to regulate the medical device industry, the FDA cannot and does not recommend specific medical devices for use in any setting. Review the instructions for use for a device you plan to use in the home before deciding on the one best for a particular patient population.

I have a patient who lives in a rural area and is being discharged from the hospital. She will be 2 hours from the nearest clinic. What medical device associated risks should I consider?

There are many risks to consider when caring for a patient who requires a medical device in their home environment, especially in rural areas. It is important to consider:

- what the device needs to operate safely and effectively (for example, electricity, running water, computer connections, backup supplies);
- power sources and outlets (for example, are they compatible with one another?);
- patient capabilities.

Where can I buy home use devices?

Home use devices are often sold to patients who have a prescription for that given device at hospitals or at pharmacies. Medical devices are also cleared or approved for sale directly to the consumer and these are called over-the-counter (OTC) products. Medical devices are also available at many online retailers. If you buy a home use device online, make sure you are buying from a reliable source. Also check the store's return policy and customer support statement before you place an order.

Who do I contact if my device breaks or doesn't work properly?

Make sure you have phone numbers for your homecare agency, doctor, or the device manufacturer to call if your device is not working properly. You should also report the problem to your doctor, to the manufacturer of your medical device, and to FDA through the Med-Watch Reporting Program (see last question in this chapter).

Who can write a prescription for a medical device?

Each state has laws and regulations that determine who can write a prescription for a medical device in that state. FDA defers to the states on determining who can write a valid prescription.

Do I need a prescription for my device?

Not all medical devices require a prescription; however, many medical devices do require a prescription (for example, contact lenses).

I can't find the instructions for use. Where can I find the information?

If you do not have the instructions, contact your healthcare provider.

How do I clean my device?

Follow the manufacturer's instructions. If you do not have the instructions, contact your healthcare provider.

Where do I dispose of hazardous waste, such as needles or tubing?

Dispose of your medical device according to the manufacturer's instructions. You may also wish to contact your pharmacist, nearest hospital, solid waste company, or state or local government for additional information about proper disposal.

Where do I report a serious injury, death, or medical device malfunction?

You may report a problem by mail, phone, fax, or online:

MedWatch [Use postage-paid FDA Form 35009]

5600 Fishers Lane
Rockville, MD 20852-9787
Toll-Free: 800-332-1088
Fax: 800-FDA-0178 (332-0178)
Website: https://www.accessdata.fda.gov/scripts/medwatch/
medwatch-online.htm

Unique Considerations in the Home

The home care setting is a challenging environment. Because it is very different from the hospital setting, it often presents additional risks to patients and providers. This text outlines environmental considerations and potential safety hazards providers and patients should be alert to when using—or considering using—a medical device in the home setting.

Geographic Location

Where a person lives makes a difference in the type of home health care services they receive. For example, home health care providers and support staff may not be readily available in a rural setting, where it may also be difficult to obtain needed back-up supplies or equipment.

Different parts of the country experience power outages more frequently than others, especially during public emergencies like Hurricane Katrina. During these uncontrollable events, patients should have back-up plans and extra supplies when using certain medical devices.

Age and Structure of a Home

A home's age and structure can affect the quality of care, especially when using medical devices. For example, older homes may not have the electrical outlets needed for some medical devices. Older homes may also have smaller doorways, hallways, and rooms that do not accommodate large medical equipment. Smaller homes may not allow for wheelchairs to pass through the entranceway, forcing patients to use walkers, crutches, or canes instead. Before a medical device goes home with a patient, check to see if the medical device is compatible with the patient's home.

In-Home Environmental Hazards

Regardless of geographic location, home settings may present other environmental challenges for the use of medical devices.

Pets: Pets may directly interfere with device operation. For example, they may chew through an electrical cord or play with an accessory, such as tubing. Pets may also contribute to unsanitary conditions where the medical device is used. They may walk over an area that is supposed to be clean, and pet fur/hair may find its way into a device.

Unsanitary conditions: Unhealthy conditions may result from dirty surface areas, wet towels on the bathroom floor, dirty dishes, and open or scattered garbage. For example, trash that is not properly contained or removed may attract insects and rodents.

The ability to manage medical waste properly and establish safe cleaning practices also requires attention. For instance, the improper disposal of sharps, such as needles, can lead to needlestick injuries in caregivers, patients, and household members. Each state or local government regulates the storage, transportation, and disposal of medical waste. Check with your local government to learn more.

Children at play: Children may interfere with medical device operation. They may change the dial, settings, and on/off switches, twist tubing, adjust machine vents, or remove electrical cords from the outlet. They can also injure themselves while playing with devices they think are toys.

Plumbing: Clean, running water is critical to the use of a medical device in the home. Some medical devices and equipment, such as dialyzers or infusion pumps, require safe water during use, cleaning, and maintenance. Even if water is not required for a device to operate, it may be necessary for cleaning its accessories.

Temperature extremes: Extreme heat and humidity can negatively affect a working device. Unusually high levels of heat and humidity may:

- cause instruments to operate in unexpected or unusual ways;

- reduce the expected life span of devices or totally destroy products;

- cause laboratory substances used in chemical analysis to lose strength; or

- compromise the cleanliness of packaged devices.

For example, high humidity becomes a problem when a low flow of air causes moisture to build up on a medical device, resulting in a malfunction. Excess moisture may also cause mold to grow on a device.

Dust: Carpets and drapes can hold allergen-containing dust. If dust gets into a medical device, it may affect the way it works.

Fire hazards: Fire hazards are a concern when considering a home use medical device. Electrical problems with device equipment such as their potential to overheat or short-circuit may increase the likelihood for home fires. Home care patients who receive supplemental oxygen therapy are also at increased risk. Wherever there is a high concentration of oxygen gas, there is also an increased risk of fire initiated from electrical faults. Taking appropriate fire safety precautions is important.

Tripping hazards: Too much clutter, loose carpeting, and slippery floor surfaces may cause people to fall. Patients who have trouble moving around without the use of a walker, crutch, or cane have a higher risk of falling when these hazards are present.

Poor lighting: Poor lighting has been shown to result in injuries, especially from patient falls. Inadequate lighting can also make it more difficult for a patient or caregiver to see and operate a medical device.

Background noise: There is a lot of noise in the home environment— from vacuum cleaners, televisions, telephones, to people arguing. Outside noise, such as trash pick-up trucks and emergency sirens, is also common. All loud noise can interfere with the ability to hear whether a medical device is operating correctly or whether an alarm has sounded.

Section 26.2

Adapting Your Living Space to Accommodate Your Disability

Excerpted from "Home Modification," by the Administration on Aging (AOA, www.aoa.gov), part of the U.S. Department of Health and Human Services, 2010.

What are home modifications?

Home modifications are changes made to adapt living spaces to meet the needs of people with physical limitations so that they can continue to live independently and safely. These modifications may include adding assistive technology or making structural changes to a home. Modifications can range from something as simple as replacing cabinet doorknobs with pull handles to full-scale construction projects that require installing wheelchair ramps and widening doorways.

Why do seniors need home modifications?

The main benefit of making home modifications is that they promote independence and prevent accidents. According to a recent AARP [American Association of Retired Persons] housing survey, "83% of older Americans want to stay in their current homes for the rest of their lives," but other studies show that most homes are not designed to accommodate the needs of people over age 65. Most older people live in homes that are more than 20 years old. As these buildings get older along with their residents, they may become harder to live in or maintain. A house that was perfectly suitable for a senior at age 55, for example, may have too many stairs or slippery surfaces for a person who is 70 or 80. Research by the national Centers for Disease Control and Prevention shows that home modifications and repairs may prevent 30% to 50% of all home accidents among seniors, including falls that take place in these older homes.

How can I tell what home modifications are right for me?

The best way to begin planning for home modifications is by defining the basic terms used and asking some simple questions. According to the Rehabilitation Engineering and Assistive Technology Society of North America (RESNA), home modifications should improve the following features of a home:

- **Accessibility:** Improving accessibility means making doorways wider, clearing spaces to make sure a wheelchair can pass through, lowering countertop heights for sinks and kitchen cabinets, installing grab bars, and placing light switches and electrical outlets at heights that can be reached easily. This remodeling must comply with the Fair Housing Amendments Act of 1988, the Americans with Disabilities Act accessibility guidelines, and American National Standards Institute regulations for accessibility. The work must also conform to state and local building codes.

- **Adaptability:** Adaptability features are changes that can be made quickly to accommodate the needs of seniors or disabled individuals without having to completely redesign the home or use different materials for essential fixtures. Examples include installing grab bars in bathroom walls and movable cabinets under the sink so that someone in a wheelchair can use the space.

- **Universal design:** Universal design features are usually built into a home when the first blueprints or architectural plans are drawn. These features include appliances, fixtures, and floor plans that are easy for all people to use, flexible enough so that they can be adapted for special needs, sturdy and reliable, and functional with a minimum of effort and understanding of the mechanisms involved.

Where do you begin?

Before you make home modifications, you should evaluate your current and future needs by going through your home room by room and answering a series of questions to highlight where changes might be made. Several checklists are available to help you conduct this review. The National Resource Center on Supportive Housing and Home Modifications is a good place to start. Go to the center's website at www.homemods.org.

You can begin your survey by examining each area of your home and asking questions about the areas in the following text.

Check your appliances, kitchen, and bathroom:

- Are cabinet doorknobs easy to use?

- Are stove controls easy to use and clearly marked?

- Are faucets easy to use?

- Are there grab bars where needed?

- Are all appliances and utensils conveniently and safely located?

- Can the oven and refrigerator be opened easily?

- Can you sit down while working?

- Can you get into and out of the bathtub or shower easily?

- Is the kitchen counter height and depth comfortable for you?

- Is the water temperature regulated to prevent scalding or burning?

- Would you benefit from having convenience items, such as a handheld showerhead, a garbage disposal, or a trash compactor?

Check your closets and storage spaces:

- Are your closets and storage areas conveniently located?

- Are your closet shelves too high?

- Can you reach items in the closet easily?

- Do you have enough storage space?

- Have you gotten the maximum use out of the storage space you have, including saving space with special closet shelf systems and other products?

Check your doors and windows:

- Are your doors and windows easy to open and close?
- Are your door locks sturdy and easy to operate?
- Are your doors wide enough to accommodate a walker or wheelchair?
- Do your doors have peepholes or viewing windows?

Check your driveway and garage:

- Does your garage door have an automatic opener?
- Is your parking space always available?
- Is your parking space close to the entrance of your home?

Check your electrical outlets, switches, and safety devices:

- Are light or power switches easy to turn on and off?
- Are electrical outlets easy to reach?
- Are the electrical outlets properly grounded to prevent shocks?
- Are your extension cords in good condition?
- Can you hear the doorbell in every part of the house?
- Do you have smoke detectors throughout your home?
- Do you have an alarm system?
- Is the telephone readily available for emergencies?
- Would you benefit from having an assistive device to make it easier to hear and talk on the telephone?

Check your floors:

- Are all of the floors in your home on the same level?
- Are steps up and down marked in some way?
- Are all floor surfaces safe and covered with non-slip or non-skid materials?
- Do you have scatter rugs or doormats that could be hazardous?

Check your hallways, steps, and stairways:

- Are hallways and stairs in good condition?
- Do all of your hallways and stairs have smooth, safe surfaces?

- Do your stairs have steps that are big enough for your whole foot?

- Do you have handrails on both sides of the stairway?

- Are your stair rails wide enough for you to grasp them securely?

- Would you benefit from building a ramp to replace the stairs or steps inside or outside of your home?

Check your lighting and ventilation:

- Do you have night lights where they are needed?

- Is the lighting in each room sufficient for the use of the room?

- Is the lighting bright enough to ensure safety?

- Is each room well-ventilated with good air circulation?

Once you have explored all the areas of your home that could benefit from remodeling, you might make a list of potential problems and possible solutions.

How can I pay for home modifications?

Many minor home modifications and repairs can be done for about $150–$2,000. For bigger projects, some financing options may be available. For instance, many home remodeling contractors offer reduced rates and charge sliding-scale fees based on a senior's income and ability to pay or the homeowner may be able to obtain a modest loan to cover urgent needs. Other possible sources of public and private financial assistance include the following:

- Home modification and repair funds from Title III of the Older Americans Act: These funds are distributed by your local area agency on aging (AAA). To contact your local AAA, call the Eldercare Locator (800-677-1116) or visit the Eldercare Locator website at www.eldercare.gov.

- Rebuilding Together, Inc., a national volunteer organization, through its local affiliates, is able to assist some low-income seniors with home modification efforts. Visit the following website to learn more: www.rebuildingtogether.org/section/initiatives/safehomes.

- Investment capital from the U.S. Department of Energy's Low-Income Home Energy Assistance Program (LIHEAP) and the Weatherization Assistance Program (WAP): Both of these programs are run by local energy and social services departments.

- Medicare and Medicaid funds: Although these programs usually cover only items that are used for medical purposes and ordered by a doctor, some types of home modifications may qualify. To find out if Medicare will help to cover the cost of a home modification ordered by a doctor, call 800-MEDICARE (800-633-4227 or TTY/TDD 877-486-2048). You can also find answers to your questions by visiting the website at www.medicare.gov on the internet.

- Community development block grants: Many cities and towns make grant funds available through the local department of community development.

- Home equity conversion mortgages: Local banks may allow a homeowner to borrow money against the value of his or her home and pay for needed improvements. The homeowner then repays the loan as part of his or her regular mortgage.

Seniors may also choose to bypass public assistance programs and hire a contractor to do their home modifications or even do the job by themselves. Keep in mind these points if you want to have a professional contractor come into your home to work on a large project:

- Ask for a written agreement that includes only a small down payment and specifies exactly what work will be done and how much it will cost (with the balance of payment to be made when the job is finished).

- Check with your local Better Business Bureau and Chamber of Commerce to see if any complaints have been filed against the contractor.

- Make sure that the contractor has insurance and is licensed to do the work required.

- Talk with your family and friends to get recommendations based on their experiences with the contractors they have hired. This step may actually be the most important one because contractors with a good reputation can usually be counted on to do a good job.

- Go to www.homemods.org and view the National Directory of Home Modification and Repair Programs for a listing of what is available in the state where you live.

Chapter 27

Technology for People with Intellectual Disabilities

What types of technology help people with intellectual disabilities?

Assistive Technology (AT) can be a device or a service. An assistive technology device is any item, piece of equipment, or product system, that is used to increase, maintain, or improve functional capabilities of individuals with disabilities. An assistive technology service means any service that helps an individual with a disability select, acquire, or use an assistive technology device (Assistive Technology Act of 2004).

Electronic and Information Technology (E&IT) includes computers and related resources and communication products such as telephones, transaction machines such as ATMs for banking, World Wide Web sites, and office copiers and faxes (Wehmeyer et al, 2004).

How can technology benefit people with intellectual disabilities?

Kelker (1997) developed the following list indicating that assistive technology may be considered appropriate when it does any or all of the following things:

- Enables an individual to perform functions that can be achieved by no other means

---

- Enables an individual to approximate normal fluency, rate, or standards—a level of accomplishment that could not be achieved by any other means

- Provides access for participation in programs or activities which otherwise would be closed to the individual

- Increases endurance or ability to persevere and complete tasks that otherwise are too laborious to be attempted on a routine basis

- Enables an individual to concentrate on learning or employment tasks, rather than mechanical tasks

- Provides greater access to information

- Supports normal social interactions with peers and adults

- Supports participation in the least restrictive educational environment

How do people with intellectual disabilities use technology?

Communication: For individuals who cannot communicate with their voices technology can help them communicate. Augmentative and alternative communication (AAC) may involve technology ranging from low-tech message boards to computerized voice output communication aids and synthesized speech.

Mobility: Simple to sophisticated computer controlled wheelchairs and mobility aids are available. Technology may be used to aid direction-finding, guiding users to destinations. Computer cueing systems and robots have also been used to guide users with intellectual disabilities.

Environmental control: Assistive technology can help people with severe or multiple disabilities to control electrical appliances, audio/video equipment such as home entertainment systems, or to do something as basic as lock and unlock doors.

Activities of daily living: Technology is assisting people with disabilities to successfully complete everyday tasks of self-care. Examples include:

- Automated and computerized dining devices allow an individual who needs assistance at mealtime to eat more independently.

- Audio prompting devices may be used to assist a person with memory difficulties to complete a task or to follow a certain sequence of steps from start to finish in such activities as making a bed or taking medication.

- Video-based instructional materials can help people learn functional life skills such as grocery shopping, writing a check, paying the bills, or using the ATM machine.

Education: Technology is used in education to aid communication, support activities of daily living, and to enhance learning. Computer-assisted instruction can help in many areas, including word recognition, math, spelling, and even social skills. Computers have also been found to promote interaction with non-disabled peers.

Employment: Technology, such as video-assisted training, is being used for job training and job skill development and to teach complex skills for appropriate job behavior and social interaction. Prompting systems using audio cassette recorders and computer-based prompting devices have been used to help workers stay on task. Computerized prompting systems can help people manage their time in scheduling job activities.

Sports and recreation: Toys can be adapted with switches and other technologies to facilitate play for children. Computer or video games provide age-appropriate social opportunities and help children learn cognitive and eye-hand coordination skills. Specially designed internet-access software can help people with intellectual disabilities access the World Wide Web. Exercise and physical fitness can be supported by video-based technology.

What are some barriers to technology use by people with intellectual disabilities?

A survey by The Arc (Wehmeyer, 1998) found that lack of information about the availability of the device and the cost of devices were the main barriers. Other barriers included the unavailability of assessment information, limited training on device use, and device complexity.

Even though it is the goal of most technology development efforts to incorporate the principles of universal design, cognitive access is not carefully considered. Universal design ensures that the technology may be used by all people without the need for adaptation or specialized design. An example of cognitive access would be if someone with disabilities is using a computer program, onscreen messages should last long enough or provide wait time to consider whether to press a computer key. Or the time should be sufficient between dialing and pressing the numerals to complete a phone call using a rechargeable phone card as payment. Because individuals with intellectual disabilities have a range of learning and processing abilities, it is difficult to develop assistive technology solutions that are appropriate for all.

Do schools have to provide assistive technology to students who need it?

The Individuals with Disabilities Education Act (IDEA) requires that the need for AT be considered for all students when developing the individualized education program. The intention of the special education law is that, if a student with disabilities needs technology in order to be able to learn, the school district will (a) evaluate the student's technology needs; (b) acquire the necessary technology; (c) coordinate technology use with other therapies and interventions; and (d) provide training for the individual, the individual's family, and the school staff in the effective use of the technology. If the student's individualized education program specifies AT is needed for home use to ensure appropriate education, the school must provide it. If the school purchases an AT device for use by the student, the school owns it. The student cannot take it when moving to another school or when leaving school.

What are some sources of information and help?

- The Alliance for Technology Access (ATA) (http://www.ataccess .org) has a network of community-based technology resource centers that provide information and support services to children and adults with disabilities.

- The Association of Assistive Technology Act Programs (ATAP) (http://www.ataporg.org) supports state AT programs in implementing the Assistive Technology Act. States may operate a state finance program or a device loan program for assistive technology devices. For a list of state programs, go to http:// www.ataporg.org.

- The Beach Center on Disability, University of Kansas, has technology resources on its website (http://www.beachcenter.org).

- The Coleman Institute for Cognitive Disabilities is another source of assistive technology information (http://www.coleman institute.org).

References

Assistive Technology Act of 2004. (October 25, 2004). Public Law 108-364.

Individuals with Disabilities Education Act (IDEA). (December 3, 2004). Public Law 108-446.

Kelker, K.A. (1997). *Family Guide to Assistive Technology*. Parents, Let's Unite for Kids (PLUK). Accessed online at http://www.pluk.org/AT1.html

Wehmeyer, M.L. (1998). National survey of the use of assistive technology by adults with mental retardation. *Mental Retardation, 36*, 44–51.

Wehmeyer, M.L., Smith, S.J., Palmer, S.B., Davies, D.K. & Stock, S.E. (2004). Technology use and people with mental retardation. *International Review of Research in Mental Retardation, 29*, 291–337.

Chapter 28

Devices for Improving Communication and Hearing

Chapter Contents

Section 28.1—Captions for Deaf and
            Hard-of-Hearing Viewers 238

Section 28.2—Cochlear Implants 242

Section 28.3—Hearing Aids 245

Section 28.4—Other Hearing Assistive Technology 249

Section 28.5—Profoundly Paralyzed Communicate
            with Brain-Computer Interface 253

Section 28.1

Captions for Deaf and Hard-of-Hearing Viewers

From "Captions for Deaf and Hard-of-Hearing Viewers," by the National Institute on Deafness and Other Communication Disorders (NIDCD, www .nidcd.nih.gov), part of the National Institutes of Health, July 2002. Updated by David A. Cooke, MD, FACP, July 14, 2011.

On August 5, 1972, Julia Child, "The French Chef," in a program televised from WGBH studios in Boston, taught viewers how to make one of her prized chicken recipes. The significance of that day stretched far beyond the details of the entree to have a profound and lasting impact on human communication. It was the first time Americans who are deaf and hard-of-hearing could enjoy the audio portion of a national television program through the use of captions.

Since then, captions have opened the world of television to people who are deaf and hard-of-hearing. At first, special broadcasts of some of the more popular programs were made accessible through the Public Broadcasting Service. Now, more than 2,000 hours of entertainment, news, public affairs, and sports programming are captioned each week on network, public, and cable television. Captions are no longer a novelty: They have become a necessity.

What Are Captions?

Captions are words displayed on a television screen that describe the audio or sound portion of a program. Captions allow viewers who are deaf or hard of hearing to follow the dialogue and the action of a program simultaneously. They can also provide information about who is speaking or about sound effects that may be important to understanding a news story, a political event, or the plot of a program.

Captions are created from the transcript of a program. A captioner separates the dialogue into captions and makes sure the words appear in sync with the audio they describe. A specially designed computer software program encodes the captioning information and combines it with the audio and video to create a new master tape or digital file of the program.

Open and closed captions: Captions may be "open" or "closed." To view closed captions, viewers need a set-top decoder or a television with built-in decoder circuitry. Open captions appear on all television sets and can be viewed without a decoder. In the past, some news bulletins, presidential addresses, or programming created by or for deaf and hard-of-hearing audiences were open captioned. With the widespread availability of closed-caption technology, open captions are rarely used.

Digital closed captioning: Closed captioning has become available for digital television sets, such as high-definition television (HDTV) sets, manufactured after July 1, 2002. Digital captioning provides greater flexibility by enabling the viewer to control the caption display, including font style, text size and color, and background color.

Real-time captioning: Real-time captions are created as an event takes place. A captioner (often trained as a court reporter or stenographer) uses a stenotype machine with a phonetic keyboard and special software. A computer translates the phonetic symbols into English captions almost instantaneously. The slight delay is based on the captioner's need to hear the word and on the computer processing time. Real-time captioning can be used for programs that have no script; live events, including congressional proceedings; news programs; and nonbroadcast meetings, such as the national meetings of professional associations.

Although most real-time captioning is more than 98 percent accurate, the audience will see occasional errors. The captioner may mishear a word, hear an unfamiliar word, or have an error in the software dictionary. Often, real-time captions are produced at a different location from the programming and are transmitted by phone lines. In addition to live, real-time captioning, captions are being put on prerecorded video, rental movies on tape and DVD, and educational and training tapes using a similar process but enabling error correction.

Electronic newsroom captions: Electronic newsroom captions (ENR) are created from a news script computer or teleprompter and are commonly used for live newscasts. Only material that is scripted can be captioned using this technique. Therefore, spontaneous commentary, live field reports, breaking news, and sports and weather updates may not be captioned using ENR, and real-time captioning is needed.

Edited and verbatim captions: Captions can be produced as either edited or verbatim captions. Edited captions summarize ideas and shorten phrases. Verbatim captions include all of what is said.

Although there are situations in which edited captions have been preferred for ease in reading (such as for children's programs), most people who are deaf or hard-of-hearing prefer the full access provided by verbatim texts.

Rear window captioning: More and more movie theaters across the country are offering this type of captioning system. An adjustable Lucite panel attaches to the viewer's seat and reflects the captions from a light-emitting diode (LED) panel on the back of the theatre.

Current Research

Researchers are studying caption features, speeds, and the effects of visual impairments on reading captions. This research will help the broadcast television industry understand which caption features should be retained and which new features should be adopted to better serve consumers. Other research is examining the potential for captions as a learning tool for acquiring English-language and reading skills. These studies are looking at how captions can reinforce vocabulary, improve literacy, and help people learn the expressions and speech patterns of spoken English.

The Law

The Americans with Disabilities Act (ADA) of 1990 requires that businesses and public accommodations ensure that disabled individuals are not excluded from or denied services because of the absence of auxiliary aids. Captions are considered one type of auxiliary aid. Since the passage of the ADA, the use of captioning has expanded. Entertainment, educational, informational, and training materials are captioned for deaf and hard-of-hearing audiences at the time they are produced and distributed.

The Television Decoder Circuitry Act of 1990 requires that all televisions larger than 13 inches sold in the United States after July 1993 have a special built-in decoder that enables viewers to watch closed-captioned programming. The Telecommunications Act of 1996 directs the Federal Communications Commission (FCC) to adopt rules requiring closed captioning of most television programming.

Captions and the FCC

The original FCC rules on closed captioning became effective January 1, 1998. They require people or companies that distribute television programs directly to home viewers to make sure those programs are captioned. The Telecommunications Act of 1996 broadened these rules to apply regardless of distribution technology. Since January 1, 2006, all new programming has been required to be closed captioned. Due to the large amount of content, requirements on older programs have been phased in gradually to provide time to generate the captioning. As of January 1, 2008, at least 75% of analog programming that first aired before January 1, 1998, and digital programming that first aired prior to July 1, 2002, must have closed captioning.

Who is required to provide closed captions?

Originally, the rules applied to people or companies that distribute television programs directly to home viewers (video program distributors). Some examples are local broadcast television stations, satellite television services, and local cable television operators. Subsequently, the Telecommunications Act of 1996 extended the requirements to all video program providers, regardless of the specific technology being used. The FCC is currently considering new rules requiring movie theaters to provide closed captioning.

What programs are exempt?

Some advertisements, public service announcements, non-English-language programs (with the exception of Spanish programs), locally produced and distributed non-news programming, textual programs, early-morning programs, and nonvocal musical programs are exempt from captioning.

Section 28.2

Cochlear Implants

Excerpted from "Cochlear Implants," by the National Institute of Deafness and Communication Disorders (NIDCD, www.nidcd.nih.gov), part of the National Institutes of Health, August 2009.

What is a cochlear implant?

A cochlear implant is a small, complex electronic device that can help to provide a sense of sound to a person who is profoundly deaf or severely hard-of-hearing. The implant consists of an external portion that sits behind the ear and a second portion that is surgically placed under the skin (see Figure 28.1). An implant has the following parts:

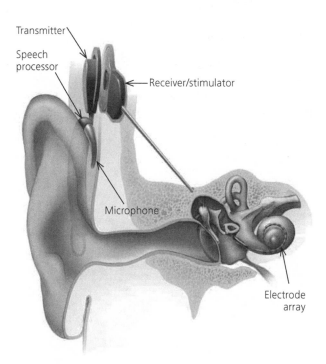

Figure 28.1. *Ear with cochlear implant.*

- A microphone, which picks up sound from the environment

- A speech processor, which selects and arranges sounds picked up by the microphone

- A transmitter and receiver/stimulator, which receive signals from the speech processor and convert them into electric impulses

- An electrode array, which is a group of electrodes that collects the impulses from the stimulator and sends them to different regions of the auditory nerve

An implant does not restore normal hearing. Instead, it can give a deaf person a useful representation of sounds in the environment and help him or her to understand speech.

How does a cochlear implant work?

A cochlear implant is very different from a hearing aid. Hearing aids amplify sounds so they may be detected by damaged ears. Cochlear implants bypass damaged portions of the ear and directly stimulate the auditory nerve. Signals generated by the implant are sent by way of the auditory nerve to the brain, which recognizes the signals as sound. Hearing through a cochlear implant is different from normal hearing and takes time to learn or relearn. However, it allows many people to recognize warning signals, understand other sounds in the environment, and enjoy a conversation in person or by telephone.

Who gets cochlear implants?

Children and adults who are deaf or severely hard of hearing can be fitted for cochlear implants. According to the U.S. Food and Drug Administration (FDA), as of December 2010, approximately 219,000 people worldwide have received implants. In the United States, roughly 42,600 adults and 28,400 children have received them.

Adults who have lost all or most of their hearing later in life often can benefit from cochlear implants. They learn to associate the signal provided by an implant with sounds they remember. This often provides recipients with the ability to understand speech solely by listening through the implant, without requiring any visual cues such as those provided by lipreading or sign language.

Cochlear implants, coupled with intensive postimplantation therapy, can help young children to acquire speech, language, and social skills. Most children who receive implants are between 2 and 6 years old. Early implantation provides exposure to sounds that can be help-ful during the critical period when children learn speech and language skills. In 2000, the FDA lowered the age of eligibility to 12 months for one type of cochlear implant.

How does someone receive a cochlear implant?

Use of a cochlear implant requires both a surgical procedure and significant therapy to learn or relearn the sense of hearing. Not ev-eryone performs at the same level with this device. The decision to receive an implant should involve discussions with medical specialists, including an experienced cochlear-implant surgeon. The process can be expensive. For example, a person's health insurance may cover the expense, but not always. Some individuals may choose not to have a cochlear implant for a variety of personal reasons. Surgical implanta-tions are almost always safe, although complications are a risk factor, just as with any kind of surgery. An additional consideration is learn-ing to interpret the sounds created by an implant. This process takes time and practice. Speech-language pathologists and audiologists are frequently involved in this learning process. Prior to implantation, all of these factors need to be considered.

Section 28.3

Hearing Aids

Excerpted from "Hearing Aids," by the National Institute of Deafness
and Communication Disorders (NIDCD, www.nidcd.nih.gov), part of the
National Institutes of Health, April 2007.

What is a hearing aid?

A hearing aid is a small electronic device that you wear in or behind your ear. It makes some sounds louder so that a person with hearing loss can listen, communicate, and participate more fully in daily activities. A hearing aid can help people hear more in both quiet and noisy situations. However, only about one out of five people who would benefit from a hearing aid actually uses one.

A hearing aid has three basic parts—a microphone, amplifier, and speaker. The hearing aid receives sound through a microphone, which converts the sound waves to electrical signals and sends them to an amplifier. The amplifier increases the power of the signals and then sends them to the ear through a speaker.

How can hearing aids help?

Hearing aids are primarily useful in improving the hearing and speech comprehension of people who have hearing loss that results from damage to the small sensory cells in the inner ear, called hair cells. This type of hearing loss is called sensorineural hearing loss. The damage can occur as a result of disease, aging, or injury from noise or certain medicines.

A hearing aid magnifies sound vibrations entering the ear. Surviving hair cells detect the larger vibrations and convert them into neural signals that are passed along to the brain. The greater the damage to a person's hair cells, the more severe the hearing loss, and the greater the hearing aid amplification needed to make up the difference. However, there are practical limits to the amount of amplification a hearing aid can provide. In addition, if the inner ear is too damaged, even large vibrations will not be converted into neural signals. In this situation, a hearing aid would be ineffective.

How can I find out if I need a hearing aid?

If you think you might have hearing loss and could benefit from a hearing aid, visit your physician, who may refer you to an otolaryngologist or audiologist.

An otolaryngologist is a physician who specializes in ear, nose, and throat disorders and will investigate the cause of the hearing loss. An audiologist is a hearing health professional who identifies and measures hearing loss and will perform a hearing test to assess the type and degree of loss.

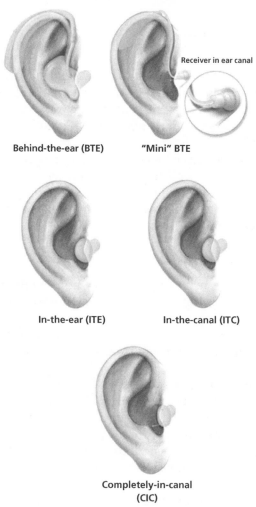

Figure 28.2. Styles of hearing aids.

Are there different styles of hearing aids?

There are three basic styles of hearing aids. The styles differ by size, their placement on or inside the ear, and the degree to which they amplify sound (see Figure 28.2).

Behind-the-ear (BTE) hearing aids consist of a hard plastic case worn behind the ear and connected to a plastic earmold that fits inside the outer ear. The electronic parts are held in the case behind the ear. Sound travels from the hearing aid through the earmold and into the ear. BTE aids are used by people of all ages for mild to profound hearing loss.

A new kind of BTE aid is an open-fit hearing aid. Small, open-fit aids fit behind the ear completely, with only a narrow tube inserted into the ear canal, enabling the canal to remain open. For this reason, open-fit hearing aids may be a good choice for people who experience a buildup of earwax, since this type of aid is less likely to be damaged by such substances. In addition, some people may prefer the open-fit hearing aid because their perception of their voice does not sound "plugged up."

In-the-ear (ITE) hearing aids fit completely inside the outer ear and are used for mild to severe hearing loss. The case holding the electronic components is made of hard plastic. Some ITE aids may have certain added features installed, such as a telecoil. A telecoil is a small magnetic coil that allows users to receive sound through the circuitry of the hearing aid, rather than through its microphone. This makes it easier to hear conversations over the telephone. A telecoil also helps people hear in public facilities that have installed special sound systems, called induction loop systems. Induction loop systems can be found in many churches, schools, airports, and auditoriums. ITE aids usually are not worn by young children because the casings need to be replaced often as the ear grows.

Canal aids fit into the ear canal and are available in two styles. The in-the-canal (ITC) hearing aid is made to fit the size and shape of a person's ear canal. A completely-in-canal (CIC) hearing aid is nearly hidden in the ear canal. Both types are used for mild to moderately severe hearing loss.

Because they are small, canal aids may be difficult for a person to adjust and remove. In addition, canal aids have less space available for batteries and additional devices, such as a telecoil. They usually are not recommended for young children or for people with severe to profound hearing loss because their reduced size limits their power and volume.

Which hearing aid will work best for me?

The hearing aid that will work best for you depends on the kind and severity of your hearing loss. If you have a hearing loss in both of your ears, two hearing aids are generally recommended because two aids provide a more natural signal to the brain. Hearing in both ears also will help you understand speech and locate where the sound is coming from.

You and your audiologist should select a hearing aid that best suits your needs and lifestyle. Price is also a key consideration because hearing aids range from hundreds to several thousand dollars. Similar to other equipment purchases, style and features affect cost. However, don't use price alone to determine the best hearing aid for you. Just because one hearing aid is more expensive than another does not necessarily mean that it will better suit your needs.

A hearing aid will not restore your normal hearing. With practice, however, a hearing aid will increase your awareness of sounds and their sources. You will want to wear your hearing aid regularly, so select one that is convenient and easy for you to use. Other features to consider include parts or services covered by the warranty, estimated schedule and costs for maintenance and repair, options and upgrade opportunities, and the hearing aid company's reputation for quality and customer service.

Section 28.4

Other Hearing Assistive Technology

What Are Hearing Assistive Technology Systems (HATS)?

Hearing assistive technology systems (HATS) are devices that can help you function better in your day-to-day communication situations. HATS can be used with or without hearing aids or cochlear implants to make hearing easier—and thereby reduce stress and fatigue. Hearing aids + HATS = better listening and better communication!

The following situations are difficult for all listeners, but they are especially difficult for people with hearing loss:

- **Distance between the listener and the sound source:** The farther away you are from a speaker, of course, the harder it is to hear the speaker. This is because the intensity, or loudness, of a sound fades rapidly as it travels over distance. So, while you may have no difficulty hearing someone in close range, you may have considerable difficulty hearing the same person across the room.

- **Competing noise in the environment:** Most rooms have background noise that competes with the spoken message or sound we want to hear. Examples of background noise include ventilation systems, others talking, paper shuffling, computers, radios, TVs, outside traffic or construction, and activities in adjacent rooms. Background noise can make hearing very challenging. For optimum hearing, speech should be at least 20–25 decibels (dB) louder than any competing noise. This is called the signal-to-noise ratio, or S/N ratio.

- **Poor room acoustics/reverberation:** A room's acoustics are the quality of sound maintained in the room, and they can affect your ability to hear effectively. Sound waves bounce off hard surfaces like windows, walls, and hard floors. This creates sound reflections and echoes (called reverberation). The result of excess reverberation is distorted speech. Large gyms, cathedrals, and open marble lobbies quickly come to mind when we think about reverberation. Reverberation also can occur in smaller spaces such as classrooms. We've all experienced how much easier it is to hear in rooms that are carpeted and have upholstered furniture (which absorbs noise) than in empty rooms with tile or cement floors.

Any one of these conditions (distance, noise, or reverberation) can create listening problems. More often than not, they occur together and have a debilitating effect on the ability to hear and process speech. HATS can help you overcome these listening difficulties.

FM Systems

Personal frequency modulation (FM) systems are like miniature radio stations operating on special frequencies. The personal FM system consists of a transmitter microphone used by the speaker (such as the teacher in the classroom, or the speaker at a lecture) and a receiver used by you, the listener. The receiver transmits the sound to your ears or, if you wear a hearing aid, directly to the hearing aid.

Personal FM systems are useful in a variety of situations, such as in a classroom lecture, in a restaurant, in a sales meeting, or in a nursing home or senior center.

FM systems are also used in theaters, places of worship, museums, public meeting places, corporate conference rooms, convention centers, and other large areas for gathering. In these situations, the microphone/transmitter is built into the overall sound system. You are provided with an FM receiver that can connect to your hearing aid or cochlear implant. The receiver can also connect to a headset if you don't wear a hearing aid.

Infrared Systems

Infrared systems are often used in the home with TV sets, but, like FM systems, they can also be used in large settings like theaters.

With an infrared system, sound from the TV is transmitted using infrared light waves. This sound is transmitted to your receiver, which you can adjust to your desired volume. The TV can be set to a volume comfortable for any other viewers with normal hearing. Thus, TV watching as a family becomes pleasurable for all.

Induction Loop Systems

Induction loop systems are most common in large group areas. They can also be purchased for individual use.

Induction loop systems work with hearing aids. An induction loop wire is permanently installed (typically under a carpet or in the ceiling) and connects to a microphone used by a speaker. The person talking into the microphone generates a current in the wire, which creates an electromagnetic field in the room. When you switch your hearing aid to the "T" (telecoil/telephone) setting, your hearing aid telecoil picks up the electromagnetic signal. You can then adjust the volume of the signal through your hearing aid.

One-to-One Communicators

Sometimes in a restaurant, nursing home situation, or riding in a car, you want to be able to easily hear just one person. Or perhaps you are delivering a lecture or running a meeting and a person in the audience has a question. You can give the person a microphone to speak into. The sound is amplified and delivered directly into your hearing aid (or headset if you don't have a hearing aid), and you can adjust the volume to your comfort level. When using the one-to-one communicator, the speaker does not have to shout, private conversations can remain private, and in a car your eyes can remain on the road!

Other Hearing Assistive Technology Systems Solutions

There are many other HATS available, such as:

- telephone amplifying devices for cordless, cell, digital, and wired phones;
- amplified answering machines;
- amplified telephones with different frequency responses;
- loud doorbells;
- computers;
- wake-up alarms (loud bell or vibrating clock).

To learn more about HATS and how they can help you, you should contact a certified audiologist.

Are there communication devices besides those that assist listening? Yes, there are visual systems that can be used alone or in combination with listening devices and hearing aids. Persons who are hard of hearing or deaf, or even persons who have no hearing loss, can benefit. There are also alerting devices that signal you when sounds such as the following occur:

- Doorbell or knock at the door
- Telephone
- Fire alarm or smoke alarm
- Baby crying
- Alarm clock

Many of these solutions use strobe light or conventional light to alert you. Others use vibrating systems to alert you. Examples of visual systems include the following:

- Text telephones, which allow phone conversations to be typed and read rather than spoken and heard
- Computerized speech recognition, which allows a computer to change a spoken message into a readable text document
- Closed-captioned TV, which allows text display of spoken dialogue and sounds. All TVs now sold with screens of at least 13 inches must have built-in captioning.
- Note taking, which allows a hard of hearing person to concentrate on listening and watching a speaker while a trained person takes notes. This has been used in schools not only for students who are deaf or hard of hearing but also for students who are unable to write.

Health Reference Series Medical Advisor's Notes and Updates

Closed-caption projection systems (Rear Window Captioning) are a form of closed captioning for movies that are becoming increasingly common at theaters. A hearing-impaired patron requests a viewing device from the service desk at the theater. The device is a piece of dark Plexiglas on a flexible arm, which clamps onto the theater chair. The Plexiglas reflects an LED (light-emitting diode) sign displaying the dialogue on the rear wall of the theater. This allows the user to see the captioning while looking forward at the movie screen. The United States government is considering a rule that would require all movie theaters to be equipped with these systems.

Section 28.5

Profoundly Paralyzed Communicate with Brain-Computer Interface

From "Connections That Count: Brain-Computer Interface Enables the Profoundly Paralyzed to Communicate," by Christopher Klose, *Medline-Plus Magazine,* National Institutes of Health, June 2007.

Most of us take the ability to communicate for granted. We talk and write. But what if you're paralyzed and can't speak? Each year, stroke silences tens of thousands of Americans. One of the most devastating consequences is "locked in" syndrome—a situation in which people are unable to move a muscle or utter a sound. Severe head injuries, spinal injuries, and amyotrophic lateral sclerosis (ALS, or Lou Gehrig disease) are also responsible for this bleak condition.

"It is hard to overestimate how much of human life is communication—being able to listen and then respond," points out William J. Heetderks, MD, director of extramural science programs at the National Institute of Biomedical Imaging and Bioengineering (NIBIB).

Since the early 1990s, Jonathan R. Wolpaw, MD, a neurologist and chief of the Wadsworth Center Laboratory of Nervous System Disorders, New York State Department of Health, Albany, has led a team of researchers in developing a brain-computer interface (BCI) system to help the profoundly paralyzed communicate. Dr. Wolpaw has received support from two NIH Institutes—NIBIB and the National Institute of Child Health and Human Development—and the James S. McDonnell Foundation.

"For the locked-in, the BCI is like being let out of jail—only better," Dr. Heetderks emphasizes.

Thought into Action

The Wadsworth BCI system works on brain power, not muscle control. It uses the team's specially developed software platform (called BCI2000) and consists of a laptop computer, portable amplifier, and a skullcap containing eight electrodes hitched to the computer. The electrodes record the user's electrical brain waves, which the computer analyzes and translates into specific commands, such as writing e-mails, selecting computer icons, or moving robotic devices. No surgery is required and users typically master the system within an hour or two.

"We are trying to use the scientific research for practical results," Dr. Wolpaw explains. "Life can be reasonable for the locked-in with the right support. That's our goal."

Currently, the Wadsworth team supports seven patients, five in the United States and two in Germany. Much time is required for system maintenance and technical support. "Our major challenge is to produce a trouble-free, reliable, affordable system that can be used at home by patients and their caregivers," Dr. Wolpaw says.

Although BCI research has been under way since the 1970s, NIBIB's Dr. Heetderks says it has taken off only in the last five years or so, thanks to substantial improvements in signal processing. In particular, he attributes such progress to "clever people like Dr. Wolpaw for making sense out of how to find and process information (the brain's electrical signals)."

The Wadsworth BCI2000 software accepts and analyzes any brain signal and can be used with a wide range of output devices—from computer icons to wheelchairs. It is now in use by more than 140 research laboratories worldwide.

"There is increased appreciation of the severely disabled and their capabilities," says Dr. Wolpaw. He predicts that "in 5 or 10 years, everything will be much clearer. We know—and are learning—much more about the brain, and the revolution in computers and electronics gives us the technology to operate BCIs in real time."

Like many physician researchers, Dr. Wolpaw combines a passion for science with the practical urges of the clinician. Of his BCI system he says, simply, "I wanted to help severely disabled people."

His greatest satisfaction? "When we got those first e-mails from the locked-in, that was great!"

Chapter 29

Therapy to Aid Communication

Chapter Contents

Section 29.1—Speech-Language Therapy.................................. 256

Section 29.2—Augmentative and Alternative
        Communication 260

Section 29.1

Speech-Language Therapy

In a recent parent-teacher conference, the teacher expressed concern that your child may have a problem with certain speech or language skills. Or perhaps while talking to your child, you noticed an occasional stutter. Could your child have a problem? And if so, what should you do?

It's wise to intervene quickly. An evaluation by a certified speech-language pathologist can help determine if your child is having difficulties.

What Is Speech-Language Therapy?

Speech-language therapy is the treatment for most kids with speech and/or language disorders. A speech disorder refers to a problem with the actual production of sounds, whereas a language disorder refers to a difficulty understanding or putting words together to communicate ideas.

Speech Disorders and Language Disorders

Speech disorders include the following problems, according to the American Speech-Language-Hearing Association (ASHA):

- Articulation disorders include difficulties producing sounds in syllables or saying words incorrectly to the point that other people can't understand what's being said.

- Fluency disorders include problems such as stuttering, the condition in which the flow of speech is interrupted by abnormal stoppages, repetitions (st-st-stuttering), or prolonging sounds and syllables (sssstuttering).

- Resonance or voice disorders include problems with the pitch, volume, or quality of the voice that distract listeners from what's being said. These types of disorders may also cause pain or discomfort for the child when speaking.

- Dysphagia/oral feeding disorders, including difficulties with eating and swallowing.

Language disorders can be either receptive or expressive:

- Receptive disorders refer to difficulties understanding or processing language.

- Expressive disorders include difficulty putting words together, limited vocabulary, or inability to use language in a socially appropriate way.

Specialists in Speech-Language Therapy

Speech-language pathologists (SLPs), often informally known as speech therapists, are professionals educated in the study of human communication, its development, and its disorders. They hold at least a master's degree and state certification/licensure in the field, as well as a certificate of clinical competency from ASHA.

By assessing the speech, language, cognitive-communication, and swallowing skills of children and adults, speech-language pathologists can identify types of communication problems and the best way to treat them.

SLPs treat problems in the areas of articulation; dysfluency; oral-motor, speech, and voice; and receptive and expressive language disorders.

Remediation

In speech-language therapy, an SLP will work with a child one-to-one, in a small group, or directly in a classroom to overcome difficulties involved with a specific disorder.

Therapists use a variety of strategies, including:

- **Language intervention activities:** In these exercises an SLP will interact with a child by playing and talking. The therapist may use pictures, books, objects, or ongoing events to stimulate language development. The therapist may also model correct pronunciation and use repetition exercises to build speech and language skills.

- **Articulation therapy:** Articulation, or sound production, exercises involve having the therapist model correct sounds and syllables for a child, often during play activities. The level of play is age-appropriate and related to the child's specific needs. The SLP will physically show the child how to make certain sounds, such as the "r" sound, and may demonstrate how to move the tongue to produce specific sounds.

- **Oral motor/feeding therapy:** The SLP will use a variety of oral exercises, including facial massage and various tongue, lip, and jaw exercises, to strengthen the muscles of the mouth. The SLP may also work with different food textures and temperatures to increase a child's oral awareness during eating and swallowing.

When Is Therapy Needed?

Kids might need speech-language therapy for a variety of reasons, including:

- hearing impairments;
- cognitive (intellectual; thinking) or other developmental delays;
- weak oral muscles;
- birth defects such as cleft lip or cleft palate;
- autism;
- motor planning problems;
- respiratory problems (breathing disorders);
- swallowing disorders;
- traumatic brain injury.

Therapy should begin as soon as possible. Children enrolled in therapy early in their development (younger than 3 years) tend to have better outcomes than those who begin therapy later.

This does not mean that older kids can't make progress in therapy; they may progress at a slower rate because they often have learned patterns that need to be changed.

Finding a Therapist

It's important to make sure that the speech-language therapist is certified by ASHA. That certification means the SLP has at least a master's degree in the field, and has passed a national examination and successfully completed a supervised clinical fellowship.

Sometimes speech assistants (who have typically earned a 2-year associate's or 4-year bachelor's degree) may assist with speech-language services under the supervision of ASHA-certified SLPs. Your child's SLP should be licensed in your state, and have experience working with kids and your child's specific disorder.

You might find a specialist by asking your child's doctor or teacher for a referral or by checking your local telephone directory. The state associations for speech-language pathology and audiology also maintain listings of licensed and certified therapists.

Helping Your Child

Speech-language experts agree that parental involvement is crucial to the success of a child's progress in speech or language therapy.

Parents are an extremely important part of their child's therapy program, and help determine whether it is a success. Kids who complete the program quickest and with the most lasting results are those whose parents have been involved.

Ask the therapist for suggestions on how you can help your child. For instance, it's important to help your child do the at-home stimulation activities that the SLP suggests to ensure continued progress and carry-over of newly learned skills.

The process of overcoming a speech or language disorder may take some time and effort, so it's important that all family members be patient and understanding with the child.

Section 29.2

Augmentative and Alternative Communication

This section contains text reprinted with permission from "Augmentative and Alternative Communication (AAC)," available on the website of the American Speech-Language-Hearing Association at www.asha.org/public/speech/disorders/AAC.htm, and "Information for AAC Users," available on the website of the American Speech-Language-Hearing Association at www.asha.org/public/speech/disorders/InfoAACUsers.htm. © American Speech-Language-Hearing Association. All rights reserved. These documents are undated. Reviewed by David A. Cooke, MD, FACP, July 14, 2011.

Augmentative and Alternative Communication (AAC)

What is AAC?

Augmentative and alternative communication (AAC) includes all forms of communication (other than oral speech) that are used to express thoughts, needs, wants, and ideas. We all use AAC when we make facial expressions or gestures, use symbols or pictures, or write.

People with severe speech or language problems rely on AAC to supplement existing speech or replace speech that is not functional. Special augmentative aids, such as picture and symbol communication boards and electronic devices, are available to help people express themselves. This may increase social interaction, school performance, and feelings of self-worth.

AAC users should not stop using speech if they are able to do so. The AAC aids and devices are used to enhance their communication.

What are the types of AAC systems?

When children or adults cannot use speech to communicate effectively in all situations, there are options.

Unaided communication systems rely on the user's body to convey messages. Examples include gestures, body language, and/or sign language.

Aided communication systems require the use of tools or equipment in addition to the user's body. Aided communication methods can range from paper and pencil to communication books or boards to devices that produce voice output (speech generating devices or SGDs) and/or written output. Electronic communication aids allow the user to use picture symbols, letters, and/or words and phrases to create messages. Some devices can be programmed to produce different spoken languages.

To contact a speech-language pathologist, visit ASHA's Find a Professional [http://www.asha.org/findpro].

What other organizations have information on AAC?

This list is not exhaustive and inclusion does not imply endorsement of the organization or the context of the website by ASHA.

- AAC Institute [www.aacinstitute.org]

- International Society for Augmentative and Alternative Communication [www.isaac-online.org]

- Rehabilitation Engineering and Assistive Technology Society of North America [www.resna.org]

- Rehabilitation Engineering Research Center on Communication Enhancement [aac-rerc.psu.edu]

Information for AAC Users

Who uses augmentative and alternative communication (AAC)?

More than 2 million people in the United States have a severe communication disorder that impairs their ability to talk.

This problem may be short or long and may be congenital (present at birth), acquired (occurring later in late), or degenerative (worsening throughout life).

Common causes of severe expressive communication disorders that may require the use of AAC are shown in the following text.

Congenital causes:

- Cerebral palsy

- Autism

- Mental retardation

- Physical disabilities

Acquired causes:

- Stroke

- Head injury

- Spinal cord injury

- Cancer

Degenerative causes:

- ALS [amyotrophic lateral sclerosis]

- Muscular dystrophy

- AIDS [acquired immunodeficiency syndrome]

- Huntington's disease

For more information about individuals who use AAC systems, see ASHA's report " Communication Facts: Special Populations: Augmentative and Alternative Communication" [http://www.asha.org/research/reports/aac.htm].

How do I know if AAC is for me or a loved one?

Selecting the best way to communicate is not as simple as getting a prescription for eyeglasses. It is important to obtain an evaluation by a group of professionals to develop the best communication system to meet your needs.

You can have an evaluation at a:

- medical facility;

- private practice;

- school district;

- center-based program.

An evaluation should involve a team of professionals working together. In addition to the AAC user and his or her family and caregivers, this team often includes the following:

- Speech-language pathologist

- Physician

- Occupational therapist

- Physical therapist

- Social worker

- Learning specialist

- Rehabilitation engineer

- Psychologist

- Vision specialist

- Vocational counselor

- AAC user and family/caregivers

Team members evaluate the person's needs, current means of communication, and potential for using different kinds of AAC. Over time, team members may change as the person's needs change.

After a decision has been made to select an AAC system, it is important to have professional follow-up. This may simply be a one-time training or may require speech-language services that focus on the development of communication using the system over a period of time.

Professionals need to help the individual and communication partners learn a variety of skills and strategies (e.g., meaning of hand signs and operating a piece of electronic equipment).

How do people use AAC systems?

There are two primary ways that people access AAC. Access is the way an individual makes selections on a communication board or speech generating device. Direct selection and scanning are two forms of access.

- Direct selection includes pointing with a body part such as a finger, hand, or toe, or through the use of a pointing device such as a beam of light, headstick, or mouthstick. Those with severe physical impairments may need to access systems by using a switch. The switches can be turned on with a body part, puff of air, or wrinkle of an eyebrow.

- Scanning one type involves the use of lights on a system that pass over each choice and the user activates a switch to stop the light and pick a choice; other types are auditory scanning and scan patterns (such as row/column, quadrant, step, and linear). Scanning requires less motor control but possibly more cognitive skill than direct selection access.

How is language represented in AAC systems?

There are three basic ways to represent language in an AAC system: Single-meaning pictures, alphabet-based systems, and semantic compaction.

- Single-meaning pictures do not require reading; the symbols are only one picture, but the group or symbol set is huge for a significant vocabulary (e.g., a 3-year-old would need a set of 1,100 pictures to represent his known vocabulary); some meaning to pictures must be taught since it is difficult to represent some words with pictures. This system is used the least compared with the others.

- Alphabet-based systems do require reading; symbol sequences are long (systems that can predict words after the first several letters can reduce the number of letter selections).

- Semantic compaction does not require reading; symbol sequences are short, typically between one and two symbols per word; symbol set is small (fitting on a single overlay to the AAC device). This system is used the most often.

Most people who rely on AAC may use more than one of these methods to communicate.

To contact a speech-language pathologist, visit ASHA's Find a Professional [http://www.asha.org/findpro].

What questions should I ask my speech-language pathologist?

The following are questions to ask a speech-language pathologist (SLP) before an AAC evaluation:

- Do you typically provide services in the area of AAC?

- How long have you worked in the area of AAC? Have you worked with anybody who has a similar problem?

- Do you work as part of a team? What members are on the team?

- After evaluation, what will you do to make the communication plan work? Will you do the follow-up treatment?

- What specific kinds of communication options (e.g., additional treatment, gesture, sign language) do you recommend?

- Where can I go to see and talk with people using AAC?

- How soon can you schedule an evaluation? What will it cost? What kinds of payment do you accept?

- If you recommend a particular device, will you help me find funding for its purchase?

- Will I be able to see actual equipment that might be recommended? If not, where else could I go to see it?

The following are questions you should be able to answer after an AAC evaluation:

- What communication approaches have been recommended?

- Which approaches will be used for various modes of communication? Quick phrases? Expressing feelings? Giving and getting information? Conversation with family and friends? Written communication?

- What symbols (e.g., letters, pictures, graphics, words, or phrases) will be used on boards or devices?

- Is there enough flexibility in the recommended communication system so that communication is possible in a variety of settings?

- Will special equipment or switches need to be bought or made?

- What body positions can be used to increase communication and function?

- Can the recommended system be modified as capabilities and needs change?

- Why were the recommended techniques chosen?

- Which professionals will be carrying out the recommended communication plan and how often must they be seen?

- Can I talk with current users of the system I am thinking about?

Chapter 30

Low Vision Devices and Services

Chapter Contents

Section 30.1—Living with Low Vision 268

Section 30.2—Reading and Vision Loss 270

Section 30.3—What Is Braille? 277

Section 30.4—Web-Braille 280

Section 30.5—Low Vision Aids for Computer Users 282

Section 30.1

Living with Low Vision

Living with low vision can be challenging, although many devices are available to help people with this condition use their remaining vision to greatest advantage.

Eye care professionals use the term "low vision" to describe significant visual impairment that cannot be corrected with standard glasses, contact lenses, medicine, or eye surgery.

Low vision includes loss of best-corrected visual acuity—to a level worse than 20/60 in the better eye, measured with a standard eye chart—or visual field loss such as tunnel vision or blind spots. It also describes legal blindness and almost total blindness.

Low vision has a variety of causes, including eye injury, diseases, and heredity. Sometimes low vision involves a lack of acuity, meaning that objects appear blurred. Other times, it involves a significant loss of peripheral vision and visual field. Other symptoms of low vision include light sensitivity, distorted vision, or loss of contrast.

The eyesight of a person with low vision may be hazy from cataracts, blurred or partially obscured in the central visual zone because of macular degeneration, or distorted and/or blurred from diabetic retinopathy. Also, people with glaucoma or retinitis pigmentosa can lose their peripheral vision and have difficulty seeing at night.

Children as well as adults can be visually impaired, sometimes as a result of a birth defect or an injury. But low vision more commonly afflicts adults and seniors. Vision loss can be very traumatic, leading to frustration and depression.

Many people who develop eye problems that cause low vision lose their jobs. According to Lighthouse International, among visually impaired Americans ages 21 to 64, only 43.7 percent are employed. Among normally sighted people in this age group, 80 percent are employed.

Not being able to drive safely, read quickly, or easily see images on a television or computer screen can cause people with low vision to feel shut off from the world. They may be unable to get around town independently, earn a living, or even shop for food and other necessities.

Some visually impaired people become completely dependent on friends and relatives, while others suffer alone.

That's a shame, because many ingenious low vision devices and strategies exist to help people overcome vision impairment and live independently.

If you have a vision impairment that interferes with your ability to perform everyday activities and enjoy life, your first step is to see an eye care professional for a complete eye exam.

Poor vision that cannot be corrected with eyeglasses or contact lenses could be the first sign of a serious eye disease such as age-related macular degeneration, glaucoma, or retinitis pigmentosa. Or it could mean you are developing a cataract that needs removal. Whatever the case, it's wise to take action before further vision loss occurs.

If your eye doctor finds that you have a vision loss that cannot be corrected with eyewear, medical treatment, or surgery, he or she can refer you to a low vision specialist.

Usually an optometrist, a low vision specialist, can evaluate the degree and type of vision loss you have, prescribe appropriate low vision aids such as magnifiers, telescopes, and video magnifiers, and help you learn how to use low vision aids.

The low vision specialist also can recommend non-optical adaptive devices, such as large-face printed material, audio tapes, special light fixtures, and signature guides for signing checks and documents.

If necessary, your specialist or eye doctor also can refer you to a counselor or mental health professional to help you cope with your vision loss.

Section 30.2

Reading and Vision Loss

If you're losing your vision, your greatest heartbreak may be the possibility of no longer being able to read. After all, literacy is a key to personal independence and self-confidence. With today's technology, however, there is a lot less to fear. Large print books, magnification tools, braille, audio texts, and a constantly growing number of products will allow you to read everything from the morning paper to the latest bestseller to your monthly phone bill.

But while there are many reading tools available to you, it's important to remember that any solution means that you will have to do things in a different way. Audio books, magnification, and other options can be very effective, but take time and patience to learn to manage effectively.

In the end, the best approach to keeping up with your reading is the hodgepodge method—that is, to try out, and mix and match, different techniques based on your own comfort level and reading habits. Not every solution is right for everyone, so do what's best for you. The URLs in the following text will give you an idea of some of the variety of available reading formats.

Bigger and Better: Large Print

The most comfortable transition to reading with vision loss, at least in the beginning, is also the simplest: Bigger print. Most major publishing houses today produce bestsellers and other materials in large print formats. Large print collections are available at most public libraries. Also, some popular periodicals such as *Reader's Digest* [https://legacy.rd.com/offer/rdlp/giftown03/index.jsp?trkid=search_ large_print&lid=20041] and a special weekly edition of *The New York Times* [http://www.thenewmagazinecity.com] are available in large, easy-to-read formats.

For more information:

- Doubleday Large Print Book Club [http://www.doubledaylarge-print.com]: A membership service that gives you access to Doubleday publications in large print.

- Random House Large Print [http://www.randomhouse.com/large print]: Your source for books published by Random House in large print.

Lend Us Your Ears: Reading by Listening

Not many people realize that the earliest phonograph records were created specifically to provide spoken recordings for people who are blind. Recorded music came later, but recording text for use by people with vision loss continues today.

Audio books and a new generation of listening devices have been a bonanza for readers with limited vision and an increasingly popular reading option for sighted audiences, as well. Think of those people you've noticed jogging or sitting next to you on the bus happily plugged into portable cassette or CD players, iPods, or even cell phones. Any one of them might just as well be listening to Stephen King as Stevie Wonder. Indeed, almost any popular novel or nonfiction book, not to mention most general interest and trade magazines and newspapers, can be experienced in a variety of accessible, inexpensive audio formats.

Even if you've always been uncomfortable with audio technology and electronics, you're almost certain to find an option you feel comfortable with.

Talking Books

Talking Books is a service provided by the National Library Service for the Blind and Physically Handicapped (NLS) [http://www.loc.gov/nls]. Launched in 1933 and sponsored by the Library of Congress, NLS is a national network of cooperating libraries that distributes books on cassettes to people with vision loss. These books are loaned and mailed free of charge, and are played on machines provided by the NLS program. The books come in special containers that can easily be mailed back with a free-of-charge postage card provided. To apply for this service, call 800-424-8567, go to the NLS website [http://www.loc.gov/nls], or visit your local library.

Commercial Audio Books

Available at all major booksellers, these are cassette and CD editions of commercial bestsellers read by their authors or by noted actors.

Completely embraced by mainstream audiences, audio books are now so popular that many publishers release the audio version of a new title simultaneously with its print counterpart. Your local library may even have an audio book section.

Digital Audio Books

Not a physical piece of hardware at all, these are digital (electronic) files that contain the same content as conventional audio books but can be downloaded onto a personal computer. Once downloaded, these files can be listened to on the computer or transferred to a portable listening device, such as an iPod or other MP3 player.

If you're not technically oriented, the digital option may sound forbidding, but it does have advantages that make it worth exploring. The main advantage is navigation. Cassettes and CDs offer no simple way to move backward or forward in the text as you would with a hard-copy print book. Digital playback is infinitely more flexible, allowing the user to jump back or forward by chapter or page. You can even set digital bookmarks that let you find a particular passage instantly.

Looking for digital books? Here's where to find them:

- Audible is the first and most widely successful source of digital books online. Here you'll find the same popular audio books that are available on cassette and CD from various publishers, usually priced at 30 percent below retail. You have the choice of simply listening to the books on your computer (this is called streaming) or you can download books in their entirety and listen to them whenever you want or transfer them to a portable MP3 player. To listen to samples of Audible books, visit www.audible.com. Remember: Not all portable devices will play Audible files or are accessible to people with vision loss. Two popular models that meet both criteria are Creative Labs' MuVo and the iPod Shuffle.

- PlayAway Books are ideal starters for older readers who have never used a digital audio book. Packaged to resemble print books—with artwork and jacket information reproduced on the front and back covers—PlayAway books are self-contained listening devices. (You don't need a separate device to play them.) Each PlayAway is about the size of a credit card and contains one featured selection. A set of earplugs, a spare battery, and operating instructions are included. While the list of available PlayAway titles isn't as extensive as other audio book formats, they earn points for their simplicity, ease of use, and affordability (most titles are priced about the same as the hardcover versions). To listen to audio samples, visit the PlayAway Books site [http://www.playaway.com].

- Public libraries in a growing number of U.S. cities are now offering audio books as digital downloads online. These books are played in Windows Media Player with the assistance of a special program called OverDrive, which you can download for free. Books are generally available on loan for a 2- or 3-week period, just like hardcopy books, except instead of having to return the title to the library it will simply vanish from your computer's hard drive when the loan period ends. The Overdrive program lets you go forward or back just a few sentences, or you can skip entire chapters. It also allows you to speed up or slow down the narrator's pace, and will keep your place even if your computer is turned off. To find out if this service is available in your area, visit OverDrive's Digital Library Reserve [http://www.overdrive .com]. You'll also need a library card from your local library.

For more information:

- AccessWorld. American Foundation for the Blind. "Product Evaluation: Kindle for PC with Accessibility Plugin." [http://www.afb .org/afbpress/pub.asp?DocID=aw120506]

- AccessWorld. American Foundation for the Blind. "An Evaluation of the Milestone 312 Digital Book Player from Bones." [http:// www.afb.org/afbpress/pub.asp?DocID=aw120507]

- AccessWorld. American Foundation for the Blind. "Product Evaluation: On the Move with MuVo." [http://www.afb.org/afbpress/ pub.asp?DocID=aw060108&select=1#1]

- AccessWorld. American Foundation for the Blind. "Product Evaluation: Read All Day with PlayAway." [http://www.afb.org/ afbpress/pub.asp?DocID=aw070409&select=1#1]

Beyond Your Local Retailer: "Specialty" Digital Players and Services

Your electronics store isn't your only choice when shopping for digital hardware for reading and listening. There are a number of specialty products—not available to the general public—exclusively designed for people with vision loss. These are in many ways superior to off-the-shelf alternatives. Here are some of the more popular ones.

Bookshare.org is a subscription service available exclusively to individuals with vision loss or who have a learning disability (you must provide proof of one or the other to join). For an annual fee of $50 (plus a $25 sign-up fee), members can download to their computers their choice of thousands of copyrighted bestsellers and periodicals. (Nonmembers can download non-copyrighted material—classics by Dickens and Jane Austen, for example—free of charge.) Unlike other talking books, Bookshare titles are not read by human narrators. Rather, they produce synthetic speech based on the written text. Most new computers come equipped with speech synthesizer software that can perform this function. As an alternative, Bookshare.org allows you to read the text onscreen with the use of a braille display or magnifier.

Material at Bookshare.org is uploaded by volunteers—most of them blind or visually impaired themselves—and sometimes contains scanning errors. These, however, are usually minor; more importantly, Bookshare.org contains a wealth of material that is easy to access. To learn more, listen to an audio sample, or become a Bookshare member, go to the Bookshare site [http://www.bookshare.org].

NFB-Newsline® is the equivalent of one of those vast, old-style newsstands, only this one is completely at your disposal . . . over your telephone. Created by the National Federation of the Blind, NFB-Newsline makes it possible for people with vision loss to read 200 different newspapers and a half-dozen magazines from any telephone. It works like this: After dialing a toll-free number and logging in with your pass code, you are welcomed by a very clear voice. From there you can use the phone's keypad to access any newspaper of your choice. With a set of easy-to-learn commands, the listening experience simulates the way most people read traditional newspapers. You can skip forward or back by section, article, or sentence. You can have unfamiliar words spelled out to you. You can speed up or slow down the reading pace. You can even skim just the headlines by phone in the same time it once took to give them the once over with your eyes. To listen to an audio sample, find out if you're eligible, and to sign up, visit the NFB-Newsline [http://www.nfb.org/nfb/Newspapers_by_Phone.asp].

Radio reading services are available in many parts of the country. Simply, these services employ volunteer readers to provide—on radio—immediate, verbatim audio access to newspapers, magazines, consumer information, and other materials that may not be readily available in braille or on tape. Listeners can tune in for the day's news, features, sports, business, opinions, advertisements, and other material from newspapers and magazines. Public affairs programs are also available on many services, as are some books or story-based shows.

Radio reading services are typically broadcast on a sub-carrier channel of an FM radio station. Listeners must have a special, pre-tuned radio receiver to pick up the closed circuit broadcast. Receivers are frequently loaned to listeners by the reading service at no cost. Some services disseminate reading services programming on television over a SAP (second audio program) channel, community cable system, or FM cable service. Many services also offer live audio streaming of their programming over the internet while others offer access to archived readings through the internet or telephone dial-in system. One popular internet radio service is ACB Radio [http://www.acbradio .org/pweb], from the American Council of the Blind; visit the site to listen to broadcasts. For more options, go to the official website of the International Association of Audio Information Services [http://www .iaais.org] to find a program near you.

Designed with You in Mind: Proprietary Players

While there are commercial audio players that work reasonably well for people with limited vision, at least three players have been designed specifically with the vision loss community in mind. There are no visual screens or prompts to deal with. All three are operated entirely by listening to audio cues and pressing easy-to-use keys. Check them out.

Victor Reader Stream

The Victor Reader Stream (VR Stream) is sold by HumanWare [http://www.humanware.com/en-usa/home]. About the size of a deck of cards, it features both text-to-speech capabilities and digital audio support. This means you can read electronic files (with synthetic speech) or digital recorded books (with human speech). This versatile device plays books in a variety of digital formats from Recording for the Blind & Dyslexic (RFB&D) [http://www.learningally.org], and digital Talking Books from NLS [http://www.loc.gov/nls] and Bookshare.org [http:// www.bookshare.org]. It can also play text files that have been loaded into it, as well as your favorite music. Simple to use, the VR Stream lets you place electronic bookmarks in any file and locate specific information or favorite passages quickly. It has variable speed playback, a time Jump feature, auto Sleep shutoff with multiple time settings, and a key lock feature. It uses a removable SD card for storage and allows file transfers from your PC to the VR Stream without file filtering software. A digital recorder accessed with one button allows you to record a note and play it back later. The VR Stream comes with a built-in rechargeable battery providing up to 15 hours of uninterrupted listening time.

It has small built-in stereo speakers, or you can use headphones or small portable speakers that plug into the headphone jack.

Book Courier

The Book Courier [http://bookcourier.com] is similar in many ways to the Book Port. Equipped with an 18-key keypad, the device is operated completely by touch and listening. The Courier can play MP3 files of audio books or music, and can "read" aloud other computer files such as web pages or Microsoft Word documents with its own built-in synthesizer that you can speed up or slow down. It can also handle files from Audible.com [http://www.audible.com] and you can set bookmarks in any file. Like the Book Port, it does not have a built-in speaker, so speakers or headphones are needed. Also, it has nearly all the same capabilities as the Book Port except the ability to act as a braille keyboard for typing in simple text notes. To listen to an audio sample, visit the Book Courier site [http://bookcourier.com].

Milestone 311

The Milestone 311 [http://www.afb.org/prodProfile.asp?ProdID=981&SourceID=69] is another handheld player designed specifically for people who are blind or visually impaired. Developed in Switzerland, it is sold in the United States by Independent Living Aids [http://www.independentliving.com/prodinfo.asp?number=757828]. About the size of a credit card, this portable player can be used for MP3 files of music or audio books. It can play books which have been recorded in an accessible format called DAISY (Digital Accessible Information System), which allows for easy skipping around within a book by chapter and heading. It has a built-in speaker so you don't need to buy headphones. It also has a recording device, and a removable secure digital card for storage of books and music. However, you cannot use it to listen to documents or web pages.

For more information:

- AccessWorld. American Foundation for the Blind. "Product Evaluation: Marking the Road to MP3 Player Accessibility: A Review of the Milestone 311" [http://www.afb.org/afbpress/pub.asp?DocID=aw070505&select=1#1]

- DAISY Consortium. Playback Tools. Includes descriptions of various players, including where to buy them. [http://www.daisy.org/tools?Cat=playback]

Section 30.3

What Is Braille?

Braille is a series of raised dots that can be read with the fingers by people who are blind or whose eyesight is not sufficient for reading printed material. Teachers, parents, and others who are not visually impaired ordinarily read braille with their eyes. Braille is not a language. Rather, it is a code by which languages such as English or Spanish may be written and read.

What does braille look like?

Braille symbols are formed within units of space known as braille cells. A full braille cell consists of six raised dots arranged in two parallel rows each having three dots. The dot positions are identified by numbers from one through six. Sixty-four combinations are possible using one or more of these six dots. A single cell can be used to represent an alphabet letter, number, punctuation mark, or even a whole word. A braille alphabet and numbers card illustrates what a cell looks like and how each dot is numbered.

How was braille invented?

Louis Braille was born in Coupvray, France, on January 4, 1809. He attended the National Institute for Blind Youth in Paris, France, as a student. While attending the Institute, Braille yearned for more books to read. He experimented with ways to make an alphabet that was easy to read with the fingertips. The writing system he invented, at age 15, evolved from the tactile "Ecriture Nocturne" (night writing) code invented by Charles Barbier for sending military messages that could be read on the battlefield at night, without light.

How is braille written?

When every letter of every word is expressed in braille, it is referred to as Grade 1 braille. Very few books or other reading material are transcribed in Grade 1 braille. However, many newly blinded adults find this useful for labeling personal or kitchen items.

The system used for reproducing most textbooks and publications is known as Grade 2 braille. In this system cells are used individually or in combination with others to form a variety of contractions or whole words. For example, in Grade 1 braille the phrase "you like him" requires 12 cell spaces. It would look like Figure 30.1.

If written in Grade 2 braille, this same phrase would take only six cell spaces. This is because the letters y and l are also used for the whole words you and like respectively. Likewise, the word him is formed by combining the letters h and m. It would look like Figure 30.2.

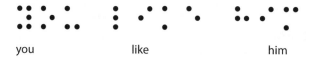

Figure 30.1. The phrase "you like him" in Grade 1 braille.

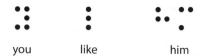

Figure 30.2. The phrase "you like him" in Grade 2 braille.

There are 189 different letter contractions and 76 short-form words used in Grade 2 braille. These "short cuts" are used to reduce the volume of paper needed for reproducing books in braille and to make the reading process easier.

Grade 1 (or uncontracted) braille has nothing to do with first grade. Most children learn grade 2 (contracted) braille from kindergarten on. In recent years, some teachers have chosen to begin teaching grade 1 braille first, transitioning to grade 2 braille by the mid-elementary years. There is currently no research that supports the superiority of one approach over the other.

Just as printed matter can be produced with a paper and pencil, typewriter, or printer, braille can also be written in several ways. The braille equivalent of paper and pencil is the slate and stylus. This consists of a slate or template with evenly spaced depressions for the dots of braille cells, and a stylus for creating the individual braille dots. With paper placed in the slate, tactile dots are made by pushing the pointed end of the stylus into the paper over the depressions. The paper bulges on its reverse side forming "dots." Because of their portability, the slate and stylus are especially helpful for taking notes during lectures and for labeling such things as file folders.

Braille is also produced by a machine known as a braillewriter. Unlike a typewriter which has more than fifty keys, the braillewriter has only six keys and a space bar. These keys are numbered to correspond with the six dots of a braille cell. In that most braille symbols contain more than a single dot, all or any of the braillewriter keys can be pushed at the same time.

Technological developments in the computer industry have provided and continue to expand additional avenues of literacy for braille users. Software programs and portable electronic braille notetakers allow users to save and edit their writing, have it displayed back to them either verbally or tactually, and produce a hard copy via a desktop computer-driven braille embosser.

Since its development in France by Louis Braille in the latter part of the nineteenth century, braille has become not only an effective means of communication, but also a proven avenue for achieving and enhancing literacy for people who are blind or have significant vision loss.

Section 30.4

Web-Braille

Excerpted from "Web-Braille," by the Library of
Congress (LOC, www.loc.gov), May 2010.

What is Web-Braille?

Web-Braille is a web-based service that provides access to thousands of braille books, magazines, and music scores produced by the National Library Service for the Blind and Physically Handicapped (NLS), Library of Congress. The service also includes a growing collection of titles transcribed locally for cooperating network libraries. The Web-Braille site is password-protected, and all files are in an electronic form of contracted braille that requires the use of special equipment for access.

Books: Nearly 10,000 press-braille books produced by NLS since 1992 are downloadable from Web-Braille or may be read online. More than 1,000 older titles are also available. Uncontracted braille, foreign-language, and print/braille books are not included. NLS adds new titles to Web-Braille upon shipment of the press-braille books to libraries serving blind and physically handicapped readers.

Magazines: NLS-produced braille magazines are available on Web-Braille. Magazine files are normally available on the download site within 1 working day after the hard-copy braille magazine is shipped to readers. A few magazine issues are available from as far back as early 2000, and every issue of the music publication *Popular Music Lead Sheets* since 1978 can be accessed.

Music Scores: Several thousand braille music scores are available on Web-Braille, and NLS adds more every month. The scores are for a range of instruments, from voice to violin, with levels of difficulty from beginning methods to advanced works, especially for the piano. The styles of music range from popular songs to standard repertoires for each instrument, with particular strength in the eighteenth-, nineteenth-, and early-twentieth-century masters.

Who is eligible to use Web-Braille?

Copyright laws require that access to Web-Braille be limited to NLS patrons and eligible institutions. Access outside the United States, except to eligible American citizens, is not permitted.

Eligible institutions include schools for the blind; public or private schools providing braille to blind children; and nonprofit organizations whose primary purpose is to produce braille books for the use of eligible readers in the United States, such as instructional materials resource centers and nonprofit transcribing agencies.

Agencies may use Web-Braille files only to produce braille copies. Under current copyright law, agencies may not make large-print or unencrypted e-text versions of books without the permission of the copyright holder.

How do eligible individuals or institutions sign up for Web-Braille service?

To register for Web-Braille, eligible program users must contact their cooperating network library and provide the library with an e-mail address and a six- to eight-character password. When the subscription is activated, the user will receive access instructions by e-mail.

How can a specific Web-Braille book be located?

Web-Braille books may be located in two ways:

- **Online catalog:** Links to Web-Braille books are included in the NLS International Union Catalog at www.loc.gov/nls. To retrieve Web-Braille titles using the quick search page, type the words "web braille" (as two words with no hyphen) in the keyword field. The results list will contain a link to each volume of a Web-Braille title. When a Web-Braille volume is selected, the user will be prompted for a Web-Braille user ID and password.

- **Online *Braille Book Review*:** The web version of each bimonthly issue of *Braille Book Review* since July–August 1999 contains links to braille books recently added to the book collection and available on Web-Braille. The online version of *Braille Book Review* may be accessed from the main Web-Braille page or from www.loc.gov/nls/bbr.

In what format are the Web-Braille files?

Web-Braille files are in contracted braille ASCII format. Each file represents one volume of a braille book or magazine. Each volume of an NLS-produced book is named with the book's BR and volume numbers and has a ".brf" file extension. For example, volume 2 of BR 12345 will have the file name "12345v02.brf." Magazine files have a two-letter magazine code, followed by the month, day (if applicable), year, and letter indicating part of the magazine. Items from the NLS Music Section are named with a BRM number but have the letter "m" preceding their volume number to distinguish them from national collection braille titles.

Items produced by cooperating network libraries have a two-letter state abbreviation followed by a three-digit book number.

What equipment is needed to access Web-Braille?

Web-Braille files may be read online or downloaded for viewing off-line or for embossing. Reading Web-Braille files requires a braille display, braille-aware notetaker, or braille embosser.

Section 30.5

Low Vision Aids for Computer Users

In general, visually impaired people can use the same low vision aids for viewing a computer screen as they do for regular reading activities. These include eyeglass-mounted magnifiers, handheld magnifiers, and stand-alone magnifiers.

But also, special software has been developed to either display computer data in large print or read the material aloud in a synthetic voice.

These adaptive low vision devices let partially sighted people do the same computer-related tasks as fully sighted people—such as word processing, creating and using spreadsheets and viewing web pages online.

Most computer operating systems and internet browsers allow you to increase the size of web pages and text on your computer screen to make them more visible to partially sighted users.

Here are a few simple tips for adjusting text size:

- In browsers such as Microsoft's Internet Explorer and Mozilla's Firefox, you can enlarge text on your screen by holding down the Control ("Ctrl") key on your keyboard and tapping the "+" key. (If you use Apple's Safari browser, use the Command key instead.)

- To return the text to its normal size, tap the "-" key while holding down the Control (or Command) key.

- You also can hold down the Control or Command key, then use the wheel on your mouse to increase or decrease the text size on your screen.

- Still another way to enlarge text on your screen is to use the "Text Size" or "Make Text Larger" command within "View" in the drop-down menu bar that appears at the top of your screen when you use popular software programs such as Microsoft Word and Outlook. On a Mac, the View menu has a "Zoom" option to enlarge text in Word and other applications.

Large-print display software goes the extra step and displays not just larger text, but also icons, mouse pointers, and other navigation items at larger sizes.

Another option is to use a screen magnifier placed in front of your display. But with the prices of LCD [liquid crystal display] coming down, you might instead consider purchasing a larger display that's 19–24 inches with a diagonal measurement.

Voice Computer Systems

People with tunnel vision from glaucoma or central blind spots from macular degeneration may find it difficult and tiring to read an entire computer screen. This is one reason that "talking computers" were invented.

Talking computers are based on optical character recognition (OCR) systems that first scan text in a word processing document or web page and then convert the text to sounds. The result is a synthetic voice that reads aloud not only the actual text but also important navigation items such as the cursor location. Voice systems are available from several major software companies.

Your Mouse

Some people with low vision prefer using keyboard commands instead of a mouse, because impaired vision can make it more much difficult to precisely position the cursor on the screen with a mouse.

Telesensory's Genie Pro offers a split screen so you can view your magnified image and your computer monitor's display at the same time. Making the effort to memorize those keyboard commands may help you work faster at the computer, with less frustration.

If you would rather use a mouse, you may want to invest in one that is ergonomically designed for comfort and ease of use.

A wireless optical mouse is another good option, because your movements aren't limited by the wire leading from the mouse to the computer. If you sometimes experience hand cramps, try using a bigger mouse that lets your hand stay in a more open position, instead of clenched up.

A common source of frustration is a mouse set at a speed that is too fast or too slow. If you're a Windows user and you can't control your mouse because it seems to "zoom" across the screen, you can adjust this by clicking on the Start menu, then Control Panel, then Mouse. There you'll find all kinds of mouse behavior settings, including the pointer speed.

Glare and Contrast Adjustments for Low Vision

If you have low vision, you should consider using higher contrast settings on your computer screen. You'll find appropriate settings this way:

1. Select Control Panel on your PC.

2. Open the Display Properties dialog box and choose Appearances or Settings.

3. Under the Appearances and Themes tab in more modern software, select the High Contrast option.

4. Under Control Panel in modern software, you also might have a tab for Accessibility Options containing tips for low vision adjustments.

If you have a Mac, select System Preferences and then Displays. You'll then find options for adjusting screen resolution to increase contrast and to change the appearance, which allows you to select colors.

Dark text displayed against light backgrounds generally is considered the best color combination for those with low vision.

To reduce glare on your computer screen, make sure you close curtains to prevent reflections from outside lighting. Also, try adjusting the position of your computer screen to reduce glare. Special screens and hoods are available to fit around your computer screen to maximize visibility.

Flickering Screens and Other Problems

If you are using an older desktop computer with a tube-style display (also called a cathode ray tube or CRT) and you notice the screen "flickers," be aware that this can cause computer eyestrain.

Usually you can eliminate the flickering sensation by adjusting the CRT display settings. If you use Windows, go to the Display menu within Control Panel. Click on the "Advanced" tab and adjust the refresh rate of the screen to 70 Hz (hertz) or higher. This should eliminate the flicker and increase viewing comfort.

Modern liquid crystal display (LCD) screens create images using different technology and don't cause flicker problems. Therefore, these "flat panel" displays tend to be more comfortable for long-term viewing and cause less eyestrain than CRT screens.

Chapter 31

Occupational and Physical Therapy

Chapter Contents

Section 31.1—Occupational Therapy for People
with Disabilities 288

Section 31.2—Physical Therapy for People
with Disabilities 290

Section 31.1

Occupational Therapy for People with Disabilities

Occupational therapy is a health and rehabilitation profession focused on helping people regain, develop, and build skills that are important for independent functioning, health, well-being, security, and happiness. Occupational therapy practitioners work with people of all ages who, because of illness, injury, or developmental or psychological impairment, require specialized assistance to [re]learn skills that enable them to lead independent and productive lives.

Occupational therapy is a major health service that can be used to manage pain, regain performance skills lost through injury, maximize independence, promote and maintain health, and prevent injury or disability.

Who Needs Occupational Therapy?

Occupational therapy is often necessary for persons who have had a stroke, arthritis, behavior problems, back injury, mental retardation, developmental delay, cerebral palsy, psychiatric disturbances, or other conditions.

Understand

Occupational therapy is used to:

- improve muscle strength and range of motion through activities;
- increase independence in daily living skills, such as dressing, eating, bathing and vocational pursuits;
- improve gross motor skills;
- develop play skills and leisure interests;
- help individuals adjust to the use of artificial limbs and adaptive devices;

- modify environments, including home and workplace accommodations;

- apply emerging technologies that contribute to independent living.

The Occupational Therapist

The occupational therapist (or O.T.) who provides treatment is a professionally-trained specialist, a graduate of a college program accredited by the Accreditation Council for Occupational Therapy Education. Extensive supervised fieldwork provides occupational therapy students opportunities for both observation and broad clinical experience.

Some occupational therapists hold master's and doctoral degrees and work as teachers, administrators, researchers, or consultants. Some specialize in a specific area, such as mental health, pediatrics, or aging.

Occupational therapists who pass a national exam given by the national board certification on occupational therapy qualify to use the initials "OTR" after their name. OTRIL means they are licensed in their state, e.g., in Illinois.

Certified occupational therapy assistants sometimes are employed to provide certain aspects of treatment included in occupational therapy programs; they use the initials "COTA" after their name.

Occupational therapy aides also may be employed to assist occupational therapists. Aides are trained on the job.

Individualized Treatment Plans

To plan a client's program, an occupational therapist evaluates a person's needs, abilities, and interests using interviews, assessments, and medical records.

Treatment may cover one or more areas, ranging from muscle strengthening and self-care to social-emotional adjustment and use of adaptive equipment and splints.

The first focus in therapy for a person with a disability is on performing daily activities, including dressing, grooming, bathing, and eating. Then an emphasis is placed on family and home responsibilities, participating in education, or seeking and maintaining employment.

Therapy goals change as treatment progresses and programs are re-evaluated. The occupational therapist consults and works very closely with a team that often includes a physician, other health care practitioners, the client, and the client's family to set treatment objectives that are realistic and consistent with the client's needs.

Section 31.2

Physical Therapy for People with Disabilities

Physical therapy is a profession provided by physical therapists (PTs) who diagnose and treat people of all ages who have medical problems or other health-related conditions that limit their ability to perform daily activities. They also help prevent conditions associated with loss of mobility through fitness and wellness programs that achieve healthy and active lifestyles.

PTs examine individuals and develop plans using treatment techniques that promote the ability to move, reduce pain, restore function, and prevent disability. They provide care in hospitals, clinics, schools, sports facilities, and more.

Understand

Physical therapy aims to:

- improve functional mobility;
- increase range of motion and strength;
- promote tissue healing;
- prevent disability and pain;
- decrease pain and swelling;
- teach patients and families self-care;
- provide prevention and education.

Physical therapy is often necessary:

- after birth, to evaluate infants suspected of having disabling conditions and to recommend corrective action;
- after operations, to restore function to affected muscles and to keep unaffected muscles strong and useful;

- following stroke, to restore movement and independent living;

- before illness, to design programs of preventive health care;

- to help people with spinal cord injuries, sports injuries, broken bones, and amputations learn to use crutches, braces, wheelchairs, and artificial limbs.

Physical Therapy is used to:

- reduce pain and improve motion in arthritic joints;

- ease the pain of sprains and strains and prevent future injuries;

- plan treatment programs, including physical education, for children who have neurological, orthopedic, and other disorders;

- test for exercise stress and design exercise programs for individuals who have coronary artery disease or are at risk for coronary artery disease;

- evaluate low-back pain and eliminate functional causes;

- rebuild self-confidence and interest in returning to an independent, active life.

The Physical Therapist's Education

PTs must have a graduate degree from an accredited physical therapy program before taking the national licensure examination. The minimum educational requirement is a master's degree, yet most educational programs now offer the doctor of physical therapy (DPT) degree. Licensure is required in each state in which a physical therapist practices.

Physical Therapist Assistants (PTAs) provide physical therapy services under the direction and supervision of a physical therapist. PTAs must complete a 2-year associate's degree and are licensed, certified, or registered in most states.

Individualized Treatment Plans

A PT consults and works closely with an individual's physician, other health care practitioners and the individual in setting treatment objectives that are realistic and consistent with the individual's needs. This includes reviewing the individual's medical records, evaluating him or her, and identifying the problem(s).

PTs perform tests and evaluations that provide information about joint motion, condition of muscles and reflexes, appearance and stability of walking, need for and use of braces and artificial limbs, function of the heart and lungs, integrity of sensation, and perception and performance of activities required in daily living.

Along with the patient and other health care practitioners, the physical therapist shares the hard work and commitment needed to accomplish each individual's successes.

Chapter 32

Art and Music Therapy

Chapter Contents

Section 32.1—The Benefits of Art Therapy for People
with Disabilities 294

Section 32.2—Music Therapy Helps People with
Disabilities.. 296

Section 32.1

The Benefits of Art Therapy for People with Disabilities

Excerpted from "Art Therapist: Making a Difference in the Lives of Children with Special Needs," by the Council for Exceptional Children (www .cec.sped.org), 1999. Reviewed by David A. Cooke, MD, FACP, July 23, 2011.

An art therapist is someone who helps people understand their problems and guides them to solutions through the creative process. He or she is concerned with the treatment and rehabilitation of persons with mental, emotional, medical, or physical disabilities. An art therapist uses art, as well as traditional means of therapy, to lessen an individual's frustration, promote healthy development, and diminish the effects of a disability. Art has also proven to be a useful tool in diagnosis and mental health evaluation, particularly for children.

Art therapists work in a number of settings from schools and residential facilities to hospitals, mental health facilities, rehabilitation centers, and even correctional institutions. Some art therapists also have their own private practices. More and more schools are recognizing the value of art therapy. Students with developmental, medical, educational, social, or psychological impairments may be assigned to an art therapist and treated individually or in groups.

What Is Art Therapy?

Art is a nonverbal form of communication. This does not mean that an art therapist is a wizard who can magically interpret everything in a drawing. Rather an art therapist draws on his or her knowledge of art, psychology, and the "artist." He or she may ask clients or students to create works of art using crayons, paints, clay, or other art media. The result—their artwork—is a container for strong emotions that often cannot be easily expressed any other way.

Art therapy is based on the principle that making or drawing an art object is an important element in the healing process. The therapist studies the artwork and determines what, if any, symbolic images or themes may be present. Anger, depression, and aggression may all be expressed through color, form, and other art elements. If the client is receptive, it is sometimes helpful, especially with children, to discuss the artwork with its creator to elicit more specific information. Children, and to a lesser extent adults, may be unwilling or unable to share their thoughts and emotions through words. The art therapist can encourage them to express themselves through art, which the therapist can use to help a client explore underlying meanings and feelings. Although any art can have many possible meanings, the possibilities are framed by the therapist's knowledge and understanding of the creator of the artwork and by the artist's verbal and non-verbal responses. It is from this total picture of art and artist that the art therapist draws conclusions.

Sometimes the process itself aids the artist. Especially with children, the line between reality and fantasy can be blurred. Although children developing normally usually learn to distinguish between the two by age 6 or so, many children who have mental or emotional disorders or who suffer from extreme stress cannot distinguish fantasy from reality or real danger from monsters. Often just drawing or otherwise artfully creating the fantasies helps to diminish their risk to the child. Vague or fuzzy images become clearer and more focused through art. These images, if positive, can then be enhanced by the therapist. If they are threatening negative images, such as monsters, the therapist can guide the child to the possibilities of a monster-free world.

Art therapists are mainly used to help children exhibiting behavioral or emotional difficulties or those with developmental disabilities. Children with autism, youth who have suffered brain damage, preschoolers through adolescents exhibiting aggressive behaviors or mutism, and students with mental retardation or schizophrenia have been helped by art therapy. The art therapist may work one on one with a young person or in small groups. The therapist may be directive in choosing projects for the students or may decide to let the students choose the direction their artwork is to take. Individual diagnosis and goal setting determine the course of action for the art therapist.

However, when working with a new student, the art therapist generally finds that the therapeutic relationship develops through several general stages: From the student testing the art therapist and the limits of the therapy; to trusting the art therapist and the art therapy process; to finally reaching a willingness to take risks and to communicate experiences, fears, and fantasies to the therapist either through the artwork, or language, or, if the student chooses, both.

Generally, the art therapist is part of an interdisciplinary team and may share his or her insights and conclusions with the team. This involves writing reports and filling out forms, attending team and staff meetings, and maintaining contact with parents if the clients are children. Art therapists are also often required to develop ongoing treatment programs for certain clients to help the team achieve its goals for that individual. They are responsible for supplying a variety of art media and materials and for keeping tools and equipment in a safe and useable condition. Art therapists may also function as supervisors, administrators, consultants, and expert witnesses.

Section 32.2

Music Therapy Helps People with Disabilities

From the U.S. Department of State (www.america.gov),
December 17, 2007.

Some stroke victims who have lost the ability to speak fluently often are able to sing, says a leading music therapist. But even when you have the beat, it is hard to play music if you cannot move.

Innovations in music technology are making it possible—and enjoyable—for people with severe physical disabilities to play and compose music. They also can help restore speech.

Research shows that music therapy is effective in promoting wellness among healthy people, and it has been shown to alleviate pain and improve the quality of life for persons with disabilities.

Singing Helps Speech Recovery

Singing and speaking are neurologically different functions, said Concetta M. Tomaino, who has a doctorate in music therapy. For example, stroke victims can sometimes sing entire lyrics of songs but are unable to speak a simple "Hello."

Clinical studies conducted by Tomaino and her colleagues, especially Dr. Oliver Sacks, author of *Musicophilia: Tales of Music and the Brain* and a British neurologist on the faculty at Columbia University in

New York, have shown that singing word phrases such as "Hello, how are you?" affects speech recovery by "rehearsing" speech. By putting regular speech and common phrases into a musical context, patients who have trouble speaking but are conscious and cognizant of what is being said to them are learning to say "Hello" and more.

Tomaino, a trained musician, is executive director of the Institute for Music and Neurologic Function and vice president of music therapy at Beth Abraham Family Health Services in New York. "Singing rehearses the speech element in the brain to become functional," Tomaino told USINFO. "We are now studying the potential effect of singing and related 'cueing' on the recovery of speech—using musical sounds that sound like phrases or putting regular speech phrases into a musical context."

Live and Digital Musical Instruments Can Improve Motor Skills

In addition to restoring speech, music therapy can improve motor skills and coordination, according to the American Music Therapy Association.

Most of the music therapy work with stroke patients and people suffering symptoms of neurologic diseases such as Parkinson disease consists of what therapists call "live and in the moment." Such therapy incorporates live and recorded music and encourages patients to play actual musical instruments.

For some patients suffering physical disabilities and people with brain injuries, therapists use software known as MIDI (Musical Interface Digital Instrument) as an important component of music therapy, Tomaino said.

Companies equip musical instruments with devices that make it possible for individuals with disabilities to hold and play instruments. But for people with little or no ability to move their arms or legs, or to move them in a coordinated way, it has been impossible to play an instrument.

Now patients who need to increase strength and range of motion in their hands and arms can use digital drumsticks, Tomaino said.

Other Innovations in Computer Music Technology Also Help Disabled

Similarly, at the REHAB school in Poughkeepsie, New York, physically disabled children and teenagers use tiny movements of their head to make music as part of a project developed by musicians and computer software designers at the Deep Listening Institute in Kingston, New York.

A digital video camera connected to a computer displays an image of the patient on a screen. A cursor placed on some part of the screen image of the head tracks even subtle head movements electronically that translate into musical notes heard through the computer's speakers. The program can be played in two modes.

In piano mode, a movement from side to side plays a piano scale; in percussion mode the same movement creates a drum roll.

The computer program Hyperscore allows people to compose music by scoring it using line graphs comprising a broad range of instrument sounds. Hyperscore was developed by Tod Machover, a professor of music and media at the Massachusetts Institute of Technology (MIT) and director of the Opera of the Future project at MIT.

Other organizations developing MIDI software include the Drake Music Project in London. At Drake Music, students with cerebral palsy, including some as young as 11, wear a Cyberlink headband that detects electrical signals from facial and eye movements and even brainwaves. Special software, called Brainfingers at Drake, turns the signals into "fingers" that move the mouse and play notes on the keyboard to create music.

Chapter 33

Service Animals and People with Disabilities

Service Animals in the Workplace

How are service animals defined?

A service animal is an animal that performs a task or tasks for a person with a disability to help overcome limitations resulting from the disability. Federal law defines service animal as "any dog that is individually trained to do work or perform tasks for the benefit of an individual with a disability, including a physical, sensory, psychiatric, intellectual, or other mental disability. Other species of animals, whether wild or domestic, trained or untrained, are not service animals for the purposes of this definition. The work or tasks performed by a service animal must be directly related to the individual's disability." (U.S. Department of Justice).

What types of services do service animals provide?

According to the Department of Justice, "examples of work or tasks include, but are not limited to, assisting individuals who are blind or have low vision with navigation and other tasks, alerting individuals who are deaf or hard of hearing to the presence of people or sounds, providing non-violent protection or rescue work, pulling a wheelchair,

---

This chapter contains excerpts from "Service Animals in the Workplace," by Linda Carter Batiste, JD, and Carmen Fullmer, MS, from the Job Accommodation Network (JAN, www.askjan.org), June 2011, and excerpts from "Commonly Asked Questions About Service Animals in Places of Business," by the U.S. Department of Justice, January 2008.

assisting an individual during a seizure, alerting individuals to the presence of allergens, retrieving items such as medicine or the telephone, providing physical support and assistance with balance and stability to individuals with mobility disabilities, and helping persons with psychiatric and neurological disabilities by preventing or interrupting impulsive or destructive behaviors. The crime deterrent effects of an animal's presence and the provision of emotional support, well-being, comfort, or companionship do not constitute work or tasks for the purposes of this definition."

What is the difference between service, therapy, companion, and social/therapy animals?

According to the Delta Society, a human-services organization dedicated to improving people's health and well-being through positive interactions with animals:

Service animals are legally defined under title III of the Americans with Disabilities Act and are trained to meet the disability-related needs of their handlers who have disabilities. The ADA protects the rights of individuals with disabilities to be accompanied by their service animals in public places. Service animals are not considered pets.

Therapy animals are not legally defined by federal law, but some states have laws defining therapy animals. They provide people with contact to animals, but are not limited to working with people who have disabilities. They are usually the personal pets of their handlers, and work with their handlers to provide services to others. Federal laws have no provisions for people to be accompanied by therapy animals in places of public accommodation that have "no pets" policies. Therapy animals usually are not service animals.

A companion animal is not legally defined, but is accepted as another term for pet.

Social/therapy animals have no legal definition. They often are animals that did not complete service animal or service dog training due to health, disposition, trainability, or other factors, and are made available as pets for people who have disabilities. These animals might or might not meet the definition of service animals.

Because more people are using service animals, employers are asking more questions about service animals in the workplace. The following text includes a summary of some of those questions. The answers are based on informal guidance from the Equal Employment Opportunity Commission (EEOC) and do not represent the EEOC's formal position on these issues or legal advice.

Does title I of the ADA require employers to automatically allow employees with disabilities to bring their service animals to work?

Title III (public access) of the ADA requires a public accommodation to modify policies, practices, or procedures to permit the use of a service animal by an individual with a disability. Title III also requires public accommodations to make reasonable modifications in policies, practices, or procedures to permit the use of a miniature horse by an individual with a disability if the miniature horse has been individually trained to do work or perform tasks for the benefit of the individual with a disability.

But what about title I (employment) of the ADA? According to the EEOC, title I does not require employers to automatically allow employees to bring their service animals to work. Instead, allowing a service animal into the workplace is a form of reasonable accommodation.

What this means for employers: Employers must consider allowing an employee with a disability to use a service animal at work unless doing so would result in an undue hardship. In addition, the ADA allows employers to choose among effective accommodations.

If an employee wants to bring his service animal to work to help with personal medical needs (e.g., an employee with diabetes wants to bring his service animal to work to help monitor his blood sugar level), can the employer deny the request and ask the employee to take care of his medical needs in another way?

According to the EEOC, if the service animal has been trained to help with the employee's medical needs, the employee has a right to ask that, as a reasonable accommodation, the service animal be allowed to accompany him to work.

The employer has a right to know that the animal is actually trained and what the animal does for the employee. However, the employer probably cannot insist that the person take care of his medical needs in a different way if this is the way the employee does it; under the ADA an employer cannot require employees to use other medical treatment/procedures.

What this means for employers: In general, employers should not be involved in employees' personal medical decisions so an employer should not deny an employee's request to use his service animal at work if the animal helps the employee with his or her personal medical needs, unless the employer can show undue hardship.

301

Who is responsible for taking care of a service animal at work?

The employee is responsible for taking care of the service animal, including making sure the animal is not disruptive, keeping it clean and free of parasites, and taking it out to relieve itself as needed.

What this means for employers: Employees are responsible for the care of their service animals, but employers may have to provide accommodations that enable the employees to do so. When an employee is allowed to bring a service animal to work, the employer should consult with the employee to find out what accommodations are needed to care for the animal. For example, an employee might need to adjust his break times to take his service animal outside.

Commonly Asked Questions about Service Animals in Places of Business

What are the laws that apply to my business?

Under the Americans with Disabilities Act (ADA), privately owned businesses that serve the public, such as restaurants, hotels, retail stores, taxicabs, theaters, concert halls, and sports facilities, are prohibited from discriminating against individuals with disabilities. The ADA requires these businesses to allow people with disabilities to bring their service animals onto business premises in whatever areas customers are generally allowed.

What must I do when an individual with a service animal comes to my business?

The service animal must be permitted to accompany the individual with a disability to all areas of the facility where customers are normally allowed to go. An individual with a service animal may not be segregated from other customers.

I have always had a clearly posted "no pets" policy at my establishment. Do I still have to allow service animals in?

Yes. A service animal is not a pet. The ADA requires you to modify your "no pets" policy to allow the use of a service animal by a person with a disability. This does not mean you must abandon your "no pets" policy altogether but simply that you must make an exception to your general rule for service animals.

302

Can I charge a maintenance or cleaning fee for customers who bring service animals into my business?

No. Neither a deposit nor a surcharge may be imposed on an individual with a disability as a condition to allowing a service animal to accompany the individual with a disability, even if deposits are routinely required for pets. However, a public accommodation may charge its customers with disabilities if a service animal causes damage so long as it is the regular practice of the entity to charge non-disabled customers for the same types of damages. For example, a hotel can charge a guest with a disability for the cost of repairing or cleaning furniture damaged by a service animal if it is the hotel's policy to charge when non-disabled guests cause such damage.

Am I responsible for the animal while the person with a disability is in my business?

No. The care or supervision of a service animal is solely the responsibility of his or her owner. You are not required to provide care or food or a special location for the animal.

What if a service animal barks or growls at other people, or otherwise acts out of control?

You may exclude any animal, including a service animal, from your facility when that animal's behavior poses a direct threat to the health or safety of others. For example, any service animal that displays vicious behavior towards other guests or customers may be excluded. You may not make assumptions, however, about how a particular animal is likely to behave based on your past experience with other animals. Each situation must be considered individually.

Although a public accommodation may exclude any service animal that is out of control, it should give the individual with a disability who uses the service animal the option of continuing to enjoy its goods and services without having the service animal on the premises.

Chapter 34

Finding Accessible Transportation

Chapter Contents

Section 34.1—Adapting Motor Vehicles for People
    with Disabilities 306

Section 34.2—Assistance and Accommodation for
    Air Travel 311

Section 34.1

Adapting Motor Vehicles for People with Disabilities

From the National Highway Traffic Safety Administration (NHTSA, www.nhtsa.gov), December 1999. Reviewed by David A. Cooke, MD, FACP, July 23, 2011.

The introduction of new technology continues to broaden opportunities for people with disabilities to drive vehicles with adaptive devices. Taking advantage of these opportunities, however, can be time consuming and, sometimes, frustrating.

The information in this text is based on the experience of driver rehabilitation specialists and other professionals who work with individuals who require adaptive devices for their motor vehicles. It is centered around a proven process—evaluating your needs, selecting the right vehicle, choosing a qualified dealer to modify your vehicle, being trained, maintaining your vehicle—that can help you avoid costly mistakes when purchasing and modifying a vehicle with adaptive equipment.

Investigate Cost-Saving Opportunities and Licensing Requirements

Cost-Saving Opportunities

The costs associated with modifying a vehicle vary greatly. A new vehicle modified with adaptive equipment can cost from $20,000 to $80,000. Therefore, whether you are modifying a vehicle you own or purchasing a new vehicle with adaptive equipment, it pays to investigate public and private opportunities for financial assistance.

There are programs that help pay part or all of the cost of vehicle modification, depending on the cause and nature of the disability. For information, contact your state's Department of Vocational Rehabilitation or another agency that provides vocational services, and, if appropriate, the Department of Veterans Affairs. You can find phone numbers for these state and federal agencies in a local phone book. Also, consider the following.

306

- Many nonprofit associations that advocate for individuals with disabilities have grant programs that help pay for adaptive devices.

- If you have private health insurance or workers' compensation, you may be covered for adaptive devices and vehicle modification. Check with your insurance carrier.

- Many manufacturers have rebate or reimbursement plans for modified vehicles. When you are ready to make a purchase, find out if there is such a dealer in your area.

- Some states waive the sales tax for adaptive devices if you have a doctor's prescription for their use.

- You may be eligible for savings when submitting your federal income tax return. Check with a qualified tax consultant to find out if the cost of your adaptive devices will help you qualify for a medical deduction.

Licensing Requirements

All states require a valid learner's permit or driver's license to receive an on-the-road evaluation. You cannot be denied the opportunity to apply for a permit or license because you have a disability. However, you may receive a restricted license, based on your use of adaptive devices.

Evaluate Your Needs

Driver rehabilitation specialists perform comprehensive evaluations to identify the adaptive equipment most suited to your needs. A complete evaluation includes vision screening and, in general, assesses the following:

- Muscle strength, flexibility, and range of motion

- Coordination and reaction time

- Judgment and decision-making abilities

- Ability to drive with adaptive equipment

Upon completion of an evaluation, you should receive a report containing specific recommendations on driving requirements or restrictions, and a complete list of recommended vehicle modifications.

Finding a Qualified Evaluator

To find a qualified evaluator in your area, contact a local rehabilitation center or call the Association for Driver Rehabilitation Specialists (ADED). The Association maintains a database of certified driver rehabilitation specialists throughout the country. Your insurance company may pay for the evaluation. Find out if you need a physician's prescription or other documentation to receive benefits.

Being Prepared for an Evaluation

Consult with your physician to make sure you are physically and psychologically prepared to drive. Being evaluated too soon after an injury or other trauma may indicate the need for adaptive equipment you will not need in the future. When going for an evaluation, bring any equipment you normally use, e.g., a walker or neck brace. Tell the evaluator if you are planning to modify your wheelchair or obtain a new one.

Evaluating Passengers with Disabilities

Evaluators also consult on compatibility and transportation safety issues for passengers with disabilities. They assess the type of seating needed and the person's ability to exit and enter the vehicle. They provide advice on the purchase of modified vehicles and recommend appropriate wheelchair lifts or other equipment for a vehicle you own. If you have a child who requires a special type of safety seat, evaluators make sure the seat fits your child properly. They also make sure you can properly install the seat in your vehicle.

Select the Right Vehicle

Selecting a vehicle for modification requires collaboration among you, your evaluator, and a qualified vehicle modification dealer. Although the purchase or lease of a vehicle is your responsibility, making sure the vehicle can be properly modified is the responsibility of the vehicle modification dealer. Therefore, take the time to consult with a qualified dealer and your evaluator before making your final purchase. It will save you time and money. Be aware that you will need insurance while your vehicle is being modified, even though it is off the road.

The following questions can help with vehicle selection. They can also help determine if you can modify a vehicle you own.

- Does the necessary adaptive equipment require a van, or will another passenger vehicle suffice?

- Can the vehicle accommodate the equipment that needs to be installed?

- Will there be enough space to accommodate your family or other passengers once the vehicle is modified?

- Is there adequate parking space at home and at work for the vehicle and for loading/unloading a wheelchair?

- Is there adequate parking space to maneuver if you use a walker?

- What additional options are necessary for the safe operation of the vehicle?

If a third party is paying for the vehicle, adaptive devices, or modification costs, find out if there are any limitations or restrictions on what is covered. Always get a written statement on what a funding agency will pay before making your purchase.

Choose a Qualified Dealer to Modify Your Vehicle

Even a half inch change in the lowering of a van floor can affect a driver's ability to use equipment or to have an unobstructed view of the road; so, take time to find a qualified dealer to modify your vehicle. Begin with a phone inquiry to find out about credentials, experience, and references. Ask questions about how they operate. Do they work with evaluators? Will they look at your vehicle before you purchase it? Do they require a prescription from a physician or other driver evaluation specialist? How long will it take before they can start work on your vehicle? Do they provide training on how to use the adaptive equipment?

If you are satisfied with the answers you receive, check references; then arrange to visit the dealer's facility. Additional information to consider is listed in the following text.

- Are they members of the National Mobility Equipment Dealers Association (NMEDA) or another organization that has vehicle conversion standards?

- What type of training has the staff received?

- What type of warranty do they provide on their work?

- Do they provide ongoing service and maintenance?

- Do they stock replacement parts?

Once you are comfortable with the dealer's qualifications, you will want to ask specific questions, such as the following:

- How much will the modification cost?
- Will they accept third party payment?
- How long will it take to modify the vehicle?
- Can the equipment be transferred to a new vehicle in the future?
- Will they need to modify existing safety features to install the adaptive equipment?

While your vehicle is being modified, you will, most likely, need to be available for fittings. This avoids additional waiting time for adjustments once the equipment is fully installed. Without proper fittings you may have problems with the safe operation of the vehicle and have to go back for adjustments.

Some state agencies specify the dealer you must use if you want reimbursement.

Obtain Training on the Use of New Equipment

Both new and experienced drivers need training on how to safely use new adaptive equipment. Your equipment dealer and evaluator should provide information and off-road instruction. You will also need to practice driving under the instruction of a qualified driving instructor until you both feel comfortable with your skills. Bring a family member or other significant person who drives to all your training sessions. It's important to have someone else who can drive your vehicle in case of an emergency.

Some state vocational rehabilitation departments pay for driver training under specified circumstances. At a minimum, their staff can help you locate a qualified instructor. If your evaluator does not provide on-the-road instruction, ask him or her for a recommendation. You can also inquire at your local motor vehicle administration office.

Maintain Your Vehicle

Regular maintenance is important for keeping your vehicle and adaptive equipment safe and reliable. It may also be mandatory for compliance with the terms of your warranty. Some warranties specify a time period during which adaptive equipment must be inspected. These checkups for equipment may differ from those for your vehicle. Make sure you or your modifier submits all warranty cards for all equipment to ensure coverage and so manufacturers can contact you in case of a recall.

Section 34.2

Assistance and Accommodation for Air Travel

Excerpted from "Travelers with Disabilities," in chapter 8 of the 2012 *Yellow Book,* by the Centers for Disease Control and Prevention (CDC, www.cdc.gov), July 1, 2011.

Travelers with disabilities are defined as travelers whose mobility is reduced because of a physical incapacity (sensory or locomotor), an intellectual deficiency, age, illness, or another cause, and who may require special attention and adaptation of the transportation services that are available to all passengers. The medical preparation of a traveler with a stable, ongoing disability does not differ from that of any other traveler. The following recommendations are key to ensuring safe, accessible travel:

- Assess each international itinerary on an individual basis, in consultation with specialized travel agencies or tour operators.

- Consult travel health providers for additional recommendations.

- Use print and internet resources.

Air Travel

Regulations and Codes

Carriers may not refuse transportation on the basis of disability. By law, U.S. air carriers must comply with highly detailed regulations that affect people with disabilities. These do not cover foreign carriers serving the United States.

All U.S. and non-U.S. carriers are required to file annual reports of disability-related complaints with the Department of Transportation (DOT). The DOT maintains a toll-free hotline (800-778-4838) to provide real-time assistance in facilitating compliance with DOT rules and to suggest customer-service solutions to the airlines. The Transportation Security Administration (TSA) has established a program for screening travelers with disabilities and their equipment, mobility aids, and devices. TSA permits prescriptions, liquid medications, and other liquids needed by people with disabilities and medical conditions. International Air Transport Association (IATA) member airlines voluntarily adhere to codes of practice that are similar to U.S. legislation based on guidance from the International Civil Aviation Organization. However, smaller airlines overseas may not be IATA members.

Airlines are obliged to accept a declaration by a passenger that he or she is self-reliant. Medical certificates can be required only in specific situations (for example, if a person intends to travel with a possible communicable disease, will require a stretcher or oxygen, or if unusual behavior is anticipated that may affect the operation of the flight).

Assistance and Accommodations

When a traveler with a disability requests assistance, the airline is obliged to provide access to the aircraft door (preferably by a level entry bridge), an aisle wheelchair, and a seat with removable armrests. Aircraft with fewer than 30 seats are generally exempt. Airline personnel are not required to transfer passengers from wheelchair to wheelchair, wheelchair to aircraft seat, or wheelchair to lavatory seat. Travelers with disabilities who cannot transfer themselves should travel with a companion or attendant, but carriers may not, without reason, require a person with a disability to travel with an attendant.

Only wide-body aircraft with two aisles are required to have fully accessible lavatories, although any aircraft with more than 60 seats must have an onboard wheelchair, and personnel must help move the wheelchair from a seat to the lavatory area. Airline personnel are not obliged to assist with feeding, visiting the lavatory, or dispensing medication to travelers.

Airlines may not require advance notice of a passenger with a disability; however, they may require up to 48 hours' advance notice and 1-hour advance check-in for certain accommodations that require preparation time, such as the following:

- Medical oxygen for use on board the aircraft, if the service is available on the flight

- Carriage of an incubator, if the service is available on the flight

- Hook-up for a respirator to the aircraft electrical power supply, if the service is available on the flight

- Accommodation for a passenger who must travel in a stretcher, if the service is available on the flight

- Transportation of an electric wheelchair on a flight scheduled on an aircraft with fewer than 60 seats

- Provision by the airline of hazardous material packaging for a battery used in a wheelchair or other assistive devices

- Accommodation for a group of 10 or more people with disabilities who make a reservation and travel as a group

- Provision of an onboard wheelchair to be used on an aircraft that does not have an accessible lavatory

Assessment and Preparation

With high incidence of cardiopulmonary disease and millions of people traveling by air, many people are at risk for significant hypoxia and respiratory symptoms while flying. Generally, patients with an oxygen saturation by pulse oximetry >95% do not require supplemental oxygen, and those with a saturation <92% will require it during air travel. The hypoxia altitude simulation test can identify those patients (with an oxygen saturation by pulse oximetry between 92% and 95%) who may benefit from oxygen supplementation during air travel, decreasing their risk for significant cardiopulmonary effects of induced hypoxia at higher altitudes.

Internationally standardized codes for classifying disabled passengers and their needs are available in all computerized reservations systems. Passengers with disabilities should use travel agents experienced in the use of the disability coding; it is critical that appropriate codes and interairline messages are sequentially entered for all flights. The delivering carrier is always responsible for a traveler with disabilities until a subsequent carrier physically accepts responsibility for that passenger.

Service Animals

Service animals are not exempt from compliance with quarantine regulations and so may not be allowed to travel to all international destinations. They are also subject to U.S. animal import regulations on return. However, carriers must permit guide dogs or other service animals with appropriate identification to accompany a person with a disability on a flight. Carriers must permit a service animal to accompany a traveler with a disability to any seat in which the person sits, unless the animal obstructs an aisle or other area that must remain clear to facilitate an emergency evacuation, in which case the passenger will be assigned another seat.

Chapter 35

Family Support Services

Chapter Contents

Section 35.1—Understanding Respite Care 316

Section 35.2—Adult Day Care.. 327

Section 35.1

Understanding Respite Care

Everyone needs a break. If you are a caregiver, you may need a break from caregiving tasks. If you have dementia, you may want a break from the daily routine and have the opportunity to meet others who share some of the same challenges. Respite care can help, by providing a new environment or time to relax. It can be for a few hours or several days or weeks depending on your particular needs and interests.

What Is Respite Care?

Respite refers to a short time of rest or relief. It provides a break from the typical care routine—allowing the caregiver some down time while the person with dementia continues to receive care from qualified individuals and has the opportunity to have different experiences.

An individual can receive respite care:

- from paid staff, volunteers, family, or friends;
- at home, a community organization, or a residential care center;
- for part of the day, evening, or overnight; or
- occasionally or on a regular basis.

Why Use Respite Care Services?

Some caregivers work or have other responsibilities in addition to providing care. Respite care can give a caregiver the time and assistance required to meet these personal needs.

Respite care can provide the caregiver with:

- a chance to spend time with other friends and family, or to just relax;

- time to take care of errands such as shopping, exercising, getting a haircut, or going to the doctor; or

- comfort or peace of mind knowing that the person with dementia is spending time with another caring individual.

The person with dementia is experiencing many changes and challenges, too, and may also need variety in his or her routine and social interactions.

Respite care services can give the person with dementia an opportunity to:

- interact with others having similar experiences;

- spend time in a safe, supportive environment; or

- participate in enjoyable activities designed to match personal abilities and needs.

What Are the Different Kinds of Respite Care Services?

There are a number of ways that respite care can be provided. Following are descriptions of five common types.

In-Home Respite Care

These respite care services are provided in the home to assist the caregiver and the person with dementia. Services vary in type and can include:

- Companion services: Help with supervision, recreational activities, and visiting

- Personal care services: Help with bathing, dressing, toileting, exercising, and other daily activities

- Homemaker services: Help with housekeeping, shopping, and meal preparation

- Skilled care services: Help with certain medical services or care

In-home aides can be employed privately, through an agency, or as part of a government program. Be sure the aide and services are appropriate for your specific needs. Cost, level of training, and specific services provided will vary among workers and agencies. Generally,

Medicare does not pay for this type of help, but financial assistance may be available.

Some respite care aides have received training about Alzheimer's disease and the unique needs of a person with the disease. It is important that the in-home aide is knowledgeable—or at least willing to learn—about Alzheimer's disease and effective approaches to care.

Adult Day Centers

An adult day center provides care outside the home and is designed to meet individual needs while supporting strengths, abilities, and independence. Participants have the opportunity to interact with others while being part of a structured environment.

Daily activities may include music, recreation, discussion, and support groups. Staff may include a nurse, social worker, and recreation or music therapist. However, staffing can vary across centers. If the person with Alzheimer's requires medical services (i.e., insulin shots, help with medication, etc.) be sure to ask if staff provides medical assistance.

Many caregivers who work during the day find this type of center very helpful as they try to balance a job with caregiving duties. Hours of service vary at each center, but some are open from seven to 10 hours per day, five days a week. Some may even offer weekend and evening hours, and most centers provide a meal or snacks.

Informal Respite Care

Many times, a family member, close friend, neighbor, or volunteer is willing to occasionally help out, giving the caregiver time to run to the store or just take a break. Caregivers should keep in mind people who have offered to help.

Put together a schedule of times when others are available. It may be in the evenings, on the weekends, or on special occasions. This can allow the caregiver some down time while the person with dementia is spending time with someone else you both trust.

Residential Respite Care

Another respite care option is a stay in a residential facility overnight, for a few days or a few weeks. Overnight care allows caregivers to take an extended break or vacation while the person with dementia stays in a supervised, safe environment designed to meet personal needs. The cost for these services varies and is usually not covered by insurance or Medicare. Be sure to make a reservation in advance, as some centers may not always have an available room.

Sometimes, a person with dementia may have difficulty adjusting to this new environment. Regular stays can allow the overall adjustment to become easier for everyone. Over time, the staff can become more familiar with the needs of the individual, and he or she will become more comfortable with the staff and the environment.

Respite Care for Emergency Situations

Accidents, surgery, or unexpected trips can create a need for emergency respite care. In case an emergency does come up, it's helpful to have done research and planning ahead of time. Call around to agencies to find out which ones offer services when the need arises. Try out a service in a non-emergency situation and see how it works. Also, talk with people you trust—including family, friends, and neighbors—about the possibility of asking for help in case of an emergency.

How to Choose a Respite Care Service

Once you've assessed your needs for type of care, skills, location, and frequency, you can:

- select a service that best meets these needs;
- prepare the aide and the person with dementia;
- evaluate the service's effectiveness or usefulness.

In some areas, respite care options may be limited. Contact your local Alzheimer's Association to find out about the respite care services that are available in your area, and talk with people in your community to gain additional information about respite care options. Then, you can call these services with specific questions or inquiries.

Describe your situation and explain what you would like from a respite care service. Ask questions over the telephone regarding qualifications, types of services offered, cost, and hours of availability. The more information you receive over the phone, the easier it will be to identify which service is best for you. You will also be able to limit the number of services you interview or visit.

Selecting the Respite Care Service

If you are selecting an in-home aide, arrange a time to meet with the person in your home. Ask plenty of questions to gain an understanding of his or her skills.

Ask prospective aides about their availability, training, background, care philosophy, and experience with dementia.

Be specific about the needs and the characteristics of the person with dementia. If possible, it is a good idea for both the person with dementia and the caregiver to participate in the interview process.

If necessary, interview several aides to find the right person for your particular situation; don't feel pressured to settle on someone who doesn't make you feel comfortable. Do be aware, however, that if the home care aide is coming from a government program, your choices may be limited.

If you are selecting an adult day center, arrange a meeting with the staff and take time to look around. Assess your overall feeling about the environment. Look to see if individuals are involved in activities and if the center looks clean.

Get a better idea of the center by attending a function there or talking with staff. Ask if they provide personalized care, and find out about both the people who work there and those who attend the center. Be direct about the needs and characteristics of the person with dementia, and find a center that is able to meet your needs.

If you are selecting a residential facility, you will be faced with additional considerations. Since you will not be around 24 hours a day to observe care, it's important to make sure that the environment and services will be a good fit for the person with dementia.

It is also important to see the care firsthand. Ask to take a look around and talk with the facility's staff, as well as residents and families who use the service. Again, examine the environment yourself to see if it's clean, if residents seem content and engaged, and to gauge your general sense of the facility.

Stop by one evening or weekend and see if the facility is any different than during the day. You may even want to make an unannounced visit.

For a complete guide of questions you may want to ask when selecting a respite care service, see the text under the heading Things to Consider When Choosing Respite Care.

Overcoming Concerns about Respite Care

It's normal to be apprehensive about trying something new. Some concerns you may have about using respite services:

Cost

You may be concerned about how to pay for services.

Look into financial assistance such as scholarships, sliding scale fees, or government programs. Contact your local Alzheimer's Association to learn what kind of financial assistance may be available.

Reliability

You may be concerned about the dependability of the aide or service.

Those who work for an agency or facility should be reliable and well trained, and are often certified. Ask each individual and facility about training and qualifications. If hiring someone independently, interview the person thoroughly and check references.

Guilt

You may believe that you should be able to "do it all."

Seeking help does not make you a failure. It's important to remember that respite services benefit the person with dementia as well as the caregiver.

Preparing the Respite Care Provider

Whatever type or combination of respite care options you choose, you will want to familiarize the aide or staff to the needs and characteristics of the person with dementia. Be honest in your discussions. Establish a relationship and learn from each other. If necessary, define the specific tasks the respite caregiver should be responsible for.

Be sure the aide or staff gets to know the person with dementia. Provide a written history of the individual; show photographs; share stories and memories.

Use the "Personal Facts and Insights" form (in the Fact Sheets/ Forms section on CareFinder at www.alz.org) to help the respite care provider get to know the person. Provide it as a quick reference for the aide when you are not available. When completed, it provides information about the individual, including:

- personality;
- personal habits;
- level of cognition;
- daily routine;
- communication skills;

- family;

- mobility;

- hobbies;

- likes and dislikes;

- occupation.

Preparing the Person with Dementia

The person with dementia will also need time to prepare for and adjust to an additional caregiver. Provide as much information as is appropriate. Some people with dementia may initially resist new situations; to help with a smooth transition to respite care, the caregiver may say someone is coming over to help around the house or refer to a day center as a social club or work. The service or aide may have valuable suggestions if the person with dementia is hesitant.

Evaluating the Service

It is important to periodically evaluate the service you use. Many times, needs will change and a particular aide or facility may no longer be suitable. In addition, the service may suggest they can no longer meet your needs.

In either case, you will want to find a different service that can better meet your specific needs. If you do decide to change services, make a list of the limitations of the current service and compare it to other options.

When evaluating your current respite care service, consider:

- Is the service meeting your needs?

- What is working best?

- What can be improved?

- What do you need that your current service doesn't offer?

- Can you help the service recognize and address your needs?

- If not, where can you find what you need?

Contact the Alzheimer's Association 24/7 Helpline at 800-272-3900 for more information on respite care options and how to evaluate what's right for your situation.

Things to Consider When Choosing Respite Care

Use the following checklist when you are screening different respite care options to find out if the provider, service, or care setting will meet your needs. If it's helpful, make copies of this list and use it to take notes about the different care options you explore.

This list is not comprehensive, but may serve as a starting point for you to think of additional ideas, preferences, and priorities.

Checklist for Help in the Home or Home Care Provider

- Offers the specific services you need:
  - Companionship: Visiting, supervision, and leisure activities
  - Personal care: Help with bathing, dressing, toileting, and exercising
  - Homemaking: Housekeeping, shopping, and cooking
  - Skilled care: Help with medication and other medical needs

- Provider is:
  - able to communicate in the preferred language, if important;
  - trained in first aid and CPR (cardiopulmonary resuscitation);
  - trained in dementia care;
  - experienced in working with someone with dementia;
  - with an agency, if important;
  - bonded (protects clients from potential losses caused by the employee), if important;
  - able to provide references;
  - available when you need them;
  - able to provide a back-up if they are sick;
  - able to manage your specific health and behavioral care needs.

Checklist for Adult Day Care Center

- Able to provide respite care
- Convenient location
- Convenient hours

- Appropriate services and programming based on your specific health and behavioral care needs
- Staff trained in dementia care
- Affordable
- Transportation available if needed
- Meals and snacks provided
- Able to dispense/monitor medications
- Enrollment in Alzheimer's Association Safe Return® program strongly encouraged

Checklist for Nursing Home, Assisted Living, or Other Type of Residential Care

Family Involvement

- Families are encouraged to participate in care planning.
- Families are informed of changes in resident's condition and care needs.
- Families are encouraged to communicate with staff.

Staffing

- Medical care is provided to the extent that it is needed.
- Personal care and assistance is provided to the extent that it is needed.
- Staff recognize persons with dementia as unique individuals, and personalize care to meet specific needs, abilities, and interests.
- Staff trained in dementia care.

Programs and Services

- Appropriate services and programming based on specific health and behavioral care needs.
- Planned activities (ask to see activity schedule; note if the activity listed at the time of your visit is occurring).
- Activities on the weekends or during evenings.
- Activities designed to meet specific needs, interests, and abilities.

- Transportation available for:
  - medical appointments;
  - shopping for personal items.

Environment

- Indoor space that allows for freedom of movement and promotes independence
- Safe and secure indoor and outdoor areas
- Easy to navigate
- Designated family visiting area

Meals

- Regular meal and snack times
- Appetizing food (ask to see the weekly menu and come for a meal)
- Pleasant dining environment
- Family and friends able to join at mealtime
- Staff have a plan for monitoring adequate nutrition
- Staff are able to provide for any special dietary needs
- Staff provide appropriate assistance based on person's abilities (for example, allow the person to drink independently, if able)
- No environmental distractions during meal time (noisy TV, etc.)

Policies and Procedures

- Family and friends able to participate in care
- Visiting hours
- Discharge policy (learn about any situation or condition that would lead to a discharge from the facility)
- Enrollment in Alzheimer's Association Safe Return® program strongly encouraged

State Inspection Results

- If the facility is licensed, ask for recent state inspection survey results—administrators are required to provide this information if asked.

Several things to note:

- Report should be dated within the last 9–15 months.

- Compare the number of deficiencies cited to the state average.

- If a facility has received a citation in a particular service area, be sure to ask questions about this area when you visit the facility.

Beware of choosing a facility with a very high number of deficiencies compared to other facilities in the area and the state average. (Adapted from National Citizens' Coalition for Nursing Home Reform: Consumer Guide to Choosing a Nursing Home)

If the facility is a nursing home, go to the Nursing Home Compare website to learn how it compares to the national average at www.medicare.gov/nhcompare/home.asp.

When contacting a provider or residential care setting, be prepared by having the following information available about the person seeking care:

- Name and Social Security number

- Physician's name and phone number

- Diagnoses, other health and behavioral care needs

- List of medications

- Insurance coverage including Medicare, Medicaid, and long-term care insurance

- Special care equipment required

Questions to ask after evaluating:

- Does the service/program meet my needs? How?

- Does the provider appear to be adequately trained? How?

- Is it convenient?

- Is it affordable?

Quick Tips

- Good dementia care includes ensuring safety and meeting basic needs—but it also means involving the person with dementia as much as possible.

- Caregivers should aim to treat a whole person, not a patient.

- When you look for a care provider, ask about special training in dementia care.

- Find out how care providers are supervised and supported in their daily work.

- A good long-term care facility should feel comfortable and homelike.

- People with dementia may be unable to express their feelings in words and behaviors may speak for them. Care providers should try to understand a behavior's cause and consider the best solution.

Section 35.2

Adult Day Care

"Adult Day Care: One Form of Respite for Older Adults," ARCH National Respite Network and Resource Center (www.archrespite.org), April 2002. Updated by David A. Cooke, MD, FACP, July 23, 2011.

Adult day care centers, also known as adult day services, have been providing a form of respite for caregivers for more than 20 years. In 1978 there were only 300 centers nationwide. By the 1980s there were 2,100 centers, and today there are about 4,000 centers nationwide, according to the National Adult Day Services Association (NADSA). NADSA reports that the need for such centers has "jumped sharply to keep pace with the mushrooming demand for home and community based services."

This growth also is due in part to new funding sources such as Medicaid waiver programs, which support alternatives to institutional long-term care and rehabilitation. According to Mary Brugger Murphy, director of NADSA, "many of the people served by adult day centers would have been institutionalized just 10 years ago."

Adult day care centers provide a break (respite) to the caregiver while providing health services, therapeutic services, and social activities for people with Alzheimer disease and related dementia, chronic illnesses, traumatic brain injuries, developmental disabilities, and other problems that increase their care needs. Some adult day care centers are dementia specific, providing services exclusively to that population. Other centers serve the broader population.

One difference between traditional adult respite, both group and in-home care, and adult day care is that adult day centers not only provide respite to family caregivers but also therapeutic care for cognitively and physically impaired older adults.

Benefits of Adult Day Care

Adult day care allows caregivers to continue working outside the home, receive help with the physical care of a loved one, avoid the guilt of placing a loved one in institutional care, and have respite from what can be a 24/7 responsibility.

The care receiver can also benefit from adult day care. He or she is able to remain at home with family but does not require 24-hour care from the primary caregiver. Adult day care participants also have an opportunity to interact socially with peers, share in stimulating activities, receive physical or speech therapy if needed, and receive assistance with the activities of daily living with dignity.

A day at an adult day care center could include supervised care; small group and individual activities such as reminiscence, sensory stimulation, music, art, and intergenerational activities; nutritious meals; transportation; case management; recreation and exercise; nursing care; education; family counseling; assistance with activities of daily living; and occupational, speech, and physical therapies. These services are customized to each participant's needs.

Types of Adult Day Care

There are three types of adult day care:

- Adult day social care provides social activities, meals, recreation, and some health-related services

- Adult day health care offers more intensive health, therapeutic, and social services for individuals with severe medical problems and for those at risk of nursing home care

- Alzheimer-specific adult day care provides social and health services only to persons with Alzheimer disease or related dementia

Who Uses Adult Day Care?

Many caregivers who work outside the home are unable to stay home to care for loved ones. In addition, caregivers who do not work outside the home may wish a break from caregiving to run errands, socialize, or simply to rest.

How Long Do Participants Stay at Day Care?

Generally, although programs vary, participants attend the program for several hours a day to a full day (8 hours), up to 5 days a week. Most programs do not offer weekend services, although a few may offer half-day services on Saturdays.

How Do I Choose an Adult Day Care Center?

Family members must do some research to determine whether the adult day care center is right for their loved ones. The components of a quality adult day care program should include the following:

- Conducts an individual needs assessment before admission to determine the person's range of abilities and needs

- Provides an active program that meets the daily social, recreational, and rehabilitative needs of the person in care

- Develops an individualized treatment plan for participants and monitors it regularly, adjusting the plan as necessary

- Provides referrals to other needed community services

- Has clear criteria for service and guidelines for termination based on the functional status of the person in care

- Provides a full range of in-house services, which may include personal care, transportation, meals, health screening and monitoring, educational programs, counseling, and rehabilitative services

- Provides a safe, secure environment

- Uses qualified and well-trained volunteers

- Adheres to or exceeds existing state and national standards and guidelines

A good place to begin searching for a program is the Yellow Pages, which will list possible options under "Day Care Centers-Adult." The Better Business Bureau may have information on for-profit adult day care centers. At the national level, contact the National Council on Aging (NCOA), National Adult Day Services Association (NADSA) for a set of guidelines for adult day service programs. Local Area Agencies on Aging can also direct you to adult day care centers in your area. Physicians are frequently familiar with area programs, and geriatric medicine programs at major medical centers can usually guide you to appropriate resources. Ultimately, word of mouth is often one of the best ways of finding quality adult day care.

Statistics from Adult Day Care Centers

An ongoing national survey from NCOA/NADSA found the following additional information:

- Approximately 80 percent of adult day care providers are nonprofit, 10 percent are for-profit, and 10 percent use only public funds.
- Fees range from $25 per day to $70 per day, with the average around $50 per day. Many facilities provide services with a sliding fee scale, meaning that family members pay a fee based on their income.
- Most adult day care centers provide transportation. Half the centers provide this service free of charge; others charge by the trip or the number of miles.
- Full-time nursing services are in place at most sites.
- A majority of centers are licensed by the state in which they are located.

Funding for Adult Day Care

Medicare does not cover day care costs, but Medicaid can pay all the costs in a licensed day care center with a medical model or an Alzheimer environment if the senior qualifies financially. Some day care centers offer need-based scholarships. Others may use a sliding fee scale based on income. Private medical insurance policies sometimes cover a portion of day care costs when registered, licensed medical personnel are involved in the care. Long-term care insurance may also pay for adult day services, depending upon the policy. Dependent care tax credits may be available to the caregiver as well.

Conclusion

Adult day care services are a welcome respite opportunity for individuals who work or who need stretches of time away from their loved one to complete tasks, socialize, or just refresh. Additionally, adult day care can be beneficial to the participant when he or she is willing and able to be part of the adult day care experience.

Part Four

Staying Healthy
with a Disability

Chapter 36

Nutrition and Weight Management Issues for People with Disabilities

Chapter Contents

Section 36.1—Nutrition and Disability 334

Section 36.2—Nutrition for Swallowing Difficulties 341

Section 36.3—Overweight and Obesity among
        People with Disabilities 343

Section 36.1

Nutrition and Disability

"Nutrition and Disability," reprinted with permission from the University of Montana Rural Institute Research and Training Center on Disability in Rural Communities (http://rtc.ruralinstitute.umt.edu). © 2002. Reviewed by David A. Cooke, MD, FACP, July 14, 2011.

A disability often can be complicated by additional medical, psychological, or environmental problems. Under an emerging framework of health promotion for persons with disabilities, these additional health problems are referred to as secondary conditions (Brandt & Pope, 1997; Marge, 1988; Pope & Tarlov, 1991).

Until recently, it was common to conceptualize these ailments as symptomatic of the primary disability; however, it is now presumed that because these conditions can be prevented or managed, they are secondary conditions distinct from the primary disability.

Although information on secondary conditions experienced by people with developmental disabilities is limited, the literature does contain descriptions of some risk factors (Eyman, Chaney, Givens, Lopez, & Lee, 1986); identification of various diseases as sources of later, additional limitation (Miller & Eyman, 1979); and suggested health practices that might lead to the prevention of some secondary conditions (e.g., Marge, 1988).

This text describes three significant nutrition-related risk factors for secondary conditions in people with developmental disabilities—malnutrition, obesity, and issues related to the support staff responsible for food planning and preparation. These risk factors have potential to respond positively to improved health practices through well-considered interventions.

Background

Nutrition is related to secondary conditions in persons with developmental disabilities in four significant ways:

1. Nutrition may be viewed as a risk factor for secondary conditions. (Poor nutrition, nutritional status, or eating habits make the secondary condition worse.)

2. Nutrition can be a protective factor. (Good nutrition, nutritional status, or eating habits can improve the secondary condition.)

3. Poor nutrition in the form of deficiencies can be a secondary condition itself.

4. Many secondary conditions can further modify one's diet and create subsequent nutritional problems.

Malnutrition

Malnutrition encompasses both under-nutrition and over-nutrition that lead to negative anthropometrical, biochemical, or clinical outcomes for an individual. Nutrition was investigated in our 1999 universal survey of adult consumers of Montana's Developmental Disability Program (DDP) services; survey items were included to help determine nutrition as a risk factor, a protective factor, or a secondary condition.

Poor nutrition may be a risk factor in this population for the following observed secondary conditions:

• Weight problems

• Bladder dysfunction

• Fatigue

• Bowel dysfunction

• Depression

• Physical fitness/conditioning problems

• Dental/oral hygiene problems

• Sleep problems/disturbances

Poor nutrition may be a risk factor for the following possible or identified medical secondary conditions:

• Gastrointestinal dysfunction

• Urinary tract infections

• Side effects from medications

• Allergies and allergic reactions

• Cardiovascular/circulatory problems

• Diabetes

- Osteoporosis

- Nutritional deficits

- Cancer

Many of the secondary conditions listed above are associated with under-nourishment or over-nourishment in the general U.S. adult population. Over-nourishment includes consumption of nutrients in a pattern that leads to the development of such diseases as cardiovascular disease, cancer, or diabetes. Under-nourishment precipitates nutrient deficiencies leading to such conditions as anemia, osteoporosis, or wasting in adults.

Over-nutrition

It may be that the most compelling nutrition issues for adults with developmental disabilities are the same ones affecting the general U.S. adult population. In our attempts to measure and assure adequacy in these diets, nutrition researchers have set aside the more relevant problem of abundance that encourages over-nutrition and leads to chronic disease.

Over-consumption of total fat, saturated fat, and cholesterol is associated with an increased risk of obesity, as well as cardiovascular disease, some cancers, diabetes, and other chronic diseases. In general, the largest contributor of fat in the American diet is added oils and fats in the form of baked goods, salad dressings, candies, gravies, sauces, fried foods, and high-fat snack foods.

A recent review of the grocery receipts, menus, and the pantry contents of three Montana living facilities for people with developmental disabilities showed that higher fat meats and other foods are available in amounts beyond those recommended for good health. Interviews indicated that consumers consider many of these foods highly desirable. Pizza is a favorite; luncheon meat is a staple product; hot dogs and Hot Pockets—processed meat and cheese in a high fat crust—are all consumed regularly; TV dinners are popular.

Such preferences may have evolved into well-established food traditions. Food traditions in a residence include what foods the consumers have grown accustomed to preparing and eating over the years, and what food-related skills and methods are passed down from experienced staff members to new ones. Tradition that is firmly set can serve as a barrier, even to the most skilled and experienced consumers and service staff, in attempts to improve nutrition.

Under-nutrition

Underweight and maintaining weight can present problems for some adults with developmental disabilities (ADA Position Paper, 1997). Feeding problems arising from neuromuscular dysfunction and distracting behavior tend to be more problematic for children's nutrient intake (Springer, 1987; Pesce, 1989; Gouge, 1975). For example, cerebral palsy is associated with underweight and under-nutrition in children who experience difficulties in swallowing, chewing, or sucking due to partial paralysis of facial, tongue, and pharyngeal muscles (Sanders et al., 1990).

These problems may not be entirely resolved in the adult, but are most often addressed through specialized diets, therapies, and other supports.

In children with developmental disability, poor nutrition is considered a risk factor for secondary learning problems, which can be expected to further affect their development (Ault, Guy et al., 1994). Poor nutrition is not considered a risk factor for learning problems in adults, but this has not been examined adequately.

Persons with developmental disabilities are more likely to be taking prescribed medication for seizure tendencies, chronic infections, gastrointestinal problems, and poor circulation. Any of the common medications prescribed for these conditions, taken under particular circumstances (e.g., long-term use, in combination with other drugs) could affect the nutritional status of an individual (W. Docktor, personal interview, June, 2001). Various medications can affect food intake through side effects such as changes in the sense of taste, decreases or increases in appetite, dry mouth, or nausea.

Obesity

Obesity can be a condition secondary to the primary developmental disability and is an example of a condition that can lead to subsequent limitations. Obesity in the general population contributes to premature death, heart disease, diabetes, cancer, breathing problems, arthritis, reproductive complications, gallbladder disease, incontinence, increased surgical risk, and depression (Surgeon General *Call to Action,* 2002).

While to date little research has been done to show the same result in adults with developmental disabilities, there is no information that indicates a different effect. Further, the Surgeon General's report states, "Obesity can affect the quality of life through limited mobility and decreased physical endurance as well as through social, academic, and job discrimination." For a population at risk for decreased mobility and physical endurance already, further stress on those quality of life indicators through obesity has an even greater potential impact.

A high prevalence of obesity in adults with developmental disabilities has been recorded in both institutional and community settings (Cunningham et al., 1990; Warpula, 1981; Stewart, 1994). Data from the most recent administration of the Inventory for Client and Agency Planning (Bruinicks, Hill, Weatherman, & Woodcock, 1986) show the rates of overweight (Body Mass Index [BMI] >25) and obesity (BMI >30) to be 55% and 26% respectively for adults with developmental disabilities in Montana. Obesity in persons with developmental disabilities is attributed to behavioral factors such as inappropriate eating practices and limited mobility (ADA Position Paper, 1997) though environmental factors contributing to high rates of overweight and obesity in the general U.S. population may be important as well.

Some studies have suggested that nutritional and physical activity interventions might help prevent the development of obesity and lessen the effects of atypical body composition caused by excess adipose tissue (Shepherd et al., 1991). A program for weight management for a person with a developmental disability must address individual characteristics of motivation, food preferences, metabolic individuality, mobility, and feeding problems, as well as environmental contributors to overweight and obesity, just as a weight management program for a person without a developmental disability must address these issues.

Staffing Issues

In assisted living situations, staff members act as gatekeepers for foods entering the households; they often influence consumer choice or directly control how to plan and prepare the food. They facilitate access to snacks and foods that are not on the menus. Group home directors and direct service staff indicated in interviews with us that dietary quality among consumers is influenced by the behavior of the staff members who interact with them during meal and menu planning, grocery list generation, grocery shopping, meal preparation, and meal and snack service. For example, a direct service staff member preparing a meal of chicken and potatoes for eight residents has the latitude to cook the food in any manner he judges appropriate. "Chicken and potatoes" on the menu could mean breaded, fried chicken with home fries or it could mean a lower fat meal of roasted chicken with baked potatoes.

Interviews also revealed that staff members who are not responsible for food planning, shopping, etc., can actually undercut health-oriented efforts of the person who is responsible. For example, as part of a goal to reduce fat and sweets, a staff member may be monitoring and limiting how much ice cream is purchased and consumed in the household. If such goals are not explicit, staff members on other shifts might go to the grocery store and purchase more ice cream because the house "ran out."

Staff turnover can prove to be a barrier to improved nutrition. High turnover rates among staff prohibit extensive training and experience in food responsibilities. In addition, stable, individualized, and healthful food habits are created over time using a long-term plan. This is difficult to achieve with unstable staffing.

Suggestions for Change

Including a dietician on the treatment/support team has been shown to improve the nutritional status of children in an institutional setting (Hogan & Evers, 1997). This finding may well have application for adults with developmental disabilities who live in an institutional setting, as well as for adults who live in community-based settings that utilize a support staff.

Litchford and Wakefield (1985) found that a short program of nutrition education for direct service staff in an institutional setting improved consumers' intake of several key nutrients.

References

Brandt, E.N. & Pope, A.M. (1997). *Enabling America: Assessing the role of rehabilitation science and engineering.* Washington, DC: National Academy Press.

Cunningham, K., Gibney, M.J., Kelly, A., Kevany, J., & Mulcahy, M. (1990). Nutrient intakes in long-stay mentally handicapped persons. *British Journal of Nutrition, 64,* 3–11.

Eyman, R.K., Chaney, R.H., Givens, C.A., Lopez, E.G., & Lee, C.K.E. (1986). Medical conditions underlying increasing mortality of institutionalized persons with mental retardation. *Mental Retardation, 24,* 301–306.

Marge, M. (1988). Health promotion for persons with disabilities: Moving beyond rehabilitation. *American Journal of Health Promotion, 2,* 29–44.

Miller, C. & Eyman, R. (1978). Hospital and community mortality rates among the retarded. *Journal of Mental Deficiency Research, 22,* 137–145.

Pesce, K.A., Wodarski, L.A., & Wang, M. (1989). Nutritional status of institutionalized children and adolescents with developmental disabilities. *Research in Developmental Disabilities,* 10, 33–52.

Stewart, L. & Beange, H. (1994). A survey of dietary problems of adults with learning disabilities in the community. *Mental Handicap Research,* 7, 41–50.

Traci, M.A., Geurts, S., Seekins, T., Burke, R., & Humphries, K. (2001). *Health Status of Adult Montanans in Supported and Semi-Independent Living Arrangements.* Missoula: The University of Montana Rural Institute, Research and Training Center on Rural Rehabilitation Services.

Warpula, D. (1981). Meeting the nutritional needs of the mentally retarded. *Journal of the Canadian Dietetic Association,* 42, 310–315.

Resources

Food and Nutrition Information Center, National Agricultural Library, U.S. Department of Agriculture, AR, www.nal.usda.gov/fnic. Provides information on nutrition and food safety.

Surgeon General *Call to Action* (2002). Available at: www.surgeon general.gov/topics/obesity.

Healthy People 2010, Office of Disease Prevention and Health Promotion, www.health.gov/healthypeople. This is a set of national health objectives for the first decade of the new century.

Prader-Willi Syndrome Association, www.pwsausa.org. Provides a network of information, support services, and research to meet the needs of children and adults affected by this genetically-based developmental disability.

Food and Drug Administration, Center for Food Safety and Applied Nutrition, www.fda.gov/Food. Offers consumer advice on food safety and products.

Tufts University Health Sciences Library, www.library.tufts.edu. Provides a guide to nutrition resources on the internet, including links to health letters, journals, and nutrition associations.

Section 36.2

Nutrition for Swallowing Difficulties

People with a variety of health issues have problems swallowing and must avoid certain foods. Following these dietary guidelines can help prevent aspiration (allowing food or liquids into the lungs), which can cause pneumonia.

Generally, your doctor or other health care provider will give specific instructions on the types of foods to eat and those to avoid. Types of diets that are often used in treatment are listed in the following text.

Pureed Diet

Foods are mixed with liquid in a blender or food processor. To prepare pureed foods, chop any food into small pieces. Add 1 tablespoon liquid to every 4 tablespoons of food. Blend until soft.

Foods that can be pureed:

- Cooked cereal
- Yogurt
- Meat
- Cottage cheese
- Vegetables
- Custard/pudding
- Fruit
- Scrambled eggs
- Mashed potatoes

Liquids to use:

- For beef: Beef broth or tomato sauce
- For chicken: Broth or gravy
- For vegetables: Tomato juice or cheese sauce
- Milk, water, or fruit juice

Ground Diet

Foods on this diet must be soft and moist:

- Cooked meat with sauce or dressing
- Well-cooked pasta
- Well-moistened pancakes
- Canned or cooked fruit
- Well-cooked vegetables that are mashable with a fork
- Soft, moist cakes with icing

Soft Diet

Foods must be soft and easy to chew:

- Breads, soft rolls not toasted
- Most hot and cold cereals (milk must be added to cold cereal to achieve soft consistency)
- Cakes, pies, pudding
- Lean, tender meats and poultry
- Cooked vegetables and fruits
- Soft cookies
- Potatoes, rice, and pasta
- Cooked or canned fish
- Cheese

Avoid anything with a noticeable crunch such as with certain vegetables or fruit, nuts, pretzels, and toasted bread.

Thin Liquids

Foods are a similar consistency to water:

- Milk
- Juice
- Soft drinks
- Jell-O
- Coffee
- Hot cocoa
- Tea
- Broth
- Soups
- Ice cream (considered a liquid because it melts quickly)

Thick Liquids

Usually nectar-thick or honey-thick liquids. Any fluids can be thickened by adding thickener powders. These products are sold at most full service pharmacies, but may require a special order.

Malts and milk shakes are not suitable on a thick liquid diet because they melt quickly and become thin liquids. Ready-made nectar-thick or honey-thick liquids are preferable. However, if preparing your own thickened beverage using thickening powder, follow the instructions on the product to achieve desired consistency.

Section 36.3

Overweight and Obesity among People with Disabilities

Excerpted from "Overweight and Obesity
Among People with Disabilities," by the Centers for Disease
Control and Prevention (CDC, www.cdc.gov), 2010.

The importance of overweight and obesity related to people with disabilities is a particular problem of public health importance. Obesity is more prevalent among people with disabilities than for people without disabilities and is an important risk factor for other health conditions.

Overweight and obesity are both labels for ranges of weight that are greater than what is generally considered healthy for a given height. The terms also identify ranges of weight that have been shown to increase the likelihood of certain diseases and other health problems. Behavior, environment, and genetic factors can affect whether a person is overweight or obese.

For adults, overweight and obesity ranges are determined by using weight and height to calculate a number called the body mass index (BMI). BMI is used because, for most people, it correlates with their amount of body fat.

An adult who has a BMI between 25 and 29.9 is considered overweight. An adult who has a BMI of 30 or higher is considered obese. Among children of the same age and sex, overweight is defined on CDC growth charts as a BMI at or above the 85th percentile and lower than the 95th percentile. Obesity is defined as having a BMI at or above the 95th percentile.

The Obesity Epidemic

Obesity rates for adults with disabilities are approximately 57% higher than adults without disabilities. Thirty-six percent of adults with disabilities are obese, compared to 23% of adults without disabilities.

Obesity rates for children age 2–17 with disabilities are approximately 38% higher than for children without disabilities. Twenty-two percent of children with disabilities are obese, compared to 16% of children without disabilities.

Obesity affects different people in different ways and may increase the risk for other health conditions among people with and without disabilities:

- Children and adults with mobility limitations and intellectual or learning disabilities are at greatest risk for obesity.

- Twenty percent of children 10 through 17 years of age who have special health care needs are obese compared with 15% of children of the same ages without special health care needs.

- Annual health care costs of obesity that are related to disability are estimated at approximately $44 billion.

Here are some facts about obesity in the United States:

- More than one third of adults—more than 72 million people—in the United States are obese.

- Obesity rates are significantly higher among racial and ethnic groups. Non-Hispanic Blacks or African Americans have a 51% higher obesity prevalence and Hispanics have a 21% higher obesity prevalence than non-Hispanic Whites.

- Annual health care costs of obesity for all adults in the United States were estimated to be as high as $147 billion dollars for 2008.

Challenges Facing People with Disabilities

People with disabilities can find it more difficult to always eat healthy, control their weight, and be physically active. This might be due to the following:

- A lack of healthy food choices

- Difficulty with chewing or swallowing food, or with the taste or texture of foods

- Medications that can contribute to weight gain, weight loss, and changes in appetite

- Physical limitations that can reduce a person's ability to exercise

- Pain

- A lack of energy

- A lack of accessible environments (for example, sidewalks, parks, and exercise equipment) that can enable exercise

- A lack of resources (for example, money; transportation; and social support from family, friends, neighbors, and community members)

Health Consequences of Overweight and Obesity

Overweight and obesity increases the risk of a number of other conditions, including the following:

- Coronary heart disease

- Type 2 diabetes

- Cancers (endometrial, breast, and colon)

- High blood pressure

- Lipid disorders (for example, high total cholesterol or high levels of triglycerides)

- Stroke

- Liver and gallbladder disease

- Sleep apnea and respiratory problems

- Osteoarthritis (a degeneration of cartilage and its underlying bone within a joint)

- Gynecological problems (abnormal periods, infertility)

Chapter 37

Physical Activity for People with Disabilities

Chapter Contents

Section 37.1—Exercise Guidelines... 348

Section 37.2—Yoga for People with Disabilities....................... 352

Section 37.1

Exercise Guidelines

General Exercise Guidelines

Exercise is for **every** body. This slogan appears in a number of places on the NCPAD (National Center on Physical Activity and Disability) website, and for a very good reason. Exercise is a key factor in maintaining and improving overall health. In 1996, the Surgeon General of the United States reported that "significant health benefits can be obtained with a moderate amount of physical activity, preferably daily." More recently, the 2008 Physical Activity Guidelines for Americans provides science-based guidance to help individuals with disabilities aged 6 and older improve their health through appropriate physical activity. These benefits are even more important if you have a disability, since people with disabilities have a tendency to live less active lifestyles. Yet, it is just as important for your body to get exercise. This text provides some general exercise guidelines you should review. Throughout the text are resources on physical activity and exercise programs of all sorts: Indoor and outdoor, sports or recreational, solitary or team. It doesn't matter what you choose, so long as you choose to get a moderate amount of physical activity each day.

Benefits of Regular Physical Activity and Exercise

- Increased cardiac (heart) and pulmonary (lung) function
- Improved ability to perform activities of daily living
- Protection against development of chronic diseases
- Decreased anxiety and depression

- Enhanced feeling of well-being
- Weight control
- Lowered cholesterol and blood pressure

Before You Begin

1. Inform your physician or primary caregiver that you are considering starting an exercise program.

2. If possible, participate in a graded exercise test to determine your current level of fitness.

3. Find out the effects of your medication on exercise.

4. If possible, consult a trained exercise professional for an individualized exercise prescription.

Safety Considerations

- Stop exercising if you experience pain, discomfort, nausea, dizziness, lightheadedness, chest pain, irregular heartbeat, shortness of breath, or clammy hands.
- Drink plenty of fluids, especially water.
- Wear appropriate clothing.
- Set realistic short-term and long-term goals.
- Find and follow an exercise program that meets your specific goals.

Kinds of Exercise

- **Cardiovascular:** Primarily benefits your heart, circulatory system, and lungs.
- **Strength and muscle endurance:** Primarily benefits you by making you stronger and/or giving you better endurance, so you can do things longer.
- **Flexibility:** Primarily aimed at giving you greater range of motion in joints and more suppleness in your body.

Common Exercise Terms

- **Heart Rate (HR):** Determine your heart rate by finding your pulse. Place a finger on the thumb side of the bottom of your forearm or against the side of your neck, and count your pulse beat for 15 seconds. Multiply this figure by four to calculate your heart rate per minute. Note that as you exercise more regularly, your heart rate should decrease.

- **Maximum Heart Rate:** Subtract your age from 220 to determine your maximum heart rate. Example: a 40-year-old person would have a maximum heart rate of 180 (220 - 40 = 180).

- **Target Heart Rate:** Calculated at 60% to 80% of your maximum heart rate. For the range's lower cutoff point, multiply .60 to your maximum heart rate; for the top cutoff point, multiply .80 to your maximum heart rate. In the previous example, this calculates a range of 108 to 144 beats per minute.

- **Blood Pressure (BP):** A measure of the blood's pressure upon the arterial walls which consists of two values; systolic blood pressure, as the heart contracts or pumps the blood to the circulatory system (90 to 140 mmHg), and diastolic blood pressure, as the heart fills up with blood following a contraction (60 to 90 mmHg). If possible, have a trained professional monitor your blood pressure throughout the exercise session.

- **Ratings of Perceived Exertion (RPE):** This is a scale of how hard you feel you are exercising. The Borg scale ranges from 6 to 20. To use the scale, monitor how you feel while exercising, with a general goal of 12 to 13 RPE.

Other Considerations

- **Intensity** (how hard?): Intensity can vary from very light to very hard and can be monitored on the basis of training heart rate or your own subjective impression of how hard you are working.

- **Frequency** (how many?): Start with 3 days a week and work towards 7 days a week.

- **Duration** (how long?): Begin with a minimum of 20 minutes throughout a day with a goal of increasing to 60 minutes a day. This can be done in multiple 10-minute sessions or in one longer session.

- **Mode** (what kind?): Structured (walking, running, cycling, swimming, resistance training) or unstructured (gardening, household cleaning, walking to work)

Exercise Routine

- **Warm-up:** Five minutes of light activity, such as slow walking or cycling

- **Activity:** Cardiovascular, muscular strength, or flexibility training

- **Cool down:** Five minutes of light activity with some flexibility exercises built in

Suggestions for Each Type of Exercise

Cardiovascular

- Vary your workout each session.

- Be creative! Enhance your exercise routine by walking throughout the day: During lunch and coffee breaks, around the house during commercials.

- Choose a pace that feels good to you; use the Ratings of Perceived Exertion scale or the "Conversation Rule"—you should be able to converse while exercising.

- Take slow, deep breaths and "think tall" to maintain good posture.

- Types of cardiovascular training: Walking (outside, treadmill), cycling (outside, stationary bicycle, ergometer), and swimming

Strength

- Perform each movement through a complete range of motion.

- Do not hold your breath while strength training. Instead, exhale or breathe out while pushing the weight up or out and inhale or breathe in while letting the weight down or in. "Think tall" to maintain your posture.

- If your goal is to increase your muscular endurance, you should use lighter weights and perform eight to 12 repetitions.

- If your goal is to increase your muscular strength, you should use heavier weights and perform five to eight repetitions.

- Types of strength training: Weight machines, free weights, plastic tubing, "toys" (medicine balls, plastic buoys), and circuit training

Flexibility/Functionality

- The focus of flexibility/functionality work is to improve range of motion, balance, coordination, and ability to carry out the regular activities of daily living.
- Flexibility training should be incorporated before and after every cardiovascular and strength workout.
- Be sure to hold stretches and progress slowly.
- Every muscle group used in a workout should be thoroughly stretched. Spend more time on tight muscle groups.
- Stretching should not be painful.
- Types of flexibility training: Stretching, yoga, Pilates

Section 37.2

Yoga for People with Disabilities

Yoga is an ancient Indian practice which involves moving the body and training the mind to achieve balance and well-being. The purpose of traditional yoga is for each individual to be healthy, both physically and mentally, and able to reach his or her highest potential as a person.

Although there are different schools of traditional yoga (i.e., Bhakti Yoga, Karma Yoga, Patanjali's Ashtanga Yoga, Jnana Yoga, Kundalini Yoga, Swara Yoga, Raja Yoga, Kriya Yoga, and Mantra Yoga), Hatha Yoga is the most popular form practiced in the West. Hatha yoga's aim is to prepare the body for meditation through breathing and physical exercises. Hatha yoga emphasizes body-mind wellness through postures or asanas which tone and strengthen our muscles and increase our flexibility. The different asanas, particularly the twists and inversions, stimulate internal organs, as well as the nervous system, and promote circulation in all the body's major organs and glands. Research has shown that the practice of yoga as a lifestyle enhances overall health and prevents and reverses disease. (See References).

Yoga can be beneficial for individuals with disabilities or chronic health conditions through both the physical postures and breathwork. Each pose can be modified or adapted to meet the needs of the student. Yoga asanas can be performed while seated in a chair or wheelchair. Chair Yoga: The Sitting Mountain Series by Voelker-Binder was developed for individuals with arthritis, chronic obstructive pulmonary disease, multiple sclerosis, Parkinson's disease, osteoporosis, or stroke. Moreover, with time, the effects of the breathwork can affect a state of calm and renewal in one's life. Brown and Gerberg (2005) concluded that Sudarshan Kriya yoga (SKY), a sequence of specific breathing techniques (ujjayi or loud breathing, Bhastrika or Bellows Breath, and Sudarshan Kriya, a powerful, rhythmic breathing technique) can alleviate anxiety, depression, everyday stress, post-traumatic stress, and stress-related medical illnesses.

Having mentioned the benefits of yoga practice, it should be noted that yoga is used to complement an individual's already established medical care, therapy program, and exercise regime.

Components of Hatha Yoga

Pranayama or breathwork: Pranayama is the science of proper breathing (Sumar, 1998). Breathing is a body process that is both autonomic and controllable. Most people find when they are anxious, their breath becomes quick and shallow. The simple process of slowing the breath down and breathing deeper has an immediate calming effect.

Belly breathing: Basic yoga breathing involves breathing in and out through the nose. Inhale, gently push the belly out, expanding the diaphragm first. Exhale, pulling the belly in at the end of the exhalation. This last movement pushes the air completely out of the lower portion of the lungs, removing all the toxins of the used air from the lungs. [From: www.hathayogalesson.com]

Asanas or physical postures: The physical movements in yoga, asanas are gentle and non-strenuous stretches of the limbs and joints. These postures are coordinated with the breath and allow blood to circulate and vitalize every organ. Many asanas are modeled after movements that occur in nature such as tree, mountain, cat, dog, and cobra. Asanas focus on moving the joints through their full range of motion and lengthening muscles. The asanas are learned over time and with regular practice. They are meant to be held and are performed slowly and meditatively, combined with deep breathing.

Dhyana or meditation: Meditation usually refers to a state of extreme relaxation and concentration in which the body is generally at rest and the mind cleared of surface thoughts. The result is self-realization, and a clearer vision of life and the world.

Benefits of Yoga

Overall health benefits can be seen in:

- **Digestive system:** Bending and stretching poses help move and stimulate the digestive system.

- **Cardiovascular and cardiopulmonary systems:** Specific types of yoga can be a good form of aerobic exercise that increases one's heart rate. The practice of pranayama helps expand lung capacity and heart strength.

- **Lymphatic system:** This is a primary component of an individual's immune system. Unlike blood, the lymphatic system has no pump. Instead it relies on muscle activity and body movement for circulation. Physical activity and stretching (yoga asanas) propels lymph, but it will also develop strong muscles that continually encourage lymph movement. Regular practice of pranayama stimulates the action of the lungs, diaphragm, and thorax which are a primary pump for the lymph fluid (Allbritton, 2003).

- **Skeletal system and muscular systems:** Asanas encourage the individual to keep his or her body in proper alignment. Regular yoga practice strengthens the muscles and increases overall flexibility.

Developmental benefits include:

- Developmental milestones are reached.

- Motor coordination is enhanced.

- Increased body awareness and orientation are achieved.

- Yoga practices develop focus and concentration.

- Yoga games encourage learning, creativity, and imagination.

Yoga Instruction for Children and Youth with Disabilities

Due to yoga's increasing popularity in the United States, numerous books, DVDs, audio tapes, and CDs are available that can aid in learning the philosophy and practice of the different types of yoga. However, for individuals with disabilities or chronic health conditions, it is best to learn yoga from a certified yoga therapist or yoga instructor who has the experience and background knowledge in teaching children and youth with disabilities.

The International Association of Yoga Therapists and Yoga for the Special Child websites are among the institutions that provide listings of yoga therapists.

In a yoga class for individuals with disabilities, yoga asanas are modified or adapted, and may be performed with the instructor's active assistance as needed. Although the instructor assists the child in getting into and out of a posture, keep in mind that the child is still doing the "work." Children should start with one-to-one yoga instruction, then progress to group classes when the child is ready—and if it is the least restrictive environment for the child, as determined by the yoga instructor and parent.

Teaching Guidelines for Yoga Instructors

Before the very first yoga session with a student, the yoga instructor needs to do an initial assessment of the student's current strength and endurance, physical challenges (i.e., spasticity, hypertonicity, hypotonicity, etc.) or barriers. An interview with the student's parent or guardian is helpful in getting information on any medications that the student is currently taking, or recently stopped taking. This may affect the student's physical, mental, and emotional states. In addition, certain medications may make it unsafe to let the student do inversion asanas. The yoga instructor should then consult with the student's physician, explain the different asanas that may be used in the student's program, and ascertain which asanas are safe for the student to practice.

In addition, knowledge of other medical conditions, such as epilepsy, prepares the instructor to handle an epileptic seizure if and when one does occur. Designing the yoga session to focus more on meditation and relaxation can aid in decreasing the frequency and duration of seizures (Yardi, 2001). Information about a student's diet at home and in school is also helpful. A student's behavior and attention span during the yoga session may be affected by the student's diet, specifically the lack of vital nutrients in the diet.

355

When designing an appropriate yoga session for the student, the personality, behavior, and attention span of the student should be taken into consideration.

If a student is agitated, hyperactive, or easily distracted, the instructor may have the student spend less time in each asana and more time doing music therapy and pranayama. Choose asanas that build focus and concentration, and are calming at the same time. Making a game or a storytelling activity incorporating the asanas keeps the student on task and involved in the yoga session. The instructor should be creative with each session, while adhering to the main structure of the class. If an instructor is leading a group class (45–50 minutes), he or she is still expected to give equal time, attention, and/or assistance to each student as much as possible.

Yoga Equipment

An advantage of incorporating yoga practice as part of an individual's exercise program is that it does not require any fancy equipment. Yoga can be practiced anywhere—indoors, outdoors on the grass, or even on sand at the beach. Typically, a yoga mat or rug is used. Latex-free and eco-friendly mats are also available. Having some facial tissue within arms' reach comes in handy during breathing exercises when the individual needs to clear his/ her nostrils. Yoga props such as blocks and straps aid in practicing an asana safely, as well as help the individual go deeper into a pose. An eye pillow and a light blanket can be used during deep relaxation.

A Typical Yoga Class for Children and Youth

A typical yoga class for infants is usually 30 minutes long. Group or one-to-one classes for children and youth last for 45 minutes. The components in a typical yoga session for children and youth with disabilities are discussed in the following sections.

Start the class by having the student sit cross-legged (independently or with assistance) on the floor.

I. Chanting or Music Therapy

Begin the yoga session with Chanting or Music therapy. This activity brings the child's focus into the yoga session. The instructor leads the student into chanting three "Oms" (or substitute "Om" with "Peace," or "Love"). This is usually followed by singing the phrase "Hari Om" (or use any short song or nursery rhyme that the child is familiar with).

This activity starts with slow singing, then progresses to faster singing of the phrase/song. Hand movements, such as clapping rhythmically to the song, can be incorporated into the activity. The chanting and the hand movements that go with it encourages concentration and attention; stimulates the diaphragm, lungs, and vocal chords; and develops motor coordination.

II. Pranayama or Breathing Exercises

The Cleansing Breath is an ideal practice for children with asthma, sinus conditions, and bronchial congestion. Place one hand on the belly to feel the movement during this particular breathing exercise. With the other hand, hold a piece of facial tissue in front of the face. Take a slow, deep breath in, followed by a very quick, forced exhalation. The student should be able to see the tissue move with the exhalation.

The Bellows Breath is a highly energizing, rapid-breathing exercise, providing many of the same benefits as the Cleansing Breath. These vigorous in-and-out movements of the abdomen strengthen the diaphragm; saturate the lungs and blood with freshly oxygenated air; and aid in digestion, thereby benefiting the entire body. Bhavanani, Madanmohan, & Udupa (2003) found that visual reaction time (VRT) and auditory reaction time (ART) significantly decreased in school-aged boys who practiced nine rounds of bellows breath or mukh bhastrika. Reaction time (RT) is an index of the processing ability of the central nervous system and a simple means of determining sensory-motor performance. The authors recommended the practice of Bellows breath to individuals with prolonged RT, such as children with intellectual disabilities and older adults. Place one hand on the belly to feel the movement during this particular breathing exercise. Start with a rapid inhalation, immediately followed with a rapid exhalation. Start with doing one set of 10. Encourage the student to clear the nose after each set. For children, a helpful cue is to have their breathing imitate that of a "choo-choo" train.

Alternate Nostril Breathing calms the mind; strengthens the entire nervous system and helps to balance the right and left hemispheres of the brain; strengthens the immune system; stimulates digestion; and develops concentration.

1. With the right hand, keep the thumb, ring, and pinkie fingers up, while the index and middle fingers are down/tucked. This hand gesture is known as Vishnu mudra. The thumb will cover the right nostril, while both the ring and pinkie fingers will cover the left nostril.

357

2. Close the right nostril with the thumb, and take a deep inhale through the left nostril.

3. Hold the breath in, closing both nostrils.

4. Keeping the left nostril closed, exhale slowly through the right nostril.

5. Take a deep inhale through the right nostril, hold the breath, and exhale slowly through the left nostril.

6. Repeat the exercise.

III. Eye Exercises

Eye exercises: These exercises strengthen and relax the eye muscles, as well as stimulate the optic nerve. The following exercise is good for beginners:

1. Sit cross-legged on the floor (or sit comfortably on a chair) with the body properly aligned; eyes are closed.

2. Slowly open the eyes and bring the right hand in front of the face (an arm's length distance). All the fingers are tucked in a fist except for the thumb, with the thumbnail facing toward the face.

3. Instruct the student to move the right hand up. With eyes wide open, track the thumb with the eyes only without blinking. Stop when the eyes cannot see the thumb anymore.

4. With the gaze relaxed and steady, follow as the right hand moves back to center.

5. Repeat this exercise, moving the hand down—back to center— right—back to center—left—back to center.

6. After this set, rub the palms together until some warmth is generated. Gently cup the hands over the eyes ("palming") and relax.

7. Do another set of eye exercises. At the last set of exercises, end with palming and gently massage the eyelids with the fingertips, then massaging other areas of the face, neck, and shoulders.

IV. Yoga Asanas

Yoga asanas: The asanas practiced in each yoga session is determined by the instructor based on the student's needs and goals. When teaching a new asana, the instructor can start by breaking down the pose into its basic components, progressing on to the next component when the student is ready.

Typically, the student warms up with a set series of specific asanas, called the Sun Salutations. Komitor and Adamson's (2000) text provides a kid-friendly reference card showing the sun salutations for children. Budilovsky & Adamson (2003) provide instruction on the Seated Sun Salutations.

The instructor then leads the student into individual asana practice after the warm-up. The asanas practiced should be a balanced set which include postures that work on balance, strength, and flexibility; twists and inversions; forward and backward bends; postures done in the following positions: Seated, standing, prone, and supine.

V. Deep Relaxation

Deep relaxation: This is an important part of the yoga session in that it helps the student learn how to relax his or her body. Deep relaxation provides an opportunity for the body to slow down and absorb all the energy from the yoga practice. It is also a practice in stillness.

With the lights dimmed, relaxing music playing, and distractions in the room removed, the student is asked to go into shavasana or the Corpse Pose. Shavasana consists of comfortably lying supine on the floor, with the arms to the side, palms facing up. The feet are about shoulders-width apart. A blanket may be placed over the body for warmth. An eye pillow may be placed over the eyes to let them relax in darkness.

To facilitate relaxation, the student is verbally cued to bring awareness to his or her breath. If the student is responsive to massage, the instructor can perform gentle massages starting from the feet and up, giving attention to areas of the body that are tense.

Another technique that can help the student relax is by facilitating progressive relaxation. Here, the instructor verbally cues the student to consciously contract or tense the muscle and then consciously relax the muscle. The exercise starts with contracting and relaxing the muscles of the feet and legs, and then progresses up the body toward the head.

Then, slowly let the student out of deep relaxation. Cue the student to deepen the breath. With eyes still closed, let the student become aware of his or her surroundings. Have the student start to move their fingers and toes, and then gently stretch their body as if they were about to get up from a brief nap. Have the student slowly roll over to the right side, in a fetal position. When the student is ready, come up to a seated position.

VI. End of the Yoga Session

End of session: End the session by chanting "Om" three times. Then have the child place the palms together in front of the body and say "Namaste," which means "I recognize and honor the divine light in you!" (Komitor & Adamson, 2000).

Resources for Teaching and Learning Yoga

Books

Heriza, N. (2004). *Dr. Yoga: A complete program for discovering the head-to-toe benefits of yoga.* New York, NY: Tarcher/Penguin.

Sumar, S. (1998). *Yoga for the special child: A therapeutic approach for infants and children with Down syndrome, cerebral palsy, learning disabilities.* Buckingham, Vermont: Special Yoga Publications; Route 1.

Websites

Yoga for the Special Child [www.specialyoga.com]: A schedule for *Yoga for the Special Child* Teacher Training Programs is posted on their website.

Chair Yoga: The Sitting Mountain Series (CD) by Lakshmi Voelker: yogawithlakshmi.com

YogaKids: www.yogakids.com

Hatha Yoga Lesson website: www.hathayogalesson.com

Instructional Video

Yoga with a Master (Hatha Yoga video recommended by Cedars-Sinai Preventive and Rehabilitative Cardiac Center): iymagazine.org/shop.html

Organizations

Yoga for the Special Child: Sarasota, Florida [www.ncpad.org/organizations/index.php?id=850&state=Florida&city=Sarasota]

Rehabilitation Institute of Chicago: Chicago, Illinois [www.ncpad.org/organizations/index.php?id=1208&state=Illinois&city=Chicago]

Books

Heriza, N. (2004). *Dr. Yoga: A complete program for discovering the head-to-toe benefits of yoga.* New York, NY: Tarcher/Penguin.

Sumar S. (1998). *Yoga for the special child: A therapeutic approach for infants and children with Down syndrome, cerebral palsy, learning disabilities.* Buckingham, Vermont: Special Yoga Publications; Route 1.

Journals

Bastille, J. V., & Gill-Body, K. M. (2004). A yoga-based exercise program for people with chronic poststroke hemiparesis. *Physical Therapy,* 84(1), 33–48.

Bhavanani, A. B., Madanmohan, & Udupa, K. (2003). Acute effect of Mukh bhastrika (a yogic bellows type breathing) on reaction time. *Indian Journal of Physiology and Pharmacology,* 47(3), 297–300.

Bijlani, R. L., Vempati, R. P., Yadav, R. K., Ray, R. B., Gupta, V., Sharma, R., et al. (2005). A brief but comprehensive lifestyle education program based on yoga reduces risk factors for cardiovascular disease and diabetes mellitus. *Journal of Alternative and Complementary Medicine,* 11(2), 267–274.

Shannahoff-Khalsa, D. S., Sramek, B. B., Kennel, M. B., & Jamieson, S. W. (2004). Hemodynamic observations on a yogic breathing technique claimed to help eliminate and prevent heart attacks: A pilot study. *Journal of Alternative and Complementary Medicine,* 10(5), 757–766.

Harinath, K., Malhotra, A. S., Pal, K., Prasad, R., Kumar, R., Kain, T. C., et al. (2004). Effects of Hatha yoga and Omkar meditation on cardiorespiratory performance, psychologic profile, and melatonin secretion. *Journal of Alternative and Complementary Medicine,* 10(2), 261–268.

Brown, R. P., & Gerberg, P. L. (2005). Sudarshan Kriya yogic breathing in the treatment of stress, anxiety, and depression: Part I-neurophysiologic model. *Journal of Alternative and Complementary Medicine,* 11(1), 189–201.

Birkel, D. A., & Edgren, L. (2000). Hatha yoga: Improved vital capacity of college students. *Alternative Therapies in Health and Medicine,* 6(6), 55–63.

DeMayo, W., Singh, B., Duryea, B., & Riley, D. (2004). Hatha yoga and meditation in patients with post-polio syndrome. *Alternative Therapies in Health and Medicine,* 10(2), 24–25.

Galantino, M. L., Bzdewka, T. M., Eissler-Russo, J. L., Holbrook, M. L., Mogck, E. P., Geigle, P., et al. (2004). The impact of modified Hatha yoga on chronic low back pain: A pilot study. *Alternative Therapies in Health and Medicine,* 10(2), 56–59.

McIver, S., O'Halloran, P., & McGartland, M. (2004). The impact of Hatha yoga on smoking behavior. *Alternative Therapies in Health and Medicine,* 10(2), 22–23.

Jacobs, B. P., Mehling, W., Avins, A. L., Goldberg, H. A., Acree, M., Lasater, J. H., et al. (2004). Feasibility of conducting a clinical trial on Hatha yoga for chronic low back pain: Methodological lessons. *Alternative Therapies in Health and Medicine,* 10(2), 80–83.

Riley, D. (2004). Hatha yoga and the treatment of illness. *Alternative Therapies in Health and Medicine,* 10(2), 20–21.

Garfinkel, M., & Schumacher, H. R., Jr. (2000). Yoga. *Rheumatic Diseases Clinics of North America,* 26(1), 125–132.

Jayasinghe, S. R. (2004). Yoga in cardiac health (a review). *European Journal of Cardiovascular Prevention and Rehabilitation,* 11(5), 369–375.

Kreitzer, M. J., Gross, C. R., Ye, X., Russas, V., & Treesak, C. (2005). Longitudinal impact of mindfulness meditation on illness burden in solid-organ transplant recipients. *Progress in Transplantation,* 15(2), 166–172.

Oken, B. S., Kishiyama, S., Zajdel, D., Bourdette, D., Carlsen, J., Haas, M., et al. (2004). Randomized controlled trial of yoga and exercise in multiple sclerosis. *Neurology,* 62(11), 2058–2064.

Ott, M. J. (2002). Yoga as a clinical intervention. *Advance for Nurse Practitioners,* 10(1), 81–83, 90.

Ripoll, E., & Mahowald, D. (2002). Hatha yoga therapy management of urologic disorders. *World Journal of Urology,* 20(5), 306–309.

Tran, M. D., Holly, R. G., Lashbrook, J., & Amsterdam, E. A. (2001). Effects of Hatha yoga practice on the health-related aspects of physical fitness. *Preventive Cardiology,* 4(4), 165–170.

Yardi, N. (2001). Yoga for control of epilepsy. *Seizure,* 10(1), 7–12.

Chapter 38

Personal Hygiene for People with Disabilities

Chapter Contents

Section 38.1—Dental Care 364

Section 38.2—How to Bathe Someone with a Disability 365

Section 38.1

Dental Care

Excerpted from "Dental Care Every Day: A Caregiver's Guide," by the National Institute of Dental and Craniofacial Research (NIDCR, www .nidcr.nih.gov), part of the National Institutes of Health, April 2011.

Taking care of someone with a developmental disability requires patience and skill. As a caregiver, you know this as well as anyone does. You also know how challenging it is to help that person with dental care. It takes planning, time, and the ability to manage physical, mental, and behavioral problems. Dental care isn't always easy, but you can make it work for you and the person you help. This text will show you how to help someone brush, floss, and have a healthy mouth.

Everyone needs dental care every day. Brushing and flossing are crucial activities that affect our health. In fact, dental care is just as important to your client's health and daily routine as taking medications and getting physical exercise. A healthy mouth helps people eat well, avoid pain and tooth loss, and feel good about themselves.

If the person you care for is unable to brush, these suggestions might be helpful.

- First, wash your hands and put on disposable gloves. Sit or stand where you can see all of the surfaces of the teeth.

- Be sure to use a regular or power toothbrush with soft bristles.

- Use a pea-size amount of toothpaste with fluoride, or none at all. Toothpaste bothers people who have swallowing problems. If this is the case for the person you care for, brush with water instead.

- Brush the front, back, and top of each tooth. Gently brush back and forth in short strokes.

- Gently brush the tongue after you brush the teeth.

- Help the person rinse with plain water. Give people who can't rinse a drink of water or consider sweeping the mouth with a finger wrapped in gauze.

Flossing cleans between the teeth where a toothbrush can't reach. Many people with disabilities need a caregiver to help them floss. Flossing is a tough job that takes a lot of practice. Waxed, unwaxed, flavored, or plain floss all do the same thing. The person you care for might like one more than another, or a certain type might be easier to use.

Section 38.2

How to Bathe Someone with a Disability

"Bathing How-To's for Parents with Alzheimer's Disease" © 2011 AgingCare, LLC. All rights reserved. Reprinted with permission. AgingCare.com is a leading online community that connects people caring for elderly parents to other caregivers, personalized information, and local resources. Aging-Care.com has become the trusted resource for exchanging ideas, sharing conversations, and finding credible information for those seeking elder care solutions. For more information, visit www.agingcare.com.

There are a wealth of questions on how to get aging parents to bathe—especially when the elderly has Alzheimer's or severe dementia.

One consideration is how often do elderly parents need to bathe? Since the United States is a melting pot of people from around the world, we have different cultures with different views on what staying clean means. In my high plains area, many of the generation now in their 80s and 90s grew up with weekly baths—sometimes because they lived out on farms and water was too precious to waste. For others, that routine was just normal behavior. We bratty "kids" would mutter under our breath they would bathe when they were "ripe enough."

All of this is to say that if your elder won't shower every single day, he or she is not going to die of some dreadful disease caused by "lack of bath" syndrome. For some elders, some fairly clean clothes and a weekly bath is what they consider enough. However, there are other issues to consider.

Watch for change in attitude. A change in attitude is a key component with bathing, as it is with many aging issues. Is the change in bathing habits due to memory loss, confusion, or fear?

If your elder has dementia, then you may have a more difficult situation on your hands. People can think they have just showered, but in reality that was last week. Or, they can become confused when they begin the process, and rather than tell someone they are confused, they just avoid it. Or they can become afraid of the shower or bath because they don't know what it's all about or they think they will get hurt.

Think about how frightening it would be to have water pouring down on your head when you can't figure out the reason. Confusion and lack of understanding are bound to lead to fear.

Tips for Getting Your Alzheimer's Parents to Take a Bath

What can caregivers do about Alzheimer's and bathing?

- If you feel that the reason your mom isn't bathing is that she thinks she has already taken a bath, or that she just doesn't see the point, try tying her bath to something fun. Say something like, "Let's both get cleaned up and pretty and we'll go for lunch." This could nudge her into thinking it's worth her while, and even fun, to spruce up.

- Make sure the shower and/or bath are safe and comfortable. If the bathroom tends to be cool, see if there is a way it can be warmed up before a bath. If a shower is the best route to go for the person, install a grab bar to for stability while getting in, a comfortable stool to sit on, and a hand-held shower head. This type of shower head keeps the water from continually coming down on the person's head, so the elder is forewarned when it's hair washing time.

- If dementia, such as Alzheimer's, is so advanced that the elder is frightened of water, or scared of the tub or shower, you may want to try a different tactic. A person can get clean with sponge baths.

- Whether you are using a sponge bath method or helping the person with a shower, talk about what you will do next, taking into consideration the person's dementia and where they are mentally. Don't surprise them. Describe your every move in a low, soothing voice. Say, "I'm going to wipe your face with this nice warm cloth, okay?" "I'm going to lift your arm and wash, but I'm keeping you warm and comfortable under this blanket."

- Find products like dry shampoos so you don't have to wash hair as often.

- Take privacy and modesty into consideration. Some people, my mother-in-law being one of them, don't want family or others close to them to bathe them. My mother-in-law was a very modest woman. We were great friends and she let me do anything for her but give her a shower. We found that hiring an in-home agency to come and bathe her worked best. I would be at her condo when the person came, but the woman who arrived for the bath looked like a nurse in a hospital. This made the nudity more bearable for her. Also, agency people are trained, so if you find a good agency, they may be able to cope much better than family members.

- Remember that a daily bath isn't necessary. Also, please ask yourself if all the fuss is because of your own standards and what people will think of you if your mom isn't pristine all the time, or if it's really about her health and comfort. Try to compromise. Yes, cleanliness is important for good health. But a complete bath or shower daily is not next to godliness. It could be closer to torture for your loved one. Try to find alternatives and a middle ground so that some sort of hygiene is maintained with a minimum of unpleasantness.

Depression Could Lead to Not Bathing: Depression Could Be at Fault

Another issue that may contribute to an elderly parent whose bathing and grooming habits take a turn for the worse is depression. My mother was a clean freak, and she loved her daily bath. Her clothes needed to be fresh daily, preferably smelling of springtime.

When she made the decision to move to the nursing home where my dad lived, she went through the expected period of depression. One of the major clues was that she would put on the same clothes every day. Some of this was simply that she saw them laying on a chair and forgot that they'd been worn. However, some of change in her behavior was because she was temporarily depressed.

Depressed people often don't care about personal hygiene. They don't care about their clothes. The just don't care in general. If you see this happening to your elder, then you have a reason to be concerned. My mother's depression lifted as she adjusted to the nursing home. I tried to hurry that along by buying her some new clothes and making good use of the nursing home beauty shop. These steps helped, and she was soon back to being to her clean-freak self.

If her depression hadn't lifted, I would have asked the doctor to consider treating her for depression. If you find your elder has changed from a very clean person to one who doesn't care about appearances at all, you may want to consider a checkup to see if depression is at the bottom of this change. This depression is especially prominent after the death of a spouse.

Chapter 39

Bowel and Bladder Problems Associated with Disability

Bowel System: Common Problems

Listed in the following text are common bowel problems, symptoms, and management techniques.

Constipation—The Inability to Have a Bowel Movement for Three or More Days

Symptoms

- Hard stools
- Inability to have a bowel movement in many days
- Feeling bloated in the stomach area

Causes

- Insufficient fluid intake (less than 1 liter per day)
- Inactivity
- Poor diet—low in fiber-containing foods such as fruit, vegetables, and whole grains

---

This chapter includes text from "Bowel System: Common Problems," May 2011, and "Urinary System Overview," July 2010, Copyright Rehabilitation Institute of Chicago. All rights reserved. Reprinted with permission. For additional information, visit the website of the LIFE Center at the Rehabilitation Center of Chicago, http://lifecenter.ric.org.

- Side effects of medicines—especially iron, codeine, and pain medication

- Repeatedly ignoring urge to move bowels

Treatment

- Drink at least six to eight glasses of fluid each day.

- Eat a diet high in fiber.

- Ask the doctor about using a stool softener or laxative.

- If constipation persists, ask your doctor about using suppositories or an enema.

Any person with a spinal cord injury who experiences the above symptoms along with abdominal pain that does not go away after removal of the stool should contact their physician immediately. This may be a sign of autonomic dysreflexia, a serious condition of overactivity of the nervous system. Autonomic dysreflexia can happen to people who have injuries at or above T6.

Impaction—Hard Stool Plugging the Rectum

Symptoms

- Hard stools
- Bloated feeling in the stomach
- Leaking of loose or liquid stool

Causes

- Insufficient fluid intake
- Inactivity
- Poor diet
- Side effect of medications
- Chronic constipation

Treatment

Many people who experience impactions are able to remove the stool by hand. Check with your physician or health care provider to find out if this is appropriate.

Diarrhea—Loose or Liquid Stool, Usually Three or More Times a Day

Symptom

- Large amounts of loose or watery stool

Causes

- Illness, such as a cold or flu
- Poor diet, including too much spicy or greasy food
- Excessive use of laxatives or stool softeners

Treatment

- Do a rectal check looking for impaction.
- Check with your health care provider regarding the use of specific fiber supplements.
- Stop all laxatives and stool softeners.
- Drink plenty of fluids.

Hemorrhoids—Swelling or Bleeding of Tissue around the Rectum

Symptoms

- Red, bulging areas inside or outside the rectum
- Pain or rectal bleeding after a bowel movement

Causes

- Long history of hard stools or constipation
- Removal of stool by hand

Treatment

- Use medications ordered by doctor such as Anusol or Preparation H.
- If stool is hard, follow guidelines for constipation in preceding text.
- Drink plenty of liquids.

Incontinence—Problems Controlling Bowel Movements

Symptoms

- Inability to start or stop bowel movements
- Lack of awareness of bowel movements

Causes

- Decreased mobility
- Inability to communicate the need to use the toilet
- Side effects of medication
- Uncontrolled diarrhea

Treatment

- Assess bowel habits to find a pattern. Some people have bowel movements every day; others have bowel movements every 2 or 3 days. Try to anticipate when a bowel movement might occur and sit on the toilet at that time.
- Sit on the toilet after eating for 30 minutes up to an hour.
- Avoid using a bed pan as much as possible; use the toilet or a commode.
- Check with your health care provider about using suppositories to regulate bowel movements.

Urinary System Overview

After a disabling event, it is common for bladder habits to change. Some people have problems emptying the bladder, while others may have urinary accidents. The first step in learning to deal with these changes is to learn how the urinary (bladder) system works.

These are some common urinary terms:

- Bladder: Balloon-like muscle that holds urine
- Kidneys: Organs that filter blood and remove waste
- Ureters: Thin tubes that drain urine from the kidneys to the bladder
- Urethra: Tube that drains urine from the bladder to the outside of the body
- Sphincter: Muscle between the bladder and the urethra

Normal Bladder Function and Urination

There are two kidneys, one on each side toward the back just below the ribs. The kidneys remove waste from the blood and turn it into urine. Once urine is made, it moves through the ureters and then into the bladder where it is stored. To keep urine from leaking out, the bladder wall stretches like a balloon and the sphincter muscle at the bottom of the bladder tightens.

When enough pressure builds up, a message is sent from the bladder to the brain. The brain then signals the bladder to hold it a little longer; or a reflex causes the bladder walls to tighten and the sphincter muscle to relax. Then, the pressure pushes urine down through the urethra and out of the body.

Effects of Disability on the Bladder

A disability may affect the bladder in these ways:

- Incontinence: Accidental loss of urine

- Urinary frequency: Needing to urinate more than once every 2 hours

- Urinary retention: Inability to empty bladder completely; increases risk of infection

- Dysuria: Problems starting the urine stream or pain during urination

- Urinary urgency: Very sudden need to empty the bladder

Bladder Program

A good way to deal with bladder problems is to develop a routine called a bladder or toileting program (see Table 39.1 for bladder management options), which includes the following:

- Drinking plenty of fluids, spaced throughout the day. It is alright to drink less after dinner to avoid urinating often at night.

- For some people, emptying the bladder completely is difficult and a catheter can be used to drain urine from the bladder. Intermittent catheterization is the process of passing a tube through the urethra into the bladder at certain times in order to drain the urine. Indwelling catheterization leaves the tube in place to drain urine all day.

Table 39.1. Bladder Management Options

Management	Description	Advantages	Disadvantages	Things to Consider
Timed voiding (Most often used in stroke care)	Urinating at set intervals to avoid accidents and retrain bladder	No risk for infection	None	If bladder empties well and can hold urine for a reasonable amount of time
Urinating without control	Urine that empties without control and is managed by a collecting device or pad	Low risk of infection; requires very little time	Wearing an external collecting device; may cause skin problems	Good option for men if bladder only; not for women as there is no collecting device other than a pad or diaper
Intermittent catheterization without urination	Emptying the bladder at specified intervals using a catheter	Less chance of infection, if followed as prescribed; no need to wear external collecting device; lower cost	Need to catheterize around the clock; waking at night; intake of fluids may need to be limited to keep the bladder from overfilling	Best for those who are independent in their care; greater commitment to follow program guidelines, such as limiting fluids, using catheter at least every 6 hours
Intermittent catheterization with urination	Emptying the bladder at specified intervals using a catheter; frequency depends on how well the bladder empties with urination	Less chance of infection; no need to limit fluids	May need to catheterize at night; requires external collecting device	Not appropriate for females due to lack of effective external collecting device
Indwelling catheter	Hollow tube from bladder attaches to a bag worn on the leg or hung on the side of the bed	None	Greater chance of infection; males may develop sores in the urethra; could interfere with sexual intercourse (there are ways to handle this); need to wear a leg bag or night drainage bag at all times	Optimally, used short term

- Those using a catheter are taught how to use it by a healthcare professional. This includes care of the catheter; transferring on and off the toilet seat; and managing clothes and hygiene.

- People with communication difficulties are taught how to alert others of the need to use the bathroom.

- Family communication is often another important part of urinary care. Although bladder changes can be very embarrassing, it is important to talk about them with family. Honest communication will make rehabilitation easier for you and your family.

Chapter 40

Pressure Sores: What They Are and How to Prevent Them

A pressure ulcer is an area of skin that breaks down when constant pressure is placed against the skin.

Causes

Pressure against the skin reduces blood supply to that area, and the affected tissue dies. This may happen when you stay in one position for too long without shifting your weight. You might get a pressure ulcer if you use a wheelchair or are confined to a bed, even for a short period of time (for example, after surgery or an injury).

The following factors increase the risk for pressure ulcers:

- Being bedridden or in a wheelchair

- Being older

- Being unable to move certain parts of your body without help, such as after a spine or brain injury or if you have a disease like multiple sclerosis

- Having a chronic condition, such as diabetes or vascular disease, that prevents areas of the body from receiving proper blood flow

- Having a mental disability from conditions such as Alzheimer disease

- Having fragile skin

"Pressure Ulcer," © 2010 A.D.A.M., Inc. Reprinted with permission.

- Having urinary incontinence or bowel incontinence
- Not getting enough nourishment (malnourishment)

Symptoms

A pressure ulcer starts as reddened skin that gets worse over time. It forms a blister, then an open sore, and finally a crater.

The most common places for pressure ulcers to form are over bones close to the skin, like the elbow, heels, hips, ankles, shoulders, back, and back of the head.

Pressure sores are categorized by how severe they are, from Stage I (earliest signs) to Stage IV (worst):

- Stage I: A reddened area on the skin that, when pressed, does not turn white. This indicates that a pressure ulcer is starting to develop.

- Stage II: The skin blisters or forms an open sore. The area around the sore may be red and irritated.

- Stage III: The skin breakdown now looks like a crater. There is damage to the tissue below the skin.

- Stage IV: The pressure ulcer has become so deep that there is damage to the muscle and bone, and sometimes to tendons and joints.

First Aid

Discuss any new or changing pressure sore with your doctor or nurse. Once a pressure ulcer is found, the following steps must be taken right away:

- Relieve the pressure on that area. Use pillows, special foam cushions, and sheepskin to reduce the pressure.

- Treat the sore based on the stage of the ulcer. Your health care provider will give you specific treatment and care instructions.

- Avoid further injury or friction to the area. Powder the sheets lightly to decrease friction in bed. (There are many items made for this purpose—check a medical supplies store.)

- Improve nutrition and other problems that may affect the healing process.

- If the pressure ulcer is at Stage II or worse, your health care provider will give you instructions on how to clean and care for open ulcers. It is very important to do this properly to prevent infection.

- Keep the area clean and free of dead tissue. Your health care provider will give you care directions. Generally, pressure ulcers are rinsed with a salt-water rinse to remove loose, dead tissue. The sore should be covered with special gauze dressing made for pressure ulcers.

- New medicines that promote skin healing are available and may be prescribed by your doctor.

Do Not

- Do **not** massage the area of the ulcer. Massage can damage tissue under the skin.

- Donut-shaped or ring-shaped cushions are **not** recommended. They interfere with blood flow to that area and cause complications.

When to Contact a Medical Professional

Contact your health care provider if an area of the skin blisters or forms an open sore. Contact the provider immediately if there are any signs of an infection. An infection can spread to the rest of the body and cause serious problems. Signs of an infected ulcer include:

- a foul odor from the ulcer;

- redness and tenderness around the ulcer;

- skin close to the ulcer is warm and swollen.

Fever, weakness, and confusion are signs that the infection may have spread to the blood or elsewhere in the body.

Prevention

If you are bedridden or cannot move due to diabetes, circulation problems, incontinence, or mental disabilities, you should be checked for pressure sores every day. You or your caregiver need to check your body from head to toe.

Pay special attention to the areas where pressure ulcers often form. Look for reddened areas that, when pressed, do not turn white. Also look for blisters, sores, or craters. In addition, take the following steps:

- Change position at least every 2 hours to relieve pressure.

- Use items that can help reduce pressure—pillows, sheepskin, foam padding, and powders from medical supply stores.

- Eat well-balanced meals that contain enough calories to keep you healthy.

- Drink plenty of water (8 to 10 cups) every day.

- Exercise daily, including range-of-motion exercises.

- Keep the skin clean and dry.

- After urinating or having a bowel movement, clean the area and dry it well. A doctor can recommend creams to help protect the skin.

Chapter 41

Managing Pain

Pain: Medications for Pain Relief

Different medications fight pain in different areas of the pain pathway. Some fight the pain in the periphery (outside the brain or spinal cord); others act at the spinal cord level and others in the brain itself. They all have benefits and side effects and are often used in combination to address pain at a number of different levels.

Medications should always be used along with non-drug pain management techniques to prevent and treat pain.

Non-Narcotic Analgesics

Some of the newer drugs are very strong and effective for pain. They act on pain in the periphery, by reducing inflammation and/or the body's chemicals that cause pain. They can be taken every day and are not addictive.

Antidepressant Medications

Although these drugs were originally only used to treat depression, now they are also used for other medical problems including pain and

This chapter includes text from "Pain: Medications for Pain Relief," and "Pain: Non-Drug Pain Management Techniques," June 2010, Copyright Rehabilitation Institute of Chicago. All rights reserved. Reprinted with permission. For additional information, visit the website of the LIFE Center at the Rehabilitation Center of Chicago, http://lifecenter.ric.org.

sleep problems. They act on pain at the spinal cord level and help with sleep problems at the brain level. They are not addictive and can be taken every day.

Narcotic Analgesics

Narcotic analgesics act on pain at the brain level. They depress the nervous system and the emotions; decrease the ability to think; and slow breathing and heart rate. People can develop both tolerance and addiction to narcotics. Tolerance means that higher doses are needed to obtain the desired effect. True addiction occurs when needing the medication becomes more important that your daily life, and it interferes with your thoughts, work, and relationships. Addiction also means that stopping the medication will lead to withdrawal.

Narcotics are effective painkillers immediately after an injury or surgery, or at the end of life, but they are not good medications to take for chronic pain. People with a history of alcoholism or other substance abuse should be very careful taking these medications.

Please consult your medical team for any questions about medications.

Pain: Non-Drug Pain Management Techniques

Pain following an injury is common and can affect life in a number of ways.

- [It can] interfere with sleep and cause fatigue.

- [It can] reduce patience and cause more irritability.

- Small stressors and hassles usually handled can become more difficult.

- Fear of the pain and worry that it means something is seriously wrong may interfere with the things you want and need to do. You may do less and less because you are hurting, tired, and cranky. This inactivity can have serious consequences. Pain can cause problems with family, friends, and coworkers.

- The effects of pain can lead to other physical problems and emotional problems, including depression.

Certain types of injuries sometimes cause predictable pain problems. For example, people with mild brain injuries often have more severe pain, especially headaches, than those with severe brain injuries. Others may have more pain in the neck and shoulders.

Pain should be treated, not ignored. The medical team can help with prescribing medications and suggestions for pain management techniques. A combination of strategies is usually best and can be individualized for each person. Talk with your doctor and health care team to determine the best treatment for you.

Pain Management Techniques

Relaxation: Relaxation is a state of physical and emotional calmness, the opposite of the stress or "fight or flight" response. The muscles of the forehead, jaw, neck, and shoulders are often very tense during headaches and other pain episodes. This tension makes the pain worse. Relaxing the muscles is a way to break this cycle and thus reduce the pain or at least make it easier to manage. During relaxation, muscles are free of tension, reducing anxiety and irritability.

For most people, relaxation must be learned. It is not just resting or watching TV; it is a deliberate reduction in mental and physical activity. There are many ways to learn relaxation, including breathing techniques, biofeedback, progressive muscle relaxation (PMR), imagery, and meditation. Your psychologist or nurse can help you learn relaxation.

The more you practice and use relaxation, the better it will work to help manage pain. Relaxation should be practiced both when in pain and when not in pain; don't wait to practice until the pain strikes. With regular practice, a relaxed state will be quicker and easier to achieve.

Distraction: Distraction is focusing the attention on something other than the pain sensation. It starts with concentrating on something external, like music, or something internal, like an image. Distraction can be used in two ways: To handle flare-ups of pain and to provide interesting things to do and think about each day.

Exercise: Prolonged inactivity causes muscles to tighten up and become weaker, both of which cause pain. Appropriate physical activity can help many people manage pain. Always follow your physical therapist's suggestions. Do your daily exercises and stay as active as possible.

Posture: Poor posture puts a strain on muscles and causes pain. Your occupational therapist will show you how to sit, stand, and move.

Nutrition: Most people feel better eating a healthy diet. If you need help learning how to eat healthfully, consult with a nutrition professional.

Caffeine (and nicotine) may increase muscle tension. They can also cause withdrawal pain, which occurs when you do not get your usual amount of coffee, soda, or cigarettes.

Alcohol can increase feeling of depression and make it harder to function. Also some medications are affected by alcohol. Make sure to talk to your doctor about the effects of alcohol on medicine.

If you or your family feels that alcohol is a problem or if you would like to cut down on caffeine, nicotine, or other stimulants, talk to your doctor or psychologist. They can help.

Maintaining activities: With chronic pain, you may not be doing activities that you used to enjoy, because of the pain or because of being too tired or depressed to want to do anything. If the pain has gone on for a long time, you may have little or nothing to do or think about except the pain.

Try the following:

- Think about all the things you used to do each day and decide which were most enjoyable.

- Continue to do the enjoyable things that you can still do or try to modify the ones you cannot do.

- Vary your activities and try to find new activities to enjoy that are within your physical limits.

Chapter 42

Coping with Depression and Anxiety

Mental health problems such as depression and anxiety can accompany an illness. The following provides information on signs, symptoms, and treatment.

Symptoms of Depression

Depression is characterized by feelings of sadness, despair, and discouragement. It often follows a personal loss or injury but is not a sign of weakness nor does it represent a moral failing.

Sadness that lasts a long time and a loss of enjoyment in almost all activities are the central features of depression. Sadness is a symptom, but not the same thing as depression. Everyone is sad sometimes. The type of sadness that occurs in depression lasts all day or most of the day, every day for at least two weeks. Other symptoms include feelings of worthlessness or guilt, suicidal thoughts, loss of concentration, decreased energy, slowed thinking and movement, appetite loss, and sleep problems.

Many of these symptoms can occur with illnesses such as brain injury or stroke or even less serious problems like a cold or flu, but may not indicate depression. Trouble sleeping, lack of appetite, and problems concentrating alone are not reasons to be concerned about a separate mental health condition unless you also feel sad most of the time or rarely find enjoyment in life.

What Is the Difference between Normal Grief and Depression?

Some symptoms of depression are normal after any kind of loss including the onset of a disability or severe illness. If these symptoms are present for a long time it may be helpful to talk with a mental health professional. It is also helpful to talk to someone if you have other symptoms such as feeling guilty or worthless, or if sadness interferes with the ability to do important life tasks (such as take medication; go to therapies, work, or school).

Symptoms of Anxiety

Following a major life-changing event like a disabling illness, it is normal to feel a great deal of stress. Stress can build up over time and lead to anxiety. Anxiety can be a response to a specific situation such as learning to walk all over again; it can also be more generalized such as not wanting to leave the house after being discharged from the hospital.

The most common symptoms of anxiety are fear and worry. Anxiety can also cause restlessness, and difficulty concentrating and sleeping.

Sometimes people express anxiety by being irritable, tired, or even stubborn. Anxiety can cause physical symptoms like muscle tension, shortness of breath, or even feelings of panic. Nearly everyone feels anxiety when faced with a bad physical problem. It becomes a concern when these feelings are very strong and interfere with important tasks in life.

Can Anxiety or Depression Be Different Depending on Age?

Children and older adults often show anxiety and depression differently. Children may misbehave either at school or at home. Older adults might report vague physical problems when there is no clear medical cause.

Treatment

Both depression and anxiety can go away over time but without treatment the symptoms last longer and may return. Chronic depression or anxiety can cause low self-esteem and poor quality of life.

Treatment usually involves medication and/or psychotherapy (counseling) by a trained professional. Treatment is usually quite successful, so there is little reason to delay seeking help. Even when family and friends are around for support, professional attention is best. A good first step is to discuss concerns with a doctor who can provide advice about the best treatment and suggest a qualified therapist. There are several types of mental health professionals: counselors, social workers, and psychologists, but any medications must be prescribed by a physician (your regular doctor or a psychiatrist). Psychotherapy can be done individually, with other family members, or in a group. Select a therapist or group with whom you feel comfortable and can talk honestly about your feelings.

It may be best to both see a therapist and take medication, but sometimes people are afraid of acting and thinking strangely, or becoming dependent on medications. When these medications are taken as prescribed by a doctor, side effects can be reduced or eliminated and there is little risk of becoming addicted. Treatment medications are not the same as street drugs used to get high.

Coping with Anxiety and Depression While in the Hospital

There is no single, simple way to adjust to a disability, but there are a few tips.

- Follow a routine including the regular therapy schedule, going to bed the same time each night, and setting aside time for relaxing and visiting (either in person or on the phone).

- Be open with staff, family, and friends regarding your needs.

- Ask questions about any aspect of your care that is unclear.

- Talk about things that worry you. Keeping feelings bottled up often makes being in the hospital more difficult. Sometimes people do not admit anything bad has happened as a way to be protected from depression and anxiety. It is healthier to admit you may not be able to do everything you used to do.

- Acknowledge that you will be sad about this for a while until you find new things to do that you enjoy. Try not to exaggerate these losses with thoughts such as "I can't do anything anymore;" or "I will never be able to find anything worthwhile to do again."

Coping with Anxiety and Depression after Leaving the Hospital

Sometimes people have prejudices about physical disability that make them feel like "second class citizens" when they become disabled themselves. Sometimes people with a disability get into the habit of letting other people do things for them and as a result they start to feel helpless. Sometimes people with a disability avoid situations that make them nervous (for example going out in public where others can see that they look or act differently). To help cope, try these suggestions:

- Set up a routine and stay with it.

- Stay involved in enjoyable activities—either ones from before or new ones.

- Acknowledge improvements. This decreases the risk of boredom and depression and boosts self-confidence.

- Be open to the support of others. Healthy relationships with family and friends can help in preventing depression and anxiety.

- A strong spiritual life can help with both health and hopefulness.

Special Tips for Parents

Parents may need to provide extra comfort and support for children. It is not unusual for a child to regress to an earlier stage of development following a traumatic event. Children may find it hard to separate from parents, become clingy or emotionally needy during a hospital stay, but then show signs of more independence by the time of discharge. Please talk to your doctor if these problems do not improve.

Additional Resources

- American Medical Association (1998). *Essential Guide to Depression.* New York: Pocket Books.

- Bourne, E.J. (2000). *The Anxiety and Phobia Workbook.* New Harbinger Press.

- Mental Health: Does therapy work? *Consumer Reports.* November, 1995.

- Sheffield, A. (1998). *How You Can Survive When They're Depressed.* New York: Harmony.

- American Psychological Association: www.apa.org

- National Institute of Mental Health: www.nimh.nih.gov

- Psychology Information Online: www.psychologyinfo.com

- For children: KidsHealth, www.kidshealth.org

Chapter 43

Health Insurance Concerns

Chapter Contents

Section 43.1—Facts about Health Insurance That
  People with Disabilities Need to Know 390

Section 43.2—Affordable Care Act for Americans
  with Disabilities 392

Section 43.3—Medicare and Nonelderly People
  with Disabilities 395

Section 43.4—Medicaid and Children's Health
  Insurance Program 399

Section 43.1

Facts about Health Insurance That People with Disabilities Need to Know

This section contains text excerpted from "People with Disabilities: Top 5 Things to Know," "People with Disabilities: Recent Improvements," and "People with Disabilities: Coming Improvements," U.S. Department of Health and Human Services (www.healthcare.gov), 2011.

Top Five Things to Know

If you're living with a disability, private health insurance may be hard to come by. Even if you can afford to buy it, it probably doesn't cover all of your needs. Worrying about where to get coverage and the cost of your care is the last thing you want to do. The Affordable Care Act is expanding your options for health insurance and making them more affordable.

1. Under the Affordable Care Act, job-based and new individual plans are no longer allowed to deny or exclude coverage to any child under age 19 based on a pre-existing condition, including a disability. Starting in 2014, these same plans won't be able to exclude anyone from coverage or charge a higher premium for a pre-existing condition including a disability.

2. Insurance companies can no longer drop you when you get sick just because you made a mistake on your coverage application.

3. Insurance companies can no longer impose lifetime dollar limits on your coverage.

4. Medicaid covers many people with disabilities now, and in the future it will provide insurance to even more Americans. Starting in 2014, most adults under age 65 with incomes up to about $15,000 per year for single individual (higher income for couples/families with children) will qualify for Medicaid in every state. State Medicaid programs will also be able to offer additional services to help those who need long-term care at home and in the community.

5. You may be able to join and get benefits from a voluntary, enrollment-based insurance program that will be available after October 2012 called the Community Living Assistance Services and Supports (CLASS) Program. It will provide assistance to people who need help with daily activities. Under this voluntary program, you'll get a cash allowance so you can get care and other supports to help you keep your independence.

Recent Improvements

Many provisions of the Affordable Care Act are already in place and making insurance better.

- Insurance companies can no longer drop you when you get sick just because you made a mistake on your coverage application.

- New health plans must now cover certain preventive services without cost sharing.

- Insurance companies can no longer include lifetime limits on coverage.

- If a new insurance plan doesn't pay for services you believe were covered, you now have new, clear options to appeal the decision.

- Job-based health plans and new individual plans can no longer deny or exclude coverage for your children (under age 19) based on health conditions, including a disability.

- States now have the option to expand Medicaid coverage programs for adults and to include additional programs and services to help those who need long-term care at home and in the community.

Coming Improvements

- Starting in 2012, all insurance papers must be written in clear and understandable language that explains what's covered and how it works. This will help you understand your choices more clearly and decide what coverage is really best for you.

- Starting in 2014, if your employer doesn't offer insurance, you will be able to buy insurance directly in an Exchange—a new transparent and competitive insurance marketplace where individuals and small businesses can buy affordable and qualified health benefit plans. Exchanges will offer you a choice of health plans that meet certain benefits and cost standards. Members of Congress will be getting their health care insurance through Exchanges, and you will be able buy your insurance through Exchanges, too.

- Job-based health plans and new individual plans won't be allowed to deny or exclude anyone or charge more for a pre-existing condition including a disability.

- If your income is less than the equivalent of about $88,000 for a family of four today, and your job doesn't offer affordable coverage, you may get tax credits to help pay for insurance.

- Essential health benefits like hospitalizations, doctor services, prescription drugs, and rehabilitation and mental health services will be covered in all new individual, small business, and Exchange plans.

Section 43.2

Affordable Care Act for Americans with Disabilities

From the U.S. Department of Health and Human Services (HHS, www.healthcare.gov), November 16, 2010.

Eliminates Insurance Company Discrimination

As of September 23, 2010, health plans cannot limit or deny benefits or deny coverage outright for a child younger than age 19 simply because the child has a preexisting condition. In 2014, the Act will prohibit insurance companies from denying coverage or charging more to any person based on their medical history.

As of September 23, 2010 the Affordable Care Act prohibits health plans from putting a lifetime dollar limit on most benefits you receive. The Act also restricts and phases out the annual dollar limits a health plan can place on most of your benefits—and does away with these limits entirely in 2014.

As of September 23, 2010, the new law helps make wellness and prevention services affordable and accessible to you by requiring health plans to cover many preventive services without charging you a copayment, coinsurance, or deductible.

On July 1, Secretary Sebelius announced the establishment of the Pre-Existing Condition Insurance Program to provide coverage for eligible Americans who have been uninsured for 6 months because of a pre-existing condition. This program helps build a bridge to 2014, when Americans will have access to quality, affordable care in health insurance exchanges.

Greater Choices and Enhanced Protections for Americans with Disabilities

- **Allows individuals to stay on parents' plan until age 26:** Health plans that cover children must make coverage available to children up to age 26. By allowing them to stay on a parent's plan, the Affordable Care Act makes it easier and more affordable for young adults to get or keep health insurance coverage.

- **Expands the Medicaid program:** Expands the Medicaid program to more Americans, including people with disabilities. States have the option to expand their programs now, and the program will be expanded nationwide in 2014. State-based health insurance exchanges will be established to provide families with the same private insurance choices that the President and Members of Congress will have, to foster competition and increase consumer choice.

- **One-stop shopping and accessibility:** The new exchanges will supply easy to understand, standard, accessible information on available health insurance plans, so people can compare and easily identify the quality, affordable option that is right for them.

- **Out-of-pocket limits:** Going forward, plans in the health insurance exchanges and all new plans will have a cap on what insurance companies can require beneficiaries to pay in out-of-pocket expenses, such as co-pays and deductibles.

New Options for Long-Term Supports and Services

- **Extends the successful Money Follows the Person Program** through 2016 with an additional $2.25 billion in funding. Supports continuation of program in participating states and

393

extension of MFP to new states seeking to rebalance their long-term care systems. Expands definition of eligible individuals.

- **Improves Medicaid Home-and-Community-Based Services (HCBS) option.**

- **Creates Community First Choice program:** Effective October 1, 2011, a new Medicaid State Plan option called Community First Choice will launch, giving states a 6% enhanced match so that they can offer community-based attendant services and supports alongside nursing home and institutional services for eligible persons with disabilities. Community First Choice will require states to make such services and supports available to individuals under a person-centered plan of care to assist them in accomplishing activities of daily living, instrumental activities of daily living, and health-related tasks.

- **Incentives for states to offer home and community-based services as a long-term care alternative to nursing homes:** Effective October 2011, $3 billion in enhanced Medicaid matches will be available to states that now fund less than 50% of long-term services in home and community-based settings, if they achieve targets set for increasing HCBS by October 2015.

Assuring Accessible, Quality, Affordable Health Care for People with Disabilities

- **Preventive care for better health:** Invests in prevention and public health to encourage innovations in health care that prevent illness and disease before they require more costly treatment.

- **Accessible examination equipment:** Improves access to medical diagnostic equipment so people with disabilities can receive routine preventive care and cancer screenings by establishing exam equipment accessibility standards. These standards will be set by the Food and Drug Administration and the Access Board.

- **Health disparities:** Improves data collection on health disparities for persons with disabilities, as well as training and cultural competency of health providers.

- **Improves care for chronic disease:** Invests in innovations such as medical homes and care coordination demonstrations in Medicare and Medicaid to prevent disabilities from occurring and progressing and to help the one in 10 Americans who experiences a major limitation in activity due to chronic conditions.

Section 43.3

Medicare and Nonelderly People with Disabilities

"Fact Sheet: Medicare and Nonelderly People With Disabilities," (#8100), The Henry J. Kaiser Family Foundation, September 2010. This information was reprinted with permission from the Henry J. Kaiser Family Foundation. The Kaiser Family Foundation is a non-profit private operating foundation, based in Menlo Park, California, dedicated to producing and communicating the best possible analysis and information on health issues.

Medicare was established in 1965 as the health insurance program for Americans age 65 and over; since 1972, it has also covered people under age 65 who receive Social Security Disability Insurance (SSDI) benefits. To qualify for SSDI, people must be unable to engage in "substantial gainful activity" because of a medically-determined physical or mental impairment expected to last at least 12 months or until death. Medicare also covers certain nonelderly disabled widows and widowers, as well as disabled adult children of retired, deceased, or disabled workers. Today, Medicare covers 8 million people who are under age 65 and disabled, or 17% of the Medicare population, up from 8% in 1975.

Qualifying for Medicare

People under age 65 become eligible for Medicare if they have received SSDI payments for 24 months. Because people must wait 5 months before receiving disability benefits, SSDI recipients must wait a total of 29 months before their Medicare coverage begins. (Nonelderly people diagnosed with end-stage renal disease (ESRD) or amyotrophic lateral sclerosis [ALS] automatically qualify for Medicare upon diagnosis without a waiting period.) Among workers who became eligible for SSDI in 2009, 31% qualified due to impairments of the musculoskeletal system and connective tissues, 22% due to mental disorders or mental retardation, 10% due to circulatory problems, 9% due to cancer, 4% due to injuries, and 24% due to other conditions (SSA, 2010).

Characteristics of Nonelderly Disabled Beneficiaries

Nonelderly Medicare beneficiaries with disabilities differ from the elderly in several ways. More than one-third (35%) of nonelderly beneficiaries lived on incomes below 100% of poverty in 2008—$10,400 for an individual that year—compared to 12% of seniors. Two-thirds (67%) had incomes below twice the poverty level, compared to 42% of seniors. A larger share of nonelderly disabled than elderly beneficiaries are black (17% versus 8%) and Hispanic (11% versus 7%), and a larger share are male.

Nearly two-thirds of all nonelderly disabled Medicare beneficiaries (64%) have a cognitive or mental impairment, compared to 23% of seniors. More than half (58%) report their health status as fair or poor (versus 21% of seniors) and nearly half (48%) report having one or more limitations in their activities of daily living, compared to 27% of seniors.

Spending, Use, and Access to Health Care

Average per capita Medicare costs were somewhat lower for nonelderly disabled than elderly beneficiaries ($7,790 versus $7,912 in 2006), even though the nonelderly disabled report higher rates of health and cognitive problems. Nonelderly beneficiaries had lower average per capita Medicare expenditures in every service category in 2006 except outpatient hospital services and prescription drugs.

Access to care is generally good for people on Medicare across a number of standard measures, but a larger share of nonelderly disabled than elderly beneficiaries report experiencing a range of access problems. One-third of nonelderly disabled beneficiaries report having a major or minor problem paying their health care bills, compared to 13% of seniors.[1]

Although a majority of beneficiaries report no problems finding a doctor who accepts Medicare, three times as many nonelderly disabled as elderly beneficiaries report having this problem (12% versus 4%). Fifteen percent of disabled beneficiaries also report difficulty finding a doctor who understands their disability or how to treat it.

Supplemental Coverage

Most Medicare beneficiaries, including the nonelderly disabled, have public or private supplemental insurance to help cover Medicare's deductibles and cost-sharing requirements. Compared to the elderly, a greater share of nonelderly disabled people on Medicare rely on

Medicaid to supplement Medicare (39% versus 10%) because of their relatively low incomes, and a smaller share on employer plans, Medicare Advantage plans, and Medigap. Just 4% of the nonelderly disabled report having a Medigap policy, versus 19% of the elderly, which may be explained in part by a provision in law that permits Medigap insurers to deny coverage to nonelderly beneficiaries with disabilities.

One in five nonelderly disabled beneficiaries has no supplemental coverage, compared with only 8% of the elderly. Lack of supplemental coverage is associated with higher rates of cost and access problems. Among nonelderly disabled beneficiaries, a larger share of those without supplemental coverage report cost-related problems compared to those with supplemental coverage, according to a recent study.[1] Yet some sources of supplemental coverage, including Medicaid and employer coverage, provide greater financial protection than others do, and merely having supplemental coverage does not eliminate access and cost-related burdens.

Prescription Drug Coverage

Nearly 70% of disabled Medicare beneficiaries are enrolled in a Medicare Part D drug plan, either a stand-alone prescription drug plan (PDP) or a Medicare Advantage drug plan, compared to 57% of elderly beneficiaries. A higher proportion of elderly than nonelderly disabled beneficiaries have drug coverage under an employer-sponsored plan, while roughly similar shares of both groups have no drug coverage whatsoever (13% versus 11%).

Having drug coverage does not eliminate access and cost-related problems in obtaining medications. Among Part D enrollees, a larger share of nonelderly disabled than elderly beneficiaries report difficulty getting medication because it was not covered by their Part D plan, needing prior authorization before getting a medication, and delaying getting or skipping medication due to cost.[1]

Policy Implications

Medicare provides important health insurance protections for people with disabilities who are under age 65 and would otherwise face significant difficulties obtaining health insurance in the private market. Yet research reveals a consistent pattern of differences in the health care experiences of nonelderly disabled and elderly Medicare beneficiaries, with the nonelderly disabled encountering significantly more access problems and cost-related barriers to care than the elderly and being more likely to report serious health consequences as a result.

With new opportunities for improving and broadening access to public and private coverage, as well as improving Medicare benefits, the Patient Protection and Affordable Care Act offers important help to people with disabilities. For those on Medicare, the 2010 health reform law will help alleviate the out-of-pocket spending burden by phasing in coverage in the Part D coverage gap and by eliminating cost sharing for certain preventive services. For SSDI recipients in the Medicare waiting period (and other uninsured people), the law expands access to health insurance coverage through high-risk pools (beginning in 2010) and through Medicaid or insurance exchanges (beginning in 2014). For those who are dually covered by Medicare and Medicaid, the law expands coverage of home- and community-based care, and creates a new federal office to help coordinate benefits and coverage under the two programs.

Even with health insurance, people with disabilities are likely to face ongoing challenges if their coverage, including Medicare, does not provide the services and supports they need to live as independently and productively as possible. Given high rates of health problems and relatively low incomes among Medicare's nonelderly disabled beneficiaries, the needs of this population require careful attention in ongoing Medicare policy discussions.

1. J Cubanski and P Neuman, "Medicare Doesn't Work As Well For Younger, Disabled Beneficiaries As It Does For Older Enrollees," *Health Affairs,* September 2010.

Section 43.4

Medicaid and Children's Health Insurance Program

"Health Coverage of Children: The Role of Medicaid and CHIP," (#7698-04), The Henry J. Kaiser Family Foundation, August 2010. This information was reprinted with permission from the Henry J. Kaiser Family Foundation. The Kaiser Family Foundation is a non-profit private operating foundation, based in Menlo Park, California, dedicated to producing and communicating the best possible analysis and information on health issues.

During the current recession, Medicaid and the Children's Health Insurance Program (CHIP) have served as an important safety-net for children in low- or moderate-income families. Together, these programs insure almost one-third of all children and target those who do not have access to affordable private coverage. Despite the success and high participation rates in Medicaid and CHIP, 8.1 million children remain uninsured, and the vast majority of them are from low- and middle-income families. Provisions to strengthen coverage for children are included in both the 2009 Children's Health Insurance Program Reauthorization Act (CHIPRA) and the Patient Protection and Affordable Care Act (ACA) of 2010.

Medicaid and CHIP Coverage of Children

Medicaid pays for a full set of services for children, including screening and treatment (EPSDT), check-ups, physician and hospital visits, and vision and dental care. In 2007, Medicaid covered 29 million children at some point in the year. Children represent half of all Medicaid enrollees, but account for only 19% of total program spending.

The broad coverage provisions of the ACA go into effect in 2014 and will set national minimum Medicaid eligibility for nearly all individuals (including children) at 133% of poverty. Until 2014, states are required to extend Medicaid eligibility to children under 6 years old living in families with incomes at or below 133% of poverty ($29,327 for a family of four in 2009), and to children ages 6–18 living in families with incomes at or below 100% of poverty. States also have authority

399

to expand Medicaid eligibility beyond these minimum standards, and many states have used this authority to reach more children.

States can also cover children beyond their Medicaid eligibility levels through CHIP, which was created in 1997 and covers about 6 million children. Within CHIP, states are allowed to set premiums and cost sharing on a sliding scale based on income and can provide a more limited set of benefits than Medicaid. States and the federal government jointly fund both programs, although the federal government pays a higher proportion of CHIP costs up to a capped total amount for each state.

The enactment of CHIP spurred states to invest heavily in outreach and improve their enrollment processes for both Medicaid and CHIP while expanding children's coverage. As the cost of private coverage has increased, many states have expanded eligibility for public coverage. Forty-seven states including the District of Columbia cover children in families with incomes at 200% of poverty or higher.

The passage of CHIPRA provided states with increased federal funding, new tools, and fiscal incentives to promote coverage for children. Prior to CHIPRA, states were precluded from using federal dollars to provide Medicaid or CHIP to legal immigrants who had been in the United States less than 5 years. States now have the option of providing this coverage to children and pregnant women who previously would have been subject to the 5-year ban.

Trends in Children's Coverage

In 2008, despite a recession and a resulting decline in employer-sponsored coverage, the uninsured rate for children continued to drop and nearly 800,000 fewer children were uninsured than in 2007. That decline was caused by an increase in public coverage, with 1.7 million children gaining coverage through Medicaid or CHIP in 2008. In contrast, from 2004 to 2006, public coverage rates for children did not increase as private coverage rates fell. These trends resulted in a rise in the number of uninsured children during this earlier period.

Medicaid and CHIP are in a strong position to prevent children from losing coverage during the current recession because many states had expanded these programs when their economies were stronger. To aid states struggling to maintain Medicaid during the recession, the American Recovery and Reinvestment Act (ARRA) provided a temporary increase in federal Medicaid funding through December 2010. To be eligible for the funds, states could not restrict eligibility or make it more difficult for individuals to enroll. In the face of continuing high unemployment, Congress later extended that additional funding at a lower rate through June 2011. The ACA extended funding for CHIP through 2015 (an additional 2 years) and also included a maintenance of eligibility for children in Medicaid and CHIP through 2019.

Uninsured Children

Almost three-quarters (72%) of the 8.1 million uninsured children in the United States live in families with household incomes below 200% of the federal poverty level (about $44,000 for a family of four). The majority of uninsured children (68%) live in families with at least one full-time worker. These families often are not offered coverage by an employer or cannot afford the premiums. The full cost of family coverage purchased through an employer has doubled since 2000, reaching $13,375 in 2009.

Public coverage targets lower income children who are more likely to be uninsured. Most of the 5.8 million uninsured children below 200% of poverty are eligible for Medicaid or CHIP, but are not enrolled. In many families with uninsured children, the parents are not eligible for Medicaid coverage. Research suggests that this may lead to confusion about eligibility rules that results in children going uninsured. Under the ACA, more parents and other adults will qualify for Medicaid in 2014.

Racial and ethnic minority children are more likely to be uninsured than white children. However, uninsured rates for black and Hispanic children decreased significantly in 2008 as more children enrolled in Medicaid and CHIP.

The risk of being uninsured also differs depending on where a child lives, as the share of children who are uninsured varies widely across states. While the uninsured rate for children is 5% or less in six states (HI, IA, MA, ME, NH, WV), in four states (FL, NM, NV, TX) more than 15% of children are uninsured. Additionally, almost half (47%) of all uninsured children live in five states (CA, FL, GA, NY, and TX).

The role of health insurance coverage in improving access to care is well documented. Uninsured children have worse access to care than those who are insured by either Medicaid or private insurance. Research also demonstrates that parents whose children are uninsured or have public coverage think highly of Medicaid and CHIP. These programs offer strong protection against high out-of-pocket costs, while private insurance may have high deductibles and co-pays.

Outlook

The ACA uses Medicaid as a base for a broad coverage expansion in 2014, but most uninsured children are currently eligible for Medicaid or CHIP and do not need to wait until 2014 to gain coverage. The

Secretary of Health and Human Services has issued a challenge to find and enroll the 5 million uninsured children who are currently eligible for public coverage. Enrolling these children will provide them with comprehensive insurance and strengthen Medicaid's base of coverage as the wider health reform effort gets underway.

Chapter 44

Dealing with Hospitalization

A trip to the hospital with a person with disabilities can be stressful for both of you. This text can relieve some of that stress by helping you prepare for both unexpected and planned hospital visits.

Hospital Emergencies: What You Can Do Now

Planning ahead is key to making an unexpected or planned trip to the hospital easier for you and your care partner. Here is what you should do now:

- Think about and discuss hospitalization before it happens and as the disease and associated memory loss progresses. Hospitalization is a choice.

- Talk about when hospice may be a better and more appropriate alternative.

- Register your relative for a MedicAlert® + Alzheimer's Association Safe Return® bracelet through your local Alzheimer's Association chapter. People who are lost may be taken to an emergency room. This bracelet will speed up the process of reconnecting you with your care partner.

Excerpted from "Hospitalization Happens: A Guide to Hospital Visits for Individuals with Memory Loss," by the National Institute on Aging (NIA, www.nia .nih.gov), part of the National Institutes of Health, November 19, 2009.

- Learn more about safety-related programs such as Project Lifesaver International (www.projectlifesaverinternational.com).

- Know whom you can depend on. You need a family member or trusted friend to stay with your care partner when he or she is admitted to the emergency room or hospital. Arrange to have at least two dependable family members, neighbors, or friends you can call on to go with you or meet you at the hospital at a moment's notice so that one person can take care of the paperwork and the other can stay with your care partner.

Pack an Emergency Bag

Pack an emergency bag containing the following:

- **Personal information sheet:** Create a document that includes the following information on your care partner:
  - Preferred name and language (some people may revert to native languages in late-stage Alzheimer disease)
  - Contact information for doctors, key family members, minister, and helpful friends (also program into cell phone, if applicable)
  - Illness or medical conditions
  - All current medicines and dosage instructions (update whenever there is a change)
  - Any medicines that have ever caused a bad reaction
  - Any allergies to medicines or foods or special diets
  - Need for glasses, dentures, or hearing aid
  - Degree of impairment and amount of assistance needed for activities
  - Family information, living situation, major life events
  - Work, leisure, and spiritual history
  - Daily schedule and patterns and self-care preferences
  - Favorite foods and music and touch and visual resources
  - Highlight behaviors of concern, such as how your relative communicates needs and expresses emotions
- **Paperwork:** Include copies of important documents such as the following:
  - Insurance cards (include policy numbers and preauthorization phone numbers)

- Medicaid and/or Medicare cards
- Durable power of attorney, health care power of attorney, living will and/or an original DNR (do not resuscitate) order

- **Supplies for the care partner:**
    - A change of clothing, toiletries, and personal medications
    - Extra adult briefs (e.g., Depends), if usually worn (these may not be available in the emergency room if needed)
    - Moist hand wipes such as Wet Ones
    - Plastic bags for soiled clothing and/or adult briefs
    - Reassuring or comforting objects
    - An iPod, MP3, or CD player and earphones or speakers

- **Supplies for the caregiver:**
    - A change of clothing, toiletries, and personal medications
    - Pain medicine such as Advil, Tylenol, or aspirin (A trip to the emergency room may take longer than you think. Stress can lead to a headache or other symptoms.)
    - A sealed snack such as a pack of crackers and a bottle of water or juice for you and your care partner (You may have to wait for quite a while.)
    - A small amount of cash
    - A note on the outside of the emergency bag to take a cell phone with you

A pad of paper and pen to write down information and directions given to you by hospital staff is also helpful. Keep a log on your care partner's symptoms and problems. You may be asked the same questions by many people. Show them what you have written instead of repeating your answers.

By taking these steps in advance, you can reduce the stress and confusion that often accompanies a hospital visit, particularly if the visit is an unplanned trip to the emergency room.

At the Emergency Room

A trip to the emergency room may fatigue or even frighten your care partner. There are some important things to remember:

- Be patient. It could be a long wait if the reason for your visit is not life-threatening.

- Recognize that results from lab tests take time.

- Offer physical and emotional comfort and verbal reassurance to your relative. Stay calm and positive. How you are feeling will get absorbed by others.

- Realize that just because you do not see staff at work does not mean they are not working.

- Be aware that emergency room staff often have limited training in Alzheimer disease and related dementias so try to help them better understand your care partner.

- Encourage hospital staff to see your relative as an individual and not just another patient with dementia who is confused and disoriented from the disease.

- Do not assume your care partner will be admitted to the hospital.

- Do not leave the emergency room to go home without a follow-up plan. If you are sent home, make sure you have all instructions for follow-up care.

- Have an emergency bag prepared for your trip to the hospital that includes items like over-the-counter pain medication, sealed snacks, and bottled water.

Chapter 45

Rehabilitation: Options for People with Disabilities

Rehabilitation focuses on function. Being able to continue to function is key to maintaining or regaining independence and quality of life, particularly after an illness or injury. Starting rehabilitation early can help you maintain function and increase your chances of returning to your previous level of function as much as possible.

In restorative rehabilitation, the goal is to restore a function that you have lost. It is often funded by Medicare or other payers. Examples include short-term rehabilitation that usually follows a stroke or a hip fracture. In maintenance rehabilitation, the goal is to maintain and strengthen a function. Maintenance rehabilitation is less intense, with physical therapy or occupational therapy continued three times a week as an outpatient. With longer-term therapy, possibly more function can be gained or more functional loss can be prevented.

Who Benefits from Rehabilitation?

When evaluating a disability, your health care provider will focus on understanding how the loss of function developed and progressed over time. Other vital factors in predicting whether function can be regained are how severe the loss of function is, what caused it, and the potential for recovery.

"Rehabilitation," reprinted with permission from the American Geriatrics Society, © 2005. For more information visit www.healthinaging.org. Reviewed by David A. Cooke, MD, FACP, July 14, 2011.

The level of function you had before a disability is an important consideration in the level of function you can expect to regain after rehabilitation. For example, if a healthy older person who walks without a cane falls and fractures a hip, he or she will likely be able to walk again after several months of a rehabilitation program. However, the same goal is not as realistic for someone of the same age who was already having a hard time walking (possibly due to arthritis or bad circulation) before suffering a hip fracture.

If a person has additional medical conditions, such as heart, lung, or joint diseases, his or her participation in an intense rehabilitation program may be limited. However, many people can still improve their ability to exercise gradually even if they have moderate to severe heart and lung disease.

Another important factor in successful rehabilitation is commitment to an ongoing program. Commitment is important not only for the person who has lost some function, but also for family members (or other caregivers) when he or she returns home after the rehabilitation program. What the older adult and his or her family expects and prefers should also be considered, because rehabilitation programs usually require everyone's participation. Another reason why everyone should be involved in the decision-making process is because many disabilities of older adults are chronic (e.g., arthritis, diabetes, hypertension, heart disease). For older adults to be able to best control their chronic diseases, they should understand the disease or injury, feel confident that they understand and can perform the activities needed to manage their disease and prevent new problems, and be able to monitor their disease status as much as possible.

The type of disability and how severe it is, as well as what the person actually needs to do at home as well as what others can do for the person are important considerations in the decision of whether a person can safely return home after rehabilitation. People living at home should, at the very least, be able to move safely from a bed to a chair, and from walking or a wheelchair to the toilet. For people who have difficulty thinking things through or who have problems with vision, 24-hour supervision may be necessary. Often, the critical factor for discharge from a rehabilitation unit is whether 24-hour support is available at home for those who need it.

Settings for Rehabilitation Programs

Rehabilitation can take place in many types of settings:

- Special units in acute care hospitals or rehabilitation hospitals

- Nursing facilities
- Outpatient centers
- Homes
- Private offices

If you have a new disability and are a good candidate for 4–12 weeks of restorative rehabilitation, you may benefit from an intensive rehabilitation program involving a multidisciplinary team of health care professionals. Such programs are usually done in a rehabilitation unit, whether within a hospital, in a separate rehabilitation hospital or building, or in a nursing facility with a designated rehabilitation program. Other people may not require or be able to do such intensive rehabilitation and may be better suited to outpatient or home rehabilitation.

Special Rehabilitation Units

Rehabilitation programs within hospitals or special rehabilitation hospitals use a multidisciplinary team approach, which involves the combined efforts of many specialists. The members of the rehabilitation team focus on different parts of health and manage different rehabilitation activities. The specific team members will vary significantly depending on the specific disability and situation.

In general, to qualify for Medicare or other insurance coverage of comprehensive rehabilitation at the hospital level, the person needs the following:

- Close medical supervision and care by a rehabilitation physician
- Rehabilitation nursing on a 24-hour basis
- Participation in more than one discipline, such as physical
- Therapy, occupational therapy, and speech therapy
- Team approach to therapy, with a coordinated rehabilitation program
- Clear, realistic goals in rehabilitation, with the expectation of significant improvement during the rehabilitation program

In general, rehabilitation programs in these settings are for a short time. Depending on the person's needs and anticipated improvement, inpatient rehabilitation programs usually last about 6–8 weeks for someone who has had a stroke, and about 2 weeks for someone who has had a hip fracture. A longer time is generally needed for those who have had more a severe injury, and a shorter time for those who have less complicated problems and were in good shape before becoming sick. Medicare reimbursement depends on documented progress as a result of therapy. The maximal length of stay is 90 days per illness.

If you cannot tolerate or do not need an intense therapy program, you may receive services at a nursing facility, in your home, or as an outpatient. These programs may also be more appropriate for ongoing maintenance therapy after an inpatient rehabilitation program.

Nursing Facilities

In this setting, maintaining function may be the goal of care. In contrast to the Medicare requirements for the hospital level of rehabilitation, the requirements for insurance coverage at the nursing level of rehabilitation do not include occupational therapy, a multidisciplinary approach, or the services of a rehabilitation physician. However, the requirements do specify that a person must need daily physical therapy and skilled nursing care and that continued, significant functional improvement must be documented. To be eligible for skilled nursing benefits through Medicare, the person must have had a hospital stay of at least 3 days in the past 30 days. The length of Medicare coverage for rehabilitation in nursing homes is limited.

Outpatient Rehabilitation

Outpatient rehabilitation offers a wide range of services from private practitioners' offices that offer fee-for-service care, to outpatient rehabilitation facilities that provide the same comprehensive team efforts as in hospital rehabilitation units. Generally, these outpatient units are appropriate for people with short-term illnesses, such as low back pain or minor trauma. Other services may be appropriate for people who need follow-up services after being discharged from a rehabilitation hospital or for whom an inpatient rehabilitation program is not suitable. Often, the availability of transportation is what determines whether the person can participate in an outpatient rehabilitation program.

Home-Based Rehabilitation

Home-care rehabilitation programs can be an important part of follow-up care for people who have been discharged from any type of inpatient rehabilitation program. In addition, home rehabilitation services can help provide short-term or maintenance therapy. Medicare provides home-health benefits to patients who need intermittent or part-time skilled nursing care and therapy services, and who are home-bound or leave the home only occasionally. Physicians must certify the person for services, but they are rarely involved in the supervision of care. There is no requirement for prior hospitalization, and there is no limit on the number of visits a person may receive but only for the time that the person needs to have a nurse come to his or her home. Home-health services provide skilled nursing and home-health aides, therapeutic services, medical and social services, and supplies.

Advantages and Disadvantages

Each site of care has advantages and disadvantages. Inpatient care is the most intense but may not be possible for frail elderly patients, because it requires 3 hours per day of active (and tiring) therapy. Skilled nursing offers 24-hour care for those who cannot care for themselves or do not have a full-time caregiver. Patients often prefer to return to their own homes for outpatient services, but the care-giving they need may not be available. Participation in a day hospital or outpatient clinic requires transportation, which can be costly and time consuming.

Rehabilitation for Specific Diseases

Several common diseases of old age usually require rehabilitation. These include stroke, hip fracture, and diseases that result in amputation being necessary (e.g., severe problems with circulation).

Stroke Rehabilitation

Most stroke therapy programs take place in a rehabilitation hospital, a rehabilitation unit in an acute-care hospital, or a nursing facility. Patients with acute stroke who receive coordinated, multidisciplinary evaluation and services do better than patients who do not. The goal of physical therapy in these programs is the ability to walk safely again, usually using a cane, walker, or other assistive device. Generally, occupational therapists address problems with weakness and coordination of the arms, as well as with difficulties in thinking or perception. For people who have difficulty speaking, speech therapists develop specific treatment programs that include trying to restore speech ability and, if necessary, developing another way to communicate.

After someone suffers a stroke, a speech or occupational therapist may evaluate how well the person can swallow. Difficulty swallowing is a common complication of strokes that frequently is not recognized.

The involvement and education of family or caregivers during the stroke rehabilitation program is crucial to the entire rehabilitation process. This is important in establishing the appropriate goals for rehabilitation and in planning for discharge. Before the patient is discharged, physical and occupational therapists generally visit the home to evaluate it for safety and the need for any adaptive equipment. Depression after a stroke is common and may also seriously affect rehabilitation.

Prevention: Someone who has had one stroke is at very high risk for a second stroke. The rehabilitation phase is a good time to make sure that risk factors for stroke have been evaluated and any preventive treatments are started. For example, narrowing of the arteries that go to the brain (e.g., carotid arteries) and certain heart conditions can lead to stroke. If someone has one or both of these conditions, the use of aspirin or other blood thinners might be considered. Other risk factors to investigate include smoking, high blood pressure, high cholesterol levels, and diabetes.

Hip Fracture Rehabilitation

The goal of rehabilitation for people who have had a hip fracture is to regain as much function as possible. Rehabilitation focuses on physical therapy to strengthen the leg muscles. Stronger leg muscles can prepare the person for walking and can also help keep a hip fracture that has been fixed with pins or screws more stable. During therapy, arm muscles are also strengthened to help with use of walking aids such as walkers. In addition, arm strength and function are important for bathing and dressing, which may be affected by the leg problems. Generally, people progress from using a walker, to using a wide-based four-prong cane, to walking with a single-point cane, and hopefully eventually to walking without any aid at all, although many people still need a walking aid even a year after a fracture.

Several factors influence both the course and outcome of rehabilitation after a hip fracture. Whether a person can stand bearing their full weight depends on the type and severity of the fracture and the surgery. Most people are allowed to put full weight on their leg the first day after surgery. People who are able to bear their full weight early on generally need less physical therapy than others. What kind of shape the person was in before the surgery is also very important. Unfortunately, some people are not able to fully recover after a hip fracture, and may need to either have someone move in with them or move to a nursing home.

Prevention: People who fracture a hip often have a tendency to all and osteoporosis (brittle bones), which puts them at increased risk of more fractures. Key parts of rehabilitation include the following:

- Treating osteoporosis

- Improving balance

- Reducing the risk of injury

Although hip protector pads reduce the rate of hip fracture, most people find them too difficult to wear.

Rehabilitation If You Need an Amputation

Seventy-five percent of all amputations are performed on people older than 65 years. About 90% of amputations involve the leg, with two-thirds of these done below the knee. Fortunately, fewer than 15% of people with amputations below the knee eventually need amputations above the knee. Approximately 75% of older adults can regain their ability to walk, with or without assistive devices, if they undergo the proper rehabilitation program before and after they receive an artificial limb (i.e., prosthesis).

Before surgery: Ordinarily, the rehabilitation process for an amputation takes longer than that for either a stroke or hip fracture. The program begins before surgery and involves not only an evaluation of the amputation site, but also a comprehensive evaluation of both your medical condition and motivation to participate in the program. Whenever possible, management before surgery should include stabilizing any medical problems, especially heart and lung disease. Your surgeon, primary care physician, physiatrist, and you and your family should discuss your care plan after surgery as well as your conditioning and training before you get a prosthesis. This includes preparing you for the possible "phantom limb" sensation, in which you feel as if the amputated limb were still present.

After surgery: The initial efforts after surgery include the following:

- Taking proper care of the stump to promote healing

- Beginning an exercise program to strengthen the muscles above the site of the amputation

- Maintaining proper position and exercising to prevent contractures (muscle stiffening) of the knee or hip

Shrinking of the stump to accommodate the socket of a temporary prosthesis is usually done by using tight elastic cuffs or by frequent wrapping with tight elastic bandages. Usually, people are measured for a temporary prosthesis 4–8 weeks after surgery and for a permanent prosthesis 8–12 weeks after surgery.

Getting around again: In preparation for an amputation, the therapy program initially involves training in transfer techniques, such as from bed to wheelchair or from chair to toilet. After an amputation, you will progress to practicing weight bearing on a temporary prosthesis, first on parallel bars, and then using a walker and eventually crutches and a cane for assistance. By the time you complete the rehabilitation program, you will probably be able to walk without any assistance.

Artificial limbs or prostheses: The list in the following text provides some guidelines for the use of prostheses:

• Age alone is never a reason to avoid use of a prosthesis.

• In general, the prosthesis should be as light as possible, and the attachment should be easy to use.

• People who have a prosthesis should be able to (or receive training so they are able to) perform simple transfer movements without the prosthesis. For example, it should not be necessary to put on a prosthesis to transfer from a bed to either a wheelchair or the bathroom in the middle of the night.

• About 75% of older adults who have had an amputation can walk with a prosthesis. Many people who have had amputations below the knee can walk independently, without a cane, walker, or other assistive device.

• Often, the person's functional ability before an amputation is one of the most reliable predictors of success in learning to use a prosthesis, both short and long term.

• If you are faced with an amputation, meeting with a person who has successfully completed a rehabilitation program and who walks independently can be very useful and motivating.

• Depression after an amputation is common. Emotional support, appropriate treatment, and involvement of family members and other caregivers are critical.

Prevention: Overall, an older adult who has had one leg amputated runs a 20% risk of needing a second amputation within 2 years. Approximately 30% of people who need an amputation because of poor circulation need an amputation on the other side within 5 years. The risk is even higher for people whose poor circulation has been further worsened by diabetes. For these reasons, rehabilitation should include programs to reduce the risk of poor circulation, including programs to stop smoking, reduce cholesterol, and control glucose (sugar) levels in the blood. Programs that include endurance exercise can also improve function and reduce pain and weakness. Daily monitoring for infection and other skin problems are essential.

Common Medical Problems during Rehabilitation

During rehabilitation, potential barriers to regaining or maintaining function are identified and removed. Medical evaluation is often ongoing throughout rehabilitation, so that significant illness and disability can be treated or prevented. Factors that have an important influence on the outcome of rehabilitation include the following:

- The nature and extent of the limitation
- The individual's motivation and commitment
- Adequate daily supervision

Blood Clots

Older adults who have had a stroke or suffered a hip fracture are at increased risk of blood clots that are painful and could travel to the lungs (pulmonary embolus). Generally, people are treated with blood thinners during rehabilitation to prevent blood clots from forming.

Heart Disease

Most physical therapy programs do not require a high level of physical activity. In fact, it may come as a surprise that occupational therapy puts more stress on the heart and lungs than physical therapy does. This is because exercising the arms increases blood pressure and pulse rate more than exercising the legs. Therapy activities for people with heart disease are generally adjusted, especially if these activities cause chest pain, shortness of breath, light-headedness, or fatigue. Blood pressure and pulse rate are checked often. Sometimes, additional tests are needed to evaluate cardiac risk.

Joint Problems

Arthritis that is already present may get worse during rehabilitation. This is because therapy usually involves progressive weight bearing, which can stress the joints. Some people may develop an inflammation or bursitis around the shoulder or hip joints. Some of this is due to the increased physical activity in their rehabilitation program. Treatment is generally the same as for arthritis.

Lung Disease

Lung function should be checked again in people who have lung disease or who become short of breath while participating in a physical or occupational therapy program. Sometimes the amount of oxygen in the blood is measured during the therapy sessions. It may be possible to include a lung rehabilitation program within the person's primary rehabilitation program. Usually, lung rehabilitation programs work on breathing techniques, pacing activities, and learning exercises and relaxation methods to help in activities of daily living.

Tools and Techniques of Rehabilitation

Rehabilitation techniques are not limited just to programs for specific conditions, such as stroke or hip fracture. They are also used when people have difficulty performing various activities of daily living, such as transferring from wheelchair to bed or toilet, eating, bathing, and dressing.

Rehabilitation of Walking Problems

Walking problems are most common when there is a problem with the muscles, joints, or nervous system. Various assistive devices for walking, such as canes, walkers, orthotics (e.g., braces), and prostheses, are designed to improve balance and support while standing or walking.

Canes

Canes are the simplest aids for walking but provide the least amount of support and balance. They can support up to 25% of body weight. Their best use is for people whose ability to walk is limited by weakness or pain on only one side.

How to use a cane: In general, you should hold the cane in the hand of your unaffected side. This allows you to form an arch between the affected side and the cane to help support your weight. This also allows a shorter period of weight bearing on the affected side when you walk.

How long should the cane be?: The length of the cane is important for ensuring stability and comfort. The best way to determine the proper cane length is to measure the distance from your "wrist crease" to the ground when you are standing straight. In other words, a cane that is the correct length will come from the ground to the crease of your wrist, when your arm is dangling beside the cane.

Walkers

A walker has four broadly spaced posts that surround the person using it. Walkers can support up to 50% of body weight, so they may be useful for people who have a lot of weakness or problems on both sides.

Modified walkers: Walkers can be modified for people who have significant weakness or loss of function in their upper arms. For example, if you have deformed upper extremities caused by rheumatoid arthritis, you can use a modified platform walker with arm rests. These platform walkers will allow you to walk, as well as to participate in active physical therapy of your lower legs. Rolling walkers can be made into "auto-stop" walkers, so that when the user presses down on the front wheels the walker stops rolling. If you are considering using a walker, your home situation needs to be evaluated carefully. If you functioned well with a walker in a rehabilitation unit, you may find new challenges at home, including thresholds, throw rugs, narrow passages, and short stair treads.

Orthotics (Orthoses) and Braces

Orthotics are another type of device used for rehabilitation. They can be applied to the arms, legs, and spine. Orthotics are braces that are designed to modify the support and functional characteristics of the musculoskeletal system. The goals of these braces include the following:

• Relieving pain by limiting motion or weight bearing

• Protecting weak, painful, or healing body parts

• Reducing weight on that body part(s)

• Preventing and correcting deformity

• Improving function

Common reasons for using an orthosis on your legs include weakness, deformity, increased muscle tone (spasticity), ankle or knee instability, or pain on weight bearing (which sometimes occurs after surgery or with inflammatory arthritis). However, orthoses are not appropriate for everyone who has a leg problem. For example, a lower-leg orthosis may aggravate rather than improve your walking if you have poor balance, strength, or coordination. In addition, a poorly fitting device, underlying skin disease, poor circulation, or swelling all increase the chances of skin sores. The principles that apply to the use of orthoses for the arms are similar to those that apply for the legs.

Rigid braces can be valuable for people who do not have enough stability in their spine. However, the areas where the brace presses on the body must be watched carefully so that sores do not develop. Similarly, people with neck problems (e.g., muscle strain, a narrowing of the spinal canal, or arthritis) can sometimes benefit from using a cervical collar. These collars are often made of soft foam or molded plastic. Regardless of material, they all provide a similar amount of support to the neck, spine, and muscles. However, neck collars and spinal supports should be used very cautiously. The following important principles should be kept in mind when using spinal supports:

- These devices should be used for only a very short time to avoid psychological dependency.

- The prolonged use of neck collars may actually weaken and eventually wither or shrink (atrophy) your neck muscles.

Wheelchairs

Wheelchairs are an easy and frequently used (if not overused) way for older adults to move about. Several factors are important in use of a wheelchair, whether it is used during the rehabilitation process or on a long-term basis.

Proper fit: You must be properly fitted and measured to your wheelchair. If this is not done correctly, a wheelchair might actually worsen rather than help your mobility. Ideally, your weight, strength, skin condition, heart function, mental capacity, and vision should all be evaluated. In the process, you need to balance your concerns about seating comfort with those for mobility and your general functional needs.

For most people, a chair with the large rear wheel is adequate. While sitting in the chair with your feet on the floor, you should be able to raise your feet off the floor.

Footrest height: Footrests need to be properly positioned. If it is too low, it may increase the pressure under the thigh and allow your foot to drag. If it is too high, it may increase the pressure on both your foot and calf, which increases the risk of pressure ulcers and blood clots in the legs.

Seat width: The chair should be as narrow as possible, with a clearance of at least 2" on each side for entering doorways. A seat that is too narrow can make it more difficult to get into and out of the chair and can increase the risk of pressure ulcers. However, the seat can be modified to reduce the risk of pressure ulcers by using low-pressure cushions made of foam or gel. A seat that is too wide can lead to unsteadiness while sitting and to difficulty in propelling the wheelchair and overcoming various barriers, such as narrow doors.

Armrest height: If the armrests are too high, your shoulder muscles can become fatigued. If the armrests are too low, you may develop poor posture (as a result of leaning forward), and your balance within the wheelchair could become affected. Arm rests can also be modified so that the arms can be raised up, down, or folded back on each other to help when transferring into and out of the chair.

Use in the home: Homes may need to be modified to add an entrance ramp. Doorways need to be 30–36" wide, and bathrooms at least 5–6 feet wide so there is enough room to turn the wheelchair. Powered or motorized wheelchairs are generally reserved for people who have not been able to get around well enough using a manual wheelchair. Generally, these people suffer from increasing disability as a result of a progressive disease, and they should be working with both a physiatrist and a physical therapist. Powered wheelchairs are made in three-wheeled and four-wheeled versions. They vary substantially in quality, adjustability, and durability, but all are quite expensive.

Transferring from One Place to Another

Transferring means moving or shifting from one surface to another, and it can begin while sitting, standing, or lying down. If you are not able to transfer alone, you may need the help of another person or an adaptive device. Being able to transfer safely requires a combination of physical and perceptual abilities, proper equipment, and training to learn techniques that are appropriate for your specific needs. In general, to transfer safely and comfortably, you must be able to stay balanced while sitting. To transfer while standing, you must also be able to stand evenly without assistance, have lower-leg stability, and have a reasonable degree of strength in your upper arms.

Bed to wheelchair transfer: A bed-to-wheelchair transfer can begin from a sitting position. You should lock the brakes on both sides of your wheelchair, grab onto the side rails of the bed to come to a sitting position, and then sit down in the wheelchair while holding the

419

front arm of the chair with your unaffected arm (if you have weakness or paralysis on one side). This type of transfer is also known as a stand-pivot transfer. Early in the course of therapy, or if you cannot stand, a board can be used to bridge the space between the bed and the wheelchair.

Wheelchair to toilet transfer: A wheelchair-to-toilet transfer is similar to the bed-to-wheelchair transfer. You must also be able to manage clothing and undergarments. Special adaptive equipment can be used to help make these transfers easier and safer. For example, toilet seats should be approximately 20" from the floor. If necessary, raised toilet seats can be attached to the standard height toilet bowl. Handrails can be attached to the wall (if it is close enough) or freestanding. Handrails should be placed on the side of the toilet that corresponds to your unaffected side if you have weakness or paralysis on one side, or on both sides of the toilet if you have weakness on both sides.

In and out of the bathtub transfer: A transfer in and out of the bathtub must be considered carefully because it is a potentially dangerous procedure. Unlike most transfers, which normally are made from your strongest side, a tub transfer usually makes use of your weaker side. Again, adaptive equipment can help. A tub transfer bench bridges the tub side and allows you to have one leg in the tub and one leg outside the tub, so you can move safely along the bench to the tub. A person with weakness or paralysis on one side may first move the affected leg into the tub and then the unaffected leg.

Assistive Devices

Assistive devices can be used to help people who have difficulty performing activities of daily living such as feeding, bathing, and dressing. An evaluation by an occupational therapist is helpful to make sure that the assistive device is the best one for the circumstances. Several important principles need to be considered:

- A person must be physically and mentally capable of using the device effectively.

- People are more likely to use aids that are not conspicuous, complicated, cumbersome, or cosmetically ugly.

- A person with perceptual problems (e.g., poor vision) may have difficulty using a device effectively.

- Assistive devices may be expensive, and they are usually not covered by insurance or other payers.

- An evaluation of a person's home or other living situation may be needed to determine the best assistive devices to improve function and ensure safety.

Eating: Older adults with weakness, deformity, or lack of coordination of the arms, or with limited range of arm motion frequently find assistive devices for eating very helpful. A rocker knife and fork, for example, may allow a person with paralysis on one side to cut and pick up food with one hand. Similar assistive devices can be used for spoons, bowls, and plates. Eating utensils can also be modified for people who have limited motion or poor grasp. For example, silverware handles can be enlarged with foam padding or other materials. A cuff that straps around the hand to hold eating utensils in place can help a person who has a weak hand.

Food preparation: Easy ways of preparing food are often helpful. Foods that do not need to be cut, chopped, or mixed are generally recommended, along with packages and containers that are easy to open. A board with a rough surface, a rubber mat, or sponges can be used to hold food steady. Using blenders, coffee pots, crock pots, microwave ovens, and electric skillets all reduce the need to use the stove or oven. All small kitchen appliances should be on a stable work surface at a comfortable height. Pizza cutters can sometimes replace knives. Oversized bowls, plate guards, and soup dishes with high rims can be used to avoid spills for people who make extra movements or have tremors. For people who have lost some manual dexterity, electric can openers and jar openers can be extremely helpful.

Washing and personal hygiene: Many bathing and grooming aids are available to help people who have limited motion or grasping ability, weakness, or difficulty with coordination. These include the following:

- Raised toilet seats
- Tub transfer benches
- Long-handled bath sponges
- "Soap-on-a-rope"
- Wash mitts
- A hand-held shower hose attached to the faucet
- A bath mat secured to the tub surface with safety-tread tape
- Combs and brushes with foam-padded enlarged handles

421

In addition, a wall mirror can be tilted downward to permit better visibility from a wheelchair.

Dressing: Assistive devices are also available to help with dressing. These include the following:

- Buttonhooks or zipper pulls

- Hook and loop (Velcro®) attachments, which are excellent substitutes for buttons or shoelaces

- Dressing sticks, which allow users to dress while sitting (users can hook or pull the cuff or sleeve of a shirt or pant leg into position)

- Devices for putting on socks, which allow users who cannot reach their feet to pull up socks or stockings themselves

- Other slip-on dressing aids

For people who have limited motion of the arms or shoulders, various reaching aids can help in pulling hats off a shelf or in picking items up off the floor.

Other Rehabilitative Techniques

People who are undergoing either restorative or maintenance rehabilitation may benefit from electrical stimulation and thermal approaches. These techniques are used to increase circulation, stimulate muscles, and ease pain.

Electrical Stimulation

Two kinds of electrical stimulation are generally available:

- Functional electrical stimulation

- Transcutaneous electrical nerve stimulation (TENS)

In functional electrical stimulation, an electrical current is used to produce a muscle contraction. This prevents muscles that have not been used for a while from withering and shrinking (atrophy). It also increases the range of muscle motion and strength, helps increase the voluntary function of a previously paralyzed muscle, and decreases muscle tone that is too great or spastic. For older adults who have severe weakness of the upper arms, functional electrical stimulation can help prevent a shoulder dislocation, which can lead to a "frozen" shoulder. Electrical stimulation has also been used to improve the strength of pelvic muscles in older women who suffer from certain forms of incontinence.

TENS involves the direct electrical stimulation of the spinal cord. It improves muscle strength and mass, and it may relieve pain. It has been used to treat pain associated with rheumatoid arthritis, poor circulation, and nerve diseases, possibly reducing the amount of pain medicine that is needed. TENS has also been used to treat older adults who have shingles (herpes zoster), to reduce muscle tone that is too great or spastic after a stroke, and to relieve the nerve pain sometimes associated with diabetes or poor circulation. While TENS is sometimes used for chronic low back pain, it has not been proved to work.

Thermal Approaches

Various thermal approaches are used primarily to treat pain, reduce inflammation, and increase muscle tone. Heat can be applied either superficially with a hot pack, or more deeply using ultrasound or diathermy. Heat can help muscles relax, relieve pain, help with tissue healing, and prepare stiff joints and tight muscles for exercise. Hot packs can be applied to most body surfaces. They may reduce muscle spasm in older adults who have arthritis involving the neck, muscular low back pain, or muscle contractions. Baths of liquid paraffin are used most often to apply heat to the hands or feet and may be particularly helpful to reduce hand stiffness and pain in people who have arthritis.

Ultrasound is a deep-heating technique that can increase temperatures deep in the tissues. This can relieve joint tightness, loosen scar tissue, and reduce pain and muscle spasm. It has been used to treat bursitis, tendonitis, and low back pain.

Hydrotherapy in the form of a whirlpool or other pool therapy may also be helpful. It has been used to treat arthritis and joint injuries or replacements. It has also been used to relieve pain, support wound healing, and help with various neurologic disorders.

Cold treatments or cold packs are commonly used to treat sudden muscle or bone injuries. They can sometimes reduce pain and muscle spasms, especially those caused by brain injury.

Chapter 46

Choosing a Long-Term Care Setting

Adult Day Care Services

Adult day care can provide respite care as well as ongoing services. Services are provided in a variety of centers around the state. Social, recreational, and health services are provided in a protective setting to individuals who cannot be left alone because of health care needs, confusion, or disability. These programs provide meals and care services in a community setting during the day when a caregiver needs time off or must work.

Adult Foster Homes

Adult foster homes offer personal and health care to individuals in private residences. Care and supervision are provided to maintain a safe and secure setting. Adult foster homes are licensed, inspected, and monitored by the Department of Human Services, Seniors and People with Disabilities and Area Agency on Aging offices. People often choose adult foster care because it is more affordable than other care facilities and care is provided in a homelike setting. These homes provide care for no more than five individuals.

All adult foster home providers and primary caregivers must:

• pass a criminal record check;

"Choosing a long-term care setting," reprinted with permission from the Oregon Department of Human Services (www.oregon.gov/DHS), © 2010.

- complete a basic training course and pass an exam;
- be physically and mentally able to provide care;
- provide care in a home that meets structural and safety requirements.

Alzheimer's Care Units

Some facilities specialize in providing care only to persons with Alzheimer's disease or other forms of dementia. A facility that specializes in the care for people with memory impairment must receive an endorsement and is governed by additional regulations that are specifically intended to support individuals with dementia.

Structural requirements in an Alzheimer's-endorsed setting:

- a secure building that alerts staff if a resident has exited;
- a secure outdoor area that provides outdoor freedom safely;
- interior finishes that are non-glare and well lit;
- visual contrasts between floors, walls, and doorways.

Program requirements: In addition to providing the services required in our other licensed settings, Alzheimer's units must also have programs, which include:

- gross motor activities;
- self-care activities;
- social activities;
- crafts;
- sensory enhancement activities;
- outdoor activities.

Assisted Living Facilities

Assisted living facilities provide housing and supportive services for six or more residents. These facilities are fully wheelchair accessible. Residents of assisted living facilities have private apartments, ranging from a studio to one or two bedrooms. Each apartment unit has a kitchenette and private bathroom with a wheelchair accessible shower. Assisted living facilities are licensed and regulated by the Department of Human Services, Seniors and People with Disabilities.

Assisted living facilities are best suited for individuals who want to remain as independent as possible and who are able to direct their own care.

Assisted living facilities are not required to have licensed registered nurses on staff 24 hours a day.

Duties and qualifications of direct caregivers will vary among facilities. Staff to resident ratio will typically be lower than what is required for nursing homes. Caregivers are not required to be certified, although training prior to providing services to residents is mandatory.

Continuing Care Retirement Communities

Continuing Care Retirement Communities are generally made up of independent living residences, assisted living/residential care facilities, and nursing facilities. These communities require an entrance fee along with monthly and/or other periodic charges. They are required to register with the state and disclose specific information about the services they provide and their finances. Only a nursing facility, residential care, or assisted living facility located on the campus must be licensed by the state. Otherwise Continuing Care Retirement Communities are not regulated.

Nursing Facilities

Nursing facilities are licensed by the Department of Human Services, Seniors and People with Disabilities and are required to meet both federal and state regulations.

Services offered in nursing facilities:

- nursing care on a 24-hour basis;
- on-site physical rehabilitation;
- recuperation after hospitalization for serious illness or surgery;
- restorative services;
- end-of-life care.

Nursing facilities are most appropriate for people who need 24-hour medical oversight and a protective/structured setting. Residents may have medical and behavioral needs that cannot be met in other care settings. Most residents must share their room. Space is limited, but residents are allowed to bring personal items to encourage a more home-like atmosphere.

Residential Care Facilities

Residential care facilities provide housing and supportive services for six or more people who don't need 24-hour nursing care. Residential care facilities offer shared and private rooms. These facilities are not required to provide private bathrooms or kitchenettes. Many residential care facilities specialize in caring for individuals with Alzheimer's or dementia. These settings are licensed and regulated by the Department of Human Services.

When considering any long-term care setting, request copies of the residents' rights, the admission contract, and price list to read closely. Residential Care facilities are not required to have licensed nurses on staff for a specific number of hours per week.

The nurse typically does not provide hands-on personal nursing care.

Duties and qualifications of direct caregivers will vary among facilities. Staff to resident ratio will typically be lower than what is required for nursing homes. Caregivers are not required to be certified, although training prior to providing services to residents is mandatory.

Respite Care

Respite care gives families and other caregivers temporary relief from providing care for frail adults. Companionship, light assistance, recreational activities, and security are provided in the resident's home, out of home in a group setting, or overnight in a residential setting. Respite care allows for a healthier and better quality of life for both the caregiver and care receiver.

Retirement Homes/Complexes/Communities

Retirement complexes are for people who desire to and are able to live independently but do not want to maintain a home. Many people prefer to live in a community with others of the same age and with similar interests.

The Department of Human Services, Seniors and People with Disabilities does not regulate or license retirement communities.

Part Five

Special Education for Children with Disabilities

Chapter 47

Balancing Academics and Disability

When your child has a serious or chronic illness, it's hard to think beyond the next treatment. While health is the first priority, education also is important. You'll want to help your child stay on top of schoolwork as much as possible and plan for when he or she can return to school.

Not only does staying connected to school bring academic, cognitive, psychological, and social benefits—it's also your child's legal right. Under federal law, kids with disabilities are entitled to educational support, and your child might qualify for free services under the Individuals with Disabilities Education Act (IDEA).

With a little planning and a lot of communication, you can help your child balance treatment and academics.

Plan Ahead

First, talk to your doctor about how long your child is likely to be away from school and whether the treatment might interfere with concentrating, doing homework, and meeting deadlines. Are there side effects that might have an academic impact? What does your doctor recommend when it comes to attendance, tutoring, or studying?

Then talk to the teachers and school staff, and encourage your child, if well enough, to do the same. It may be necessary to set a reduced schedule or shift due dates for papers and tests. With your help, your son or daughter can work with teachers to help plan the workload. The more notice teachers have, the easier it will be to come up with a flexible solution.

Some kids who spend a lot of time away from school or in the hospital have Individual Education Programs (IEPs). These are customized goals and learning strategies created by the teachers, school psychologists (or other specialists), and counselors.

IEPs take a child's individual needs into account. Under the IDEA, kids who qualify for an IEP will receive one at no cost, in addition to receiving free support services (such as a tutor) to help them reach educational milestones.

IEPs can be requested by you or anyone on your child's education team.

Seek Out Hospital-Based Support

If your child will be spending long stretches in the hospital, ask a doctor, nurse, or child-life specialist about onsite schooling. Many hospitals provide this service free of charge to their patients.

The two most common types of educational support include bedside schooling and classroom schooling. Typically, bedside schooling is for children who are too ill to leave their hospital rooms or have weakened immune systems due to chemotherapy. Other kids who are well enough might be educated individually or in small groups in an onsite hospital classroom.

Licensed teachers who are K-12-certified in a variety of subjects and special education work intensively with students to make sure that they don't fall behind in their studies. To stay on track, hospital-based teachers work closely with teachers from a child's school to maintain curriculum continuity and ease reentry into the classroom when the child is well again. School is scheduled around medical tests and therapies, and always takes a child's medical condition and strength into consideration.

Whether your child is being educated at school, in the hospital, or at home, remember that getting better is the main priority. So be realistic about what he or she can handle. Kids may feel an unspoken pressure from parents, teachers, and themselves to continue with schoolwork, and this anxiety could hurt their recovery.

Stay Connected

Maintaining ties with classmates and teachers can help your child maintain a sense of normalcy during this difficult time. Your child might even be able to listen to a lesson or join a class over the computer. Programs nationwide offer free or low-cost laptops for use in the hospital; check with your doctor or medical staff to see if this service is available to you.

In addition to academic isolation, your child may feel cut off socially from friends and classmates. Online social networking sites, email, instant messaging (IM), text messaging, and talking on the phone can help kids stay connected. Also consider encouraging a letter-writing, email, or care package campaign from classmates—you might even set up a collection box at school where they can deposit notes and pictures. Arrange for visits from your child's friends and, if your son or daughter is up to it, take the group out to school plays, sports events, classroom parties, and other social gatherings.

Staying connected will make for a smoother transition socially and academically when your child returns to school after treatment.

Chapter 48

The Parent's Role in the Education Process

When your child with disabilities begins attending school, you will have the opportunity to become involved in your child's special education program, to become his or her educational advocate. Many school systems recommend or require that, before an individualized evaluation of a child is conducted, his or her teacher meet with an assistance team to discuss the nature of the problem and what possible modifications to instruction or the classroom might be made. These procedures are known as prereferral.

The Special Education Cycle

A number of activities make up the special education cycle:

- **Referral:** When a parent or teacher notices that a child is not making progress in school, he or she gives that information in writing to the school system so that an evaluation can be done.

- **Evaluation:** An evaluation is a careful look by a team of teachers and specialists at a child's abilities, strengths, and problems. It provides information about the child's capabilities and educational needs and helps to determine whether a special education program is necessary for the child.

Excerpted from "Parent Role in the Education Process," *ACS Exceptional Families Handbook*, by the Walter Reed Army Medical Center (www.walterreed.amedd .army.mil), U.S. Army, October 7, 2009.

- **Eligibility:** In order for a child to receive special educational services, the child must first qualify according to guidelines. An eligibility meeting is held and a decision is made as to whether a child meets the program requirements to receive special education services.

- **Individualized Education Program (IEP):** Every child in special education must have an Individualized Education Program. The IEP is a written statement describing the specially designed program developed to meet the unique needs of the child. Parents have a right to participate with the school in the development of the child's EP.

- **Placement:** The placement decision identities the appropriate school program and services needed to meet each child's educational goals. Related services may include speech therapy, occupational therapy, and transportation.

- **Instruction:** After the goals and objectives of the IEP have been written and a child has been placed in his or her school setting, learning activities begin in the classroom. Parents and school people must work together to make the IEP and placement work for the child by sharing information about the child's progress. Frequent communication is the key to success.

- **Annual review:** Every year the IEP is reviewed and a new IEP is developed for the next year. In addition, any time there is a change, or proposed change in a child's school program, parents must be informed and be a part of the decision-making process. Every 3 years, a new evaluation is completed and an eligibility decision must be made. This is called the triennial review.

Every school system in the United States has a set of regulations governing special education that include the activities listed in the preceding text. Some large school systems have very detailed, lengthy documents, while others have just a few pages.

You may have observed that your child cannot do some things that others his/her age have mastered, or you may have known that your child would need special education services from the time your child was an infant. Perhaps a teacher, pediatrician, or another professional may suggest your child be evaluated for special services. Any of these individuals can make a referral to the school system for your child to be evaluated. This must be in writing. Once a referral is made, a screening committee meets to discuss whether or not there is enough evidence to indicate that a child should be thoroughly evaluated. Screening committees are usually based in your child's home school. They may determine that there is not enough evidence to suggest special help or they may indicate a full evaluation is needed. Parents may be invited to participate in the screening committee, but in some schools, they may not be notified unless a decision has been made that the child needs to be evaluated.

Under federal and state laws, school systems must notify parents of their wish to evaluate the child and the parent's permission must be granted before the testing begins. School systems use many different tests and materials to evaluate children. Basically, tests and materials can be grouped into the following categories:

- **Educational:** An educational diagnostician or the classroom teacher, when qualified, gives various tests to measure a child's current levels of performance in academic subjects.

- **Medical:** A licensed physician assesses the child's medical history and health problems that might affect the child's learning.

- **Sociocultural:** A report is prepared by the school social worker from interviews with parents, teachers, and others describing the child's background and behavior at home and at school.

- **Psychological:** The school psychologist writes a report summarizing the test results that measure the child's general intelligence, eye-hand coordination, social skills, emotional development, and thinking skills. An evaluation by a clinical psychologist or psychiatrist might also be included.

- **Other:** This might include such evaluations as an assessment of the child's speech, language, or muscle development.

After you have been notified in writing that the school system wishes to evaluate your child, you must decide whether to give permission for your child to be tested. You may feel uncertain how to best help your child. The following suggestions are intended to help you become more confident about your decisions and actions:

- Talk to someone—share your feelings about the evaluation.

- Get parent handbooks and pamphlets on evaluations.

- Make a list of all your questions.

- Identify the school person responsible for your child's evaluation.

- Ask school officials to talk to you and/or put in writing the reasons for the evaluation.

When you have given your permission for the school to evaluate your child, you may want to do several things to prepare yourself and your child for this experience. You may want to do the following:

- Talk with your child about the reasons for the evaluation.

- Explain to your child how the evaluation will be done.

- Visit the place where the evaluation will be given.

- Give your child the chance to make some choices about the evaluation (such as what to wear).

While the evaluation is in progress you can continue to put your child at ease by doing the following:

- Review the day's plan with your child (including a celebration when it's over).

- Let your child know you will be there if appropriate.

- Watch to make sure your child's needs are met (fatigue, hunger, and bathroom needs).

- Observe the evaluation if you can and write down your thoughts concerning your child's responses.

- Make sure your child is in good health.

After the evaluation has been completed you may want to do the following:

- Ask your child which activities and people he liked and disliked.

- Praise him for his successes.

- Plan a celebration activity for your child (and for you).

- Write down any additional thoughts you have regarding the evaluation experience.

- Get a copy of the evaluation report and read it to see if you understand it and it is accurate.

- Meet with school people so they can explain to you the results of the evaluation.

Chapter 49

Laws about Educating Children with Disabilities

Chapter Contents

Section 49.1—Individuals with Disabilities
          Education Act (IDEA) 440

Section 49.2—No Child Left Behind Act................................. 441

Section 49.3—Section 504 of the Rehabilitation Act................ 445

Section 49.1

Individuals with Disabilities Education Act (IDEA)

"IDEA: The Individuals with Disabilities Education Act,"
by the National Dissemination Center for Children with Disabilities
(NICHCY, www.nichcy.org), September 2010.

IDEA (The Individuals with Disabilities Education Act) was originally enacted by Congress in 1975 to ensure that children with disabilities have the opportunity to receive a free appropriate public education, just like other children. The law has been revised many times over the years.

The most recent amendments were passed by Congress in December 2004, with final regulations published in August 2006. So, in one sense, the law is very new, even as it has a long, detailed, and powerful history. IDEA 2004 is divided into four parts, as follows:

- Part A: General Provisions, which includes findings of Congress, the purposes of IDEA, and key definitions

- Part B: Assistance for Education of All Children with Disabilities, which describes the processes that schools systems and states must use to identify children with disabilities and educate them, including preschoolers, as well as such other critical areas as parent and student rights

- Part C: Infants and Toddlers with Disabilities, which describes the responsibilities that states have for providing early intervention services to babies and toddlers with disabilities or developmental delays

- Part D: National Activities to Improve Education of Children with Disabilities, which authorizes programs meant to improve outcomes for children with disabilities, including teacher training programs, parent information and training centers in every state (PTIs), and the TA&D (Technical Assistance & Dissemination) network of projects that help states, locales, and families implement IDEA

Section 49.2

No Child Left Behind Act

What is the No Child Left Behind Act?

The No Child Left Behind Act of 2001 (NCLB) is the current version of the Elementary and Secondary Education Act (ESEA)—the principal federal law affecting public education from kindergarten through high school in the United States. The ESEA was originally passed in 1965. NCLB is important legislation for students with learning disabilities (LD), because it ensures that they reach high levels of academic standards, just like other children in America's public schools today.

NCLB is based on four principles of educational reform:

1. Stronger accountability for results

2. Increased flexibility and local control

3. Expanded options for parents

4. An emphasis on teaching qualifications and methods

Of these four, accountability for results is the principle that has the potential to greatly improve the educational results for children with LD.

How does NCLB hold schools accountable for results?

Several critical elements in NCLB ensure that schools are held accountable for educational results so that the best education possible is provided to each and every student. The three most critical elements to understand are:

- academic content standards (what students should learn);

- academic achievement standards (how well they should learn);

- state assessments (whether a school is teaching all students successfully).

441

Academic content standards and academic achievement standards in reading/language arts, mathematics, and science have been defined by each state. These standards define what all children should know and be able to do to be considered "proficient." Information about each state's standards should be available on the state's education department website and in print materials.

State assessments are the way schools must prove that they have successfully taught their students. Beginning in 2005–2006, all states must provide annual assessments that are appropriate for all students in grades 3 through 8 and once in high school in both reading/language arts and math (science assessments must be added beginning in 2007–2008). These assessments must include students with disabilities. Schools must also provide the accommodations and alternate assessments that may be needed by students with disabilities. Accommodations are changes to the assessment materials or procedures that allow for students to demonstrate their knowledge and skills rather than the effects of their disabilities. Students with learning disabilities should be participating in the regular state assessments with or without accommodations. Alternate assessments are assessments designed to measure the performance of students with disabilities who are unable to participate in state and district assessments even with appropriate accommodations. These alternate assessments are typically designed for students with complex disabilities and probably would not be appropriate for most students with learning disabilities.

How does NCLB work with the Individuals with Disabilities Education Act (IDEA)?

IDEA (Individuals with Disabilities Education Act) specifically provides services to students with disabilities. Each student served under IDEA has an Individualized Education Program (IEP) that defines the special education and related services needed by the student. NCLB holds schools accountable for the educational outcomes of those children, as well as all others. In the past, students with disabilities were frequently left out of state and district level assessment and accountability systems; and in many cases did not have access to the general curriculum on which these assessments are based. Because this type of access and assessment did not happen, there was no external measure to indicate whether special education students were learning enough to move on to a post-secondary education or to get a job.

The IEP that is designed for each individual IDEA-eligible student must address how that student will participate in state assessments.

Students with disabilities may participate in state assessments in the same way as other students, or with accommodations or by participating in alternate assessments. The IEP team should not be deciding whether a student will participate in state assessments, but how, so as to hold the educational system responsible for the student's learning. If the IEP team determines that an accommodation or modification needed by a child will invalidate a test's results for state accountability (such as, perhaps, having questions read aloud to the student), the team should decide how that student can appropriately be assessed through alternate methods.

Why is it so important that children with learning disabilities be included in state assessments?

No Child Left Behind is intended to improve the education of all children. As part of the law, all states are required to release easy-to-read, detailed report cards every year that provide parents and the general public with a measure of how schools are doing. These report cards must include information on how students in each district, as well as each school, performed on state assessments. The report cards must state student performance on three levels—basic, proficient, and advanced. The data must also be broken down by various student subgroups, including students with disabilities. Just like all other subgroups, NCLB requires that students with disabilities reach proficient levels of achievement. This is not extra pressure on the children. This is a mandate for schools to provide a better education for students with disabilities, including learning disabilities.

In addition, each state is required to set Adequate Yearly Progress (AYP) standards that schools must meet. In defining AYP, each state must set the minimum levels of improvement, measurable in terms of student performance that school districts and schools must achieve within the time frame specified by the law. Basically, states have to continue to raise the bar on academic achievement, and by 2013–2014 all subgroups in all schools in all states must be achieving proficient levels in reading and math on state assessments. This includes students with learning disabilities. Unlike in the past, NCLB is setting a way (the state assessments) for schools to be held accountable for what their students with learning disabilities are learning and achieving.

How else does NCLB set out to improve public education?

Here is a brief summary of other ways NCLB will ensure a better education for students with LD:

443

- **Increased flexibility and local control:** NCLB gives both states and local school districts greater flexibility in the use of federal funds than they previously had. This flexibility allows for the reallocation of certain funds to programs dedicated to teacher quality improvement, technology, safe and drug-free schools, and many others. This flexibility is dependent on improved results on state assessments and does not include IDEA funds, or the possibility of transferring money out of Title 1 programs.

- **Expanded options for parents:** Under NCLB, all parents must receive local and district report cards before the beginning of every school year. If a Title 1 school fails to meet its AYP goal for two consecutive years, parents may choose to place their children in non-failing schools in their district. Under NCLB, school districts must pay the cost of transporting students to the other public school. After 3 years of failure to meet AYP goals, schools must also offer supplemental services to the children remaining there, including tutoring, after-school programs, and summer school paid for by the district.

- **Improved teaching qualifications:** NCLB requires that all teachers be highly qualified. That means they hold at least a bachelor's degree and have passed a state test of subject knowledge. Elementary school teachers must demonstrate knowledge of teaching math and reading; while teachers in higher grades must demonstrate knowledge of the subject they teach, or must have majored in the subject. Special education teachers must be knowledgeable about the content area(s) they teach as well as special education, unless they provide consultative services to highly qualified general education teachers.

Section 49.3

Section 504 of the Rehabilitation Act

From "Your Rights under Section 504 of The Rehabilitation Act," by the
U.S. Department of Health and Human Services (DHHS, www.hhs.gov),
June 2006. Reviewed by David A. Cooke, MD, FACP, July 23, 2011.

What is Section 504?

Section 504 of the Rehabilitation Act of 1973 is a national law that
protects qualified individuals from discrimination based on their disability. The nondiscrimination requirements of the law apply to employers and organizations that receive financial assistance from any
federal department or agency, including the U.S. Department of Health
and Human Services (DHHS). These organizations and employers
include many hospitals, nursing homes, mental health centers, and
human service programs.

Section 504 forbids organizations and employers from excluding or
denying individuals with disabilities an equal opportunity to receive
program benefits and services. It defines the rights of individuals with
disabilities to participate in, and have access to, program benefits and
services.

Who is protected from discrimination?

Section 504 protects qualified individuals with disabilities. Under
this law, individuals with disabilities are defined as persons with a
physical or mental impairment that substantially limits one or more
major life activities. People who have a history of, or who are regarded
as having a physical or mental impairment that substantially limits
one or more major life activities, are also covered. Major life activities
include caring for one's self, walking, seeing, hearing, speaking, breathing, working, performing manual tasks, and learning. Some examples
of impairments that may substantially limit major life activities, even
with the help of medication or aids/devices, are AIDS [acquired immunodeficiency syndrome], alcoholism, blindness or visual impairment,
cancer, deafness or hearing impairment, diabetes, drug addiction, heart
disease, and mental illness.

445

In addition to meeting the above definition, for purposes of receiving services, education, or training, qualified individuals with disabilities are persons who meet normal and essential eligibility requirements.

For purposes of employment, qualified individuals with disabilities are persons who, with reasonable accommodation, can perform the essential functions of the job for which they have applied or have been hired to perform. (Complaints alleging employment discrimination on the basis of disability against a single individual will be referred to the U.S. Equal Employment Opportunity Commission for processing.)

Reasonable accommodation means an employer is required to take reasonable steps to accommodate your disability unless it would cause the employer undue hardship.

What are prohibited discriminatory acts in health care and human services settings?

Section 504 prohibitions against discrimination apply to service availability, accessibility, delivery, employment, and the administrative activities and responsibilities of organizations receiving federal financial assistance. A recipient of federal financial assistance may not, on the basis of disability:

- deny qualified individuals the opportunity to participate in or benefit from federally funded programs, services, or other benefits;

- deny access to programs, services, benefits, or opportunities to participate as a result of physical barriers;

- deny employment opportunities, including hiring, promotion, training, and fringe benefits, for which they are otherwise entitled or qualified.

These and other prohibitions against discrimination based on disability can be found in the DHHS Section 504 regulation.

Chapter 50

Evaluating Children for Disability

Evaluation is an essential beginning step in the special education process for a child with a disability. Before a child can receive special education and related services for the first time, a full and individual initial evaluation of the child must be conducted to see if the child has a disability and is eligible for special education. Informed parent consent must be obtained before this evaluation may be conducted.

The evaluation process is guided by requirements in our nation's special education law, the Individuals with Disabilities Education Act (IDEA). This text will help you learn more about what these requirements are.

Purposes of Evaluation

The initial evaluation of a child is required by IDEA before any special education and related services can be provided to that child. The purposes of conducting this evaluation are straightforward:

- To see if the child is a "child with a disability," as defined by IDEA
- To gather information that will help determine the child's educational needs
- To guide decision making about appropriate educational programming for the child.

From "Evaluating Children for Disability," by the National Dissemination Center for Children with Disabilities (NICHCY, www.nichcy.org), 2008.

IDEA's Definition of a "Child with a Disability"

IDEA lists different disability categories under which a child may be found eligible for special education and related services. These categories are the following:

- Autism
- Deafness
- Deaf-blindness
- Developmental delay
- Emotional disturbance
- Hearing impairment
- Mental retardation
- Multiple disabilities
- Orthopedic impairment
- Other health impairment
- Specific learning disability
- Speech or language impairment
- Traumatic brain injury
- Visual impairment, including blindness

Having a disability, though, does not necessarily make a child eligible for special education. Consider this language from the IDEA regulations: Child with a disability means a child evaluated in accordance with §§300.304 through 300.311 as having [one of the disabilities listed in the preceding text] and who, by **reason thereof**, needs special education and related services. [emphasis added]

This provision includes the very important phrase " . . . and who, by reason thereof . . . ." This means that, because of the disability, the child needs special education and related services. Many children have disabilities that do not bring with them the need for extra educational assistance or individualized educational programming. If a child has a disability but is not eligible under IDEA, he or she may be eligible for the protections afforded by other laws—such as Section 504 of the Rehabilitation Act of 1973, as amended. It's not uncommon for a child to have a 504 plan at school to address disability-related educational needs. Such a child will receive needed assistance but not under IDEA.

Identifying Children for Evaluation

Before a child's eligibility under IDEA can be determined, however, a full and individual evaluation of the child must be conducted. There are at least two ways in which a child may be identified to receive an evaluation under IDEA:

1. Parents may request that their child be evaluated. Parents are often the first to notice that their child's learning, behavior, or development may be a cause for concern. If they're worried about their child's progress in school and think he or she might need extra help from special education services, they may call, email, or write to their child's teacher, the school's principal, or the Director of Special Education in the school district. If the school agrees that an evaluation is needed, it must evaluate the child at no cost to parents.

2. The school system may ask to evaluate the child. Based on a teacher's recommendation, observations, or results from tests given to all children in a particular grade, a school may recommend that a child receive further screening or assessment to determine if he or she has a disability and needs special education and related services. The school system must ask parents for permission to evaluate the child, and parents must give their informed written permission before the evaluation may be conducted.

Giving Parents Notice

It is important to know that IDEA requires the school system to notify parents in writing that it would like to evaluate their child (or that it is refusing to evaluate the child). This is called giving prior written notice. It is not enough for the agency to tell parents that it would like to evaluate their child or that it refuses to evaluate their child. The school must also:

- explain why it wants to conduct the evaluation (or why it refuses);

- describe each evaluation procedure, assessment, record, or report used as a basis for proposing the evaluation (or refusing to conduct the evaluation);

- where parents can go to obtain help in understanding IDEA's provisions;

- what other options the school considered and why those were rejected; and

449

- a description of any other factors that are relevant to the school's proposal (or refusal) to evaluate the child.

The purpose behind this thorough explanation is to make sure that parents are fully informed, understand what is being proposed (or refused), understand what evaluation of their child will involve (or why the school system is refusing to conduct an evaluation of the child), and understand their right to refuse consent for evaluation, or to otherwise exercise their rights under IDEA's procedural safeguards if the school refuses to evaluate.

All written communication from the school must be in a form the general public can understand. It must be provided in parents' native language if they do not read English, or in the mode of communication they normally use (such as Braille or large print) unless it is clearly not feasible to do so. If parents' native language or other mode of communication is not a written language, the school must take steps to ensure:

- that the notice is translated orally (or by other means) to parents in their native language or other mode of communication,

- that parents understand the content of the notice, and

- that there is written evidence that the above two requirements have been met.

Parental Consent

Before the school may proceed with the evaluation, parents must give their informed written consent. This consent is for the evaluation only. It does not mean that the school has the parents' permission to provide special education services to the child. That requires a separate consent.

If parents refuse consent for an initial evaluation (or simply don't respond to the school's request), the school must carefully document all its attempts to obtain parent consent. It may also continue to pursue conducting the evaluation by using the law's due process procedures or its mediation procedures, unless doing so would be inconsistent with state law relating to parental consent.

However, if the child is home-schooled or has been placed in a private school by parents (meaning, the parents are paying for the cost of the private school), the school may not override parents' lack of consent for initial evaluation of the child. As the Department of Education (2006) notes: Once parents opt out of the public school system, States and school districts do not have the same interest in requiring parents to agree to the evaluation of their children. In such cases, it would be overly intrusive for the school district to insist on an evaluation over a parent's objection. (71 Fed. Reg. at 46635)

Timeframe for Initial Evaluation

Let's move on from the prerequisites for initial evaluation (parent notification and parent consent) to the actual process of initial evaluation and what the law requires. Let us assume that parents' informed consent has been given, and it's time to evaluate the child. Must this evaluation be conducted within a certain period of time after parents give their consent? Yes. In its reauthorization of IDEA in 2004, Congress added a specific timeframe: The initial evaluation must be conducted within 60 days of receiving parental consent for the evaluation—or if the state establishes its own timeframe for conducting an initial evaluation, within that timeframe. (In other words: Any timeframe established by the state takes precedence over the 60-day timeline required by IDEA.)

The Scope of Evaluation

A child's initial evaluation must be full and individual, focused on that child and only that child. This is a longstanding provision of IDEA. An evaluation of a child under IDEA means much more than the child sitting in a room with the rest of his or her class taking an exam for that class, that school, that district, or that state. How the child performs on such exams will contribute useful information to an IDEA-related evaluation, but large-scale tests or group-administered instruments are not enough to diagnose a disability or determine what, if any, special education or related services the child might need, let alone plan an appropriate educational program for the child.

The evaluation must use a variety of assessment tools and strategies to gather relevant functional, developmental, and academic information about the child, including information provided by the parent. When conducting an initial evaluation, it's important to examine all areas of a child's functioning to determine not only if the child is a child with a disability, but also determine the child's educational needs. This full and individual evaluation includes evaluating the child's:

- health,

- vision and hearing,

- social and emotional status,

- general intelligence,

- academic performance,

- communicative status, and

- motor abilities.

As IDEA states, the school system must ensure that the evaluation is sufficiently comprehensive to identify all of the child's special education and related service needs, whether or not commonly linked to the disability category in which the child has been classified.

Review Existing Data

Evaluation (and particularly reevaluation) typically begins with a review of existing evaluation data on the child, which may come from the child's classroom work, his or her performance on State or district assessments, information provided by the parents, and so on.

The purpose of this review is to decide if the existing data is sufficient to establish the child's eligibility and determine educational needs, or if additional information is needed. If the group determines there is sufficient information available to make the necessary determinations, the public agency must notify parents:

- of that determination and the reason for it; and

- that parents have the right to request assessment to determine the child's eligibility and educational needs.

Unless the parents request an assessment, the public agency is not required to conduct one.

If it is decided that additional data is needed, the group then identifies what is needed to determine:

- whether your son or daughter has a particular category of disability (e.g., "other health impairment," "specific learning disability");

- your child's present levels of performance (that is, how he or she is currently doing in school) and his or her academic and developmental needs;

- whether your child needs special education and related services; and

- if so, whether any additions or modifications are needed in the special education and related services to enable your child to meet the goals set out in the IEP to be developed and to participate, as appropriate, in the general curriculum.

An example may help crystallize the comprehensive scope of evaluations: Consider a first-grader with suspected hearing and vision impairments who's been referred for an initial evaluation. In order to fully gather relevant functional, developmental, and academic information and identify all of the child's special education and related service needs, evaluation of this child will obviously need to focus on hearing and vision, as well as, cognitive, speech/language, motor, and social/behavioral skills, to determine:

- the degree of impairment in vision and hearing and the impact of these impairments on the child;

- if there are additional impairments in other areas of functioning (including those not commonly linked to hearing and/or vision) that impact the child's aptitude, performance, and achievement; and

- what the child's educational needs are that must be addressed.

With this example, any of the following individuals might be part of this child's evaluation team—audiologist, psychologist, speech-language pathologist, social worker, occupational or physical therapist, vision specialist, regular classroom teacher, educational diagnosticians, or others.

Variety, Variety

The evaluation must use a variety of assessment tools and strategies. This has been one of the cornerstones of IDEA's evaluation requirements from its earliest days. Under IDEA, it is inappropriate and unacceptable to base any eligibility decision upon the results of only one procedure. Tests alone will not give a comprehensive picture of how a child performs or what he or she knows or does not know. Only by collecting data through a variety of approaches (e.g., observations, interviews, tests, curriculum-based assessment, and so on) and from a variety of sources (parents, teachers, specialists, child) can an adequate picture be obtained of the child's strengths and weaknesses.

IDEA also requires schools to use technically sound instruments and processes in evaluation. Technically sound instruments generally refers to assessments that have been shown through research to be valid and reliable (71 Fed. Reg. at 46642). Technically sound processes require that assessments and other evaluation materials be:

- administered by trained and knowledgeable personnel;

- administered in accordance with any instructions provided by the producer of the assessments; and

- used for the purposes for which the assessments or measures are valid and reliable.

In conjunction with using a variety of sound tools and processes, assessments must include those that are tailored to assess specific areas of educational need (for example, reading or math) and not merely those that are designed to provide a single general intelligence quotient, or IQ.

Taken together, all of this information can be used to determine whether the child has a disability under IDEA, the specific nature of the child's special needs, whether the child needs special education and related services, and, if so, to design an appropriate program.

Consider Language, Communication Mode, and Culture

Another important component in evaluation is to ensure that assessment tools are not discriminatory on a racial or cultural basis. Evaluation must also be conducted in the child's typical, accustomed mode of communication (unless it is clearly not feasible to do so) and in a form that will yield accurate information about what the child knows and can do academically, developmentally, and functionally. For many, English is not the native language; others use sign to communicate, or assistive or alternative augmentative communication devices. To assess such a child using a means of communication or response not highly familiar to the child raises the probability that the evaluation results will yield minimal, if any, information about what the child knows and can do.

Specifically, consideration of language, culture, and communication mode means the following: If your child has limited English proficiency, materials and procedures used to assess your child must be selected and administered to ensure that they measure the extent to which your child has a disability and needs special education, rather than measuring your child's English language skills.

This provision in the law is meant to protect children of different racial, cultural, or language backgrounds from misdiagnosis. For example, children's cultural backgrounds may affect their behavior or test responses in ways that teachers or other personnel do not understand. Similarly, if a child speaks a language other than English or has limited English proficiency, he or she may not understand directions or words on tests and may be unable to answer correctly. As a result, a child may mistakenly appear to be a slow learner or to have a hearing or communication problem.

- If an assessment is not conducted under standard conditions— meaning that some condition of the test has been changed (such as the qualifications of the person giving the test or the method of giving the test)—a description of the extent to which it varied from standard conditions must be included in the evaluation report.

- If your child has impaired sensory, manual, or speaking skills, the law requires that tests are selected and administered so as best to ensure that test results accurately reflect his or her aptitude or achievement level (or whatever other factors the test claims to measure), and not merely reflect your child's impaired sensory, manual, or speaking skills (unless the test being used is intended to measure those skills).

What about Evaluation for Specific Learning Disabilities?

IDEA's regulations specify additional procedures required to be used for determining the existence of a specific learning disability. Sections 300.307 through 300.311 spell out what these procedures are. It's important to note, though, that IDEA 2004 made dramatic changes in how children who are suspected of having a learning disability are to be evaluated.

- States must not require the use of a severe discrepancy between intellectual ability and achievement.

- States must permit the use of a process based on the child's response to scientific, research-based intervention.

- States may permit the use of other alternative research-based procedures for determining whether a child has a specific learning disability.

- The team that makes the eligibility determination must include a regular education teacher and at least one person qualified to conduct individual diagnostic examinations of children, such as a school psychologist, speech-language pathologist, or remedial reading teacher.

Determining Eligibility

Parents were not always included in the group that determined their child's eligibility and, in fact, were often excluded. Since the IDEA Amendments of 1997, parents are to be part of the group that determines their child's eligibility and are also to be provided a copy of the evaluation report, as well as documentation of the determination of the child's eligibility.

Some school systems will hold a meeting where they consider only the eligibility of the child for special education and related services. At this meeting, your child's assessment results should be explained. The specialists who assessed your child will explain what they did, why they used the tests they did, your child's results on those tests or other evaluation procedures, and what your child's scores mean when compared to other children of the same age and grade.

It is important to know that the group may not determine that a child is eligible if the determinant factor for making that judgment is the child's lack of instruction in reading or math or the child's limited English proficiency. The child must otherwise meet the law's definition of a "child with a disability"—meaning that he or she has one of the disabilities listed in the law and, because of that disability, needs special education and related services.

If the evaluation results indicate that your child meets the definition of one or more of the disabilities listed under IDEA and needs special education and related services, the results will form the basis for developing your child's IEP (individualized education program).

What Happens If You Don't Agree with the Evaluation Results?

If you, as parents of a child with a disability, disagree with the results of your child's evaluation as obtained by the public agency, you have the right to obtain what is known as an Independent Educational Evaluation, or IEE. An IEE means an evaluation conducted by a qualified examiner who is not employed by the public agency responsible for the education of your child. If you ask for an IEE, the public agency must provide you with, among other things, information about where an IEE may be obtained.

Who pays for the independent evaluation? The answer is that some IEEs are at public expense and others are paid for by the parents. For example, if you are the parent of a child with a disability and you disagree with the public agency's evaluation, you may request an IEE at public expense. "At public expense" means that the public agency either pays for the full cost of the evaluation or ensures that the evaluation is otherwise provided at no cost to you as parents. The public agency may grant your request and pay for the IEE, or it may initiate a hearing to show that its own evaluation was appropriate. The public agency may ask why you object to the public evaluation. However, the agency may not require you to explain, and it may not unreasonably delay either providing the IEE at public expense or initiating a due process hearing to defend the public evaluation.

If the public agency initiates a hearing and the final decision of the hearing officer is that the agency's evaluation was appropriate, then you still have the right to an IEE but not at public expense. As part of a due process hearing, a hearing officer may also request an IEE; if so, that IEE must be at public expense. Whenever an IEE is publicly funded, that IEE must meet the same criteria that the public agency uses when it initiates an evaluation. The public agency must tell you what these criteria are—such as location of the evaluation and the qualifications of the examiner—and they must be the same criteria the public agency uses when it initiates an evaluation, to the extent they are consistent with your right to an IEE. However, the public agency may not impose other conditions or timelines related to your obtaining an IEE at public expense.

Of course, you have the right to have your child independently evaluated at any time at your own expense. (Note: When the same tests are repeated within a short time period, the validity of the results can be seriously weakened.) The results of this evaluation must be considered by the public agency, if it meets agency criteria, in any decision made with respect to providing your child with FAPE (Free Appropriate Public Education). The results may also be presented as evidence at a hearing regarding your child.

What Happens down the Road?

After the initial evaluation, evaluations must be conducted at least every 3 years (generally called a triennial evaluation) after your child has been placed in special education. Reevaluations can also occur more frequently if conditions warrant, or if you or your child's teacher requests a reevaluation. Informed parental consent is also necessary for reevaluations.

As with initial evaluations, reevaluations begin with the review of existing evaluation data, including evaluations and information provided by you, the child's parents. Your consent is not required for the review of existing data on your child. As with initial evaluation, this review is to identify what additional data, if any, are needed to determine whether your child continues to be a "child with a disability" and continues to need special education and related services. If the group determines that additional data are needed, then the public agency must administer tests and other evaluation materials as needed to produce the data. Prior to collecting this additional information, the agency must obtain your informed written consent.

Or, if the group determines that no additional data are needed to determine whether your child continues to be a "child with a disability," the public agency must notify you:

- of this determination and the reasons for it; and

- of your right, as parents, to request an assessment to determine whether, for the purposes of services under IDEA, your child continues to be a "child with a disability."

A final note with respect to reevaluations: Before determining that your child is no longer a "child with a disability" and, thus, no longer eligible for special education services under IDEA, the public agency must evaluate your child in accordance with all of the provisions described above. This evaluation, however, is not required before terminating your child's eligibility due to graduation with a regular high school diploma or due to exceeding the age eligibility for FAPE under State law.

Chapter 51

Early Intervention Services

Early intervention services are concerned with all the basic and brand new skills that babies typically develop during the first 3 years of life, such as:

- physical (reaching, rolling, crawling, and walking);
- cognitive (thinking, learning, solving problems);
- communication (talking, listening, understanding);
- social/emotional (playing, feeling secure and happy); or
- self-help (eating, dressing).

Early intervention services are designed to meet the needs of infants and toddlers who have a developmental delay or disability. Sometimes it is known from the moment a child is born that early intervention services will be essential in helping the child grow and develop. Often this is so for children who are diagnosed at birth with a specific condition or who experience significant prematurity, very low birth weight, illness, or surgery soon after being born. Even before heading home from the hospital, this child's parents may be given a referral to their local early intervention office.

Some children have a relatively routine entry into the world, but may develop more slowly than others, experience setbacks, or develop in ways that seem very different from other children. For these children,

From "Overview of Early Intervention," by the National Dissemination Center for Children with Disabilities (NICHCY, www.nichcy.org), September 2010.

a visit with a developmental pediatrician and a thorough evaluation may lead to an early intervention referral. However a child comes to be referred, assessed, and determined eligible—early intervention services provide vital support so that children with developmental needs can thrive and grow. Eligible children can receive early intervention services from birth through the third birthday.

Let's take a closer look at the early intervention process, beginning with "so you're concerned about your child's development." This overview will discuss actions you can take to find help for your child, including contacting the early intervention program in your community.

Part 1: So You're Concerned about Your Child's Development

It's not uncommon for parents and family members to become concerned when their beautiful baby or growing toddler doesn't seem to be developing according to the normal schedule of "baby" milestones—"He hasn't rolled over yet," or "the little girl next door is already sitting up on her own!" or "she should be saying a few words by now." And while it's true that children develop differently, at their own pace, and that the range of what's "normal" development is quite broad, it's hard not to worry and wonder.

If you think that your child is not developing at the same pace or in the same way as most children his or her age, it is often a good idea to talk first to your child's pediatrician. Explain your concerns. Tell the doctor what you have observed with your child. Your child may have a disability or a developmental delay, or he or she may be at risk of having a disability or delay. You can also get in touch with your community's early intervention program, and ask to have your little one evaluated to see if he or she has a developmental delay or disability. This evaluation is free of charge, won't hurt your child, and looks at his or her basic skills. Based on that evaluation, your child may be eligible for early intervention services, which will be designed to address your child's special needs or delays.

Where do I go for help?

There are several ways you can find help for your child. Since you are reading this text, we recommend that you go to the NICHCY State-Specific Resources page, select your state, and find the listing for the early intervention program in your state. It'll be in the first section of the State Resource Sheet, under "State Agencies." Look for a title such as "Programs for Infants and Toddlers with Disabilities: Ages Birth through 2" or "Early Intervention." Call the agency listed. Explain that you want to find out about early intervention services for your child. Ask for the name of a contact person in your area.

If you don't have a State Resource Sheet for your state, visit www .nichcy.org/state-organization-search-by-state. All State Resource Sheets are available there. You can also call NICHCY at 800-695-0285 and ask an information specialist to give you the number for early intervention services in your state.

How else might you find out about early intervention services in your community?

Here are two ways:

- Ask your child's pediatrician to put you in touch with the early intervention system in your community or region.

- Contact the Pediatrics branch in a local hospital and ask where you should call to find out about early intervention services in your area.

It is very important to write down the names and phone numbers of everyone you talk to. You can use the Parent's Record-Keeping Worksheet (see the following text) to keep track of this important information. Having this information available will be helpful to you later on.

Parent's record-keeping worksheet: A sample record-keeping worksheet can help you start a file of information about your child. As you contact different people and places, it's a good idea to keep records of people you've talked with and what was said. As time goes by, you will want to add other information to your file, such as letters and notes (from doctors, therapists, etc.); medical records and reports; results of tests and evaluations; notes from meetings about your child; therapist reports; IFSP (individualized family service plan) and IEP (individualized education program) records; your child's developmental history, including personal notes or diaries on your child's development; records of shots and vaccinations; and family medical histories.

The Parent's Record-Keeping Worksheet is available online at: www .nichcy.org/wp-content/uploads/docs/recordkeeping.pdf.

Make sure you get copies of all written information about your child (records, reports, etc.). This will help you become an important coordinator of services and a better advocate for your child. Remember, as time goes on, you'll probably have more information to keep track of, so it's a good idea to keep it together in one place.

461

What do I say to the early intervention contact person?

Explain that you are concerned about your child's development. Say that you think your child may need early intervention services. Explain that you would like to have your child evaluated under IDEA (Individuals with Disabilities Education Act, the nation's special education law). Write down any information the contact person gives you.

The person may refer you to what is known as Child Find. One of Child Find's purposes is to identify children who need early intervention services. Child Find operates in every state and conducts screenings to identify children who may need early intervention services. These screenings are provided free of charge.

Each state has one agency that is in charge of the early intervention system for infants and toddlers with special needs. This agency is known as the lead agency. It may be the state education agency or another agency, such as the health department. Each state decides which agency will serve as the lead agency. The agency listed on the NICHCY State Resource Sheet under the heading "Programs for Infants and Toddlers: Birth Through 2" is your state's lead agency.

What happens next?

Once you are in contact with the early intervention system, the system will assign someone to work with you and your child through the evaluation and assessment process. This person will be your temporary service coordinator. He or she should have a background in early childhood development and ways to help young children who may have developmental delays. The service coordinator should also know the policies for early intervention programs and services in your state.

The early intervention system will need to determine if your child is eligible for early intervention services. To do this, the staff will set up and carry out a multidisciplinary evaluation and assessment of your child. Read on for more information about this process.

Part 2: Your Child's Evaluation

What is a multidisciplinary evaluation and assessment?

The law IDEA requires that your child receive a timely, comprehensive, multidisciplinary evaluation and assessment. The purposes of the evaluation and assessment are to find out:

- the nature of your child's strengths, delays, or difficulties; and
- whether or not your child is eligible for early intervention services.

Multidisciplinary means that the evaluation group is made up of qualified people who have different areas of training and experience. Together, they know about children's speech and language skills, physical abilities, hearing and vision, and other important areas of development. They know how to work with children, even very young ones, to discover if a child has a problem or is developing within normal ranges. Group members may evaluate your child together or individually.

Evaluation refers to the procedures used by these professionals to find out if your child is eligible for early intervention services. As part of the evaluation, the team will observe your child, ask your child to do things, talk to you and your child, and use other methods to gather information. These procedures will help the team find out how your child functions in five areas of development—cognitive development, physical development, communication, social-emotional development, and adaptive development.

Following your child's evaluation, you and a team of professionals will meet and review all of the data, results, and reports. The people on the team will talk with you about whether your child meets the criteria under IDEA and state policy for having a developmental delay, a diagnosed physical or mental condition, or being at risk for having a substantial delay. If so, your child is generally found to be eligible for services.

If found eligible, he or she will then be assessed. Assessment refers to the procedures used throughout the time your child is in early intervention. The purposes of these ongoing procedures are to:

- identify your child's unique strengths and needs; and

- determine what services are necessary to meet those needs.

With your consent, your family's needs will also be identified. This process, which is family-directed, is intended to identify the resources, priorities, and concerns of your family. It also identifies the supports and services you may need to enhance your family's capacity to meet your child's developmental needs.

The family assessment is usually conducted through an interview with you, the parents. When conducting the evaluation and assessment, team members may get information from some or all of the following:

- Doctor's reports

- Results from developmental tests and performance assessments given to your child

- Your child's medical and developmental history
- Direct observations and feedback from all members of the multidisciplinary team, including you, the parents
- Interviews with you and other family members or caretakers
- Any other important observations, records, and/or reports about your child

Who pays for the evaluation and assessment?

Under IDEA, evaluations and assessments are provided at no cost to parents. They are funded by state and federal monies.

Who is eligible for services?

Under the IDEA, "infants and toddlers with disabilities" are defined as children from birth to the third birthday who need early intervention services because they are experiencing developmental delays, as measured by appropriate diagnostic instruments and procedures, in one or more of the following areas:

- Cognitive development
- Physical development, including vision and hearing
- Communication development
- Social or emotional development
- Adaptive development
- Who have a diagnosed physical or mental condition that has a high probability of resulting in developmental delay

The term may also include, if a state chooses, children from birth through age 2 who are at risk of having substantial developmental delays if early intervention services are not provided." (34 Code of Federal Regulations 303.16)

My child has been found eligible for services. What's next?

If your child and family are found eligible, you and a team will meet to develop a written plan for providing early intervention services to your child and, as necessary, to your family. This plan is called the Individualized Family Service Plan, or IFSP. It is a very important document, and you, as parents, are important members of the team that develops it.

Part 3: Your Child's Early Intervention Services

What is an individualized family service plan, or IFSP?

The IFSP is a written document that, among other things, outlines the early intervention services that your child and family will receive. One guiding principal of the IFSP is that the family is a child's greatest resource, that a young child's needs are closely tied to the needs of his or her family. The best way to support children and meet their needs is to support and build upon the individual strengths of their family. So, the IFSP is a whole family plan with the parents as major contributors in its development. Involvement of other team members will depend on what the child needs. These other team members could come from several agencies and may include medical people, therapists, child development specialists, social workers, and others.

Your child's IFSP must include the following:

- Your child's present physical, cognitive, communication, social/emotional, and adaptive development levels and needs

- Family information (with your agreement), including the resources, priorities, and concerns of you, as parents, and other family members closely involved with the child

- The major results or outcomes expected to be achieved for your child and family; the specific services your child will be receiving

- Where in the natural environment (e.g., home, community) the services will be provided (if the services will not be provided in the natural environment, the IFSP must include a statement justifying why not)

- When and where your son or daughter will receive services

- The number of days or sessions he or she will receive each service and how long each session will last

- Whether the service will be provided on a one-on-one or group basis

- Who will pay for the services

- The name of the service coordinator overseeing the implementation of the IFSP

- The steps to be taken to support your child's transition out of early intervention and into another program when the time comes

The IFSP may also identify services your family may be interested in, such as financial information or information about raising a child with a disability.

The IFSP is reviewed every 6 months and is updated at least once a year. The IFSP must be fully explained to you, the parents, and your suggestions must be considered. You must give written consent before services can start. If you do not give your consent in writing, your child will not receive services. Each state has specific guidelines for the IFSP. Your service coordinator can explain what the IFSP guidelines are in your state.

What's included in early intervention services?

Under IDEA, early intervention services must include a multidisciplinary evaluation and assessment, a written individualized family service plan, service coordination, and specific services designed to meet the unique developmental needs of the child and family. Early intervention services may be simple or complex depending on the child's needs. They can range from prescribing glasses for a 2-year-old to developing a comprehensive approach with a variety of services and special instruction for a child, including home visits, counseling, and training for his or her family. Depending on your child's needs, his or her early intervention services may include:

- family training, counseling, and home visits;
- special instruction;
- speech-language pathology services (sometimes referred to as speech therapy);
- audiology services (hearing impairment services);
- occupational therapy;
- physical therapy;
- psychological services;
- medical services (only for diagnostic or evaluation purposes);
- health services needed to enable your child to benefit from the other services;
- social work services;
- assistive technology devices and services;
- transportation;
- nutrition services; and

- service coordination services.

How are early intervention services delivered?

Early intervention services may be delivered in a variety of ways and in different places. Sometimes services are provided in the child's home with the family receiving additional training. Services may also be provided in other settings, such as a clinic, a neighborhood daycare center, hospital, or the local health department. To the maximum extent appropriate, the services are to be provided in natural environments or settings. Natural environments, broadly speaking, are where the child lives, learns, and plays. Services are provided by qualified personnel and may be offered through a public or private agency.

Will I have to pay for services?

Whether or not you, as parents, will have to pay for any services for your child depends on the policies of your state. Under IDEA, the following services must be provided at no cost to families:

- Child Find services

- Evaluations and assessments

- The development and review of the IFSP

- Service coordination

Depending on your state's policies, you may have to pay for certain other services. You may be charged a "sliding-scale" fee, meaning the fees are based on what you earn. Check with the contact person in your area or state. Some services may be covered by your health insurance, by Medicaid, or by Indian Health Services. Every effort is made to provide services to all infants and toddlers who need help, regardless of family income. Services cannot be denied to a child just because his or her family is not able to pay for them.

Chapter 52

Individualized Education Programs (IEPs)

What's an IEP?

Kids with delayed skills or other disabilities might be eligible for special services that provide individualized education programs in public schools, free of charge to families. Understanding how to access these services can help parents be effective advocates for their kids.

The passage of the updated version of the Individuals with Disabilities Education Act (IDEA 2004) made parents of kids with special needs even more crucial members of their child's education team.

Parents can now work with educators to develop a plan—the individualized education program (IEP)—to help kids succeed in school. The IEP describes the goals the team sets for a child during the school year, as well as any special support needed to help achieve them.

Who Needs an IEP?

A child who has difficulty learning and functioning and has been identified as a special needs student is the perfect candidate for an IEP.

Kids struggling in school may qualify for support services, allowing them to be taught in a special way, for reasons such as:

- learning disabilities;
- attention deficit hyperactivity disorder (ADHD);
- emotional disorders;
- cognitive challenges;
- autism;
- hearing impairment;
- visual impairment;
- speech or language impairment;
- developmental delay.

How Are Services Delivered?

In most cases, the services and goals outlined in an IEP can be provided in a standard school environment. This can be done in the regular classroom (for example, a reading teacher helping a small group of children who need extra assistance while the other kids in the class work on reading with the regular teacher) or in a special resource room in the regular school. The resource room can serve a group of kids with similar needs who are brought together for help.

However, kids who need intense intervention may be taught in a special school environment. These classes have fewer students per teacher, allowing for more individualized attention.

In addition, the teacher usually has specific training in helping kids with special educational needs. The children spend most of their day in a special classroom and join the regular classes for nonacademic activities (like music and gym) or in academic activities in which they don't need extra help.

Because the goal of IDEA is to ensure that each child is educated in the least restrictive environment possible, effort is made to help kids stay in a regular classroom. However, when needs are best met in a special class, then kids might be placed in one.

The Referral and Evaluation Process

The referral process generally begins when a teacher, parent, or doctor is concerned that a child may be having trouble in the classroom, and the teacher notifies the school counselor or psychologist.

The first step is to gather specific data regarding the student's progress or academic problems. This may be done through:

- a conference with parents;
- a conference with the student;
- observation of the student;
- analysis of the student's performance (attention, behavior, work completion, tests, classwork, homework, etc.).

This information helps school personnel determine the next step. At this point, strategies specific to the student could be used to help the child become more successful in school. If this doesn't work, the child would be tested for a specific learning disability or other impairment to help determine qualification for special services.

It's important to note, though, that the presence of a disability doesn't automatically guarantee a child will receive services. To be eligible, the disability must affect functioning at school.

To determine eligibility, a multidisciplinary team of professionals will evaluate the child based on their observations; the child's performance on standardized tests; and daily work such as tests, quizzes, classwork, and homework.

Who's on the Team?

The professionals on the evaluation team can include:

- a psychologist;
- a physical therapist;
- an occupational therapist;
- a speech therapist;
- a special educator;
- a vision or hearing specialist;
- others, depending on the child's specific needs.

As a parent, you can decide whether to have your child assessed. If you choose to do so, you'll be asked to sign a permission form that will detail who is involved in the process and the types of tests they use. These tests might include measures of specific school skills, such as reading or math, as well as more general developmental skills, such as speech and language. Testing does not necessarily mean that a child will receive services.

Once the team members complete their individual assessments, they develop a comprehensive evaluation report (CER) that compiles their findings, offers an educational classification, and outlines the skills and support the child will need.

The parents then have a chance to review the report before the IEP is developed. Some parents will disagree with the report, and they will have the opportunity to work together with the school to come up with a plan that best meets the child's needs.

Developing an IEP

The next step is an IEP meeting at which the team and parents decide what will go into the plan. In addition to the evaluation team, a regular teacher should be present to offer suggestions about how the plan can help the child's progress in the standard education curriculum.

At the meeting, the team will discuss your child's educational needs—as described in the CER—and come up with specific, measurable short-term and annual goals for each of those needs. If you attend this meeting, you can take an active role in developing the goals and determining which skills or areas will receive the most attention.

The cover page of the IEP outlines the support services your child will receive and how often they will be provided (for example, occupational therapy twice a week). Support services might include special education, speech therapy, occupational or physical therapy, counseling, audiology, medical services, nursing, vision or hearing therapy, and many others.

If the team recommends several services, the amount of time they take in the child's school schedule can seem overwhelming. To ease that load, some services may be provided on a consultative basis. In these cases, the professional consults with the teacher to come up with strategies to help the child but doesn't offer any hands-on instruction. For instance, an occupational therapist may suggest accommodations for a child with fine-motor problems that affect handwriting, and the classroom teacher would incorporate these suggestions into the handwriting lessons taught to the entire class.

Other services can be delivered right in the classroom, so the child's day isn't interrupted by therapy. The child who has difficulty with handwriting might work one on one with an occupational therapist while everyone else practices their handwriting skills. When deciding how and where services are offered, the child's comfort and dignity should be a top priority.

The IEP should be reviewed annually to update the goals and make sure the levels of service meet your child's needs. However, IEPs can be changed at any time on an as-needed basis. If you think your child needs more, fewer, or different services, you can request a meeting and bring the team together to discuss your concerns.

Your Legal Rights

Specific timelines ensure that the development of an IEP moves from referral to providing services as quickly as possible. Be sure to ask about this timeframe and get a copy of your parents' rights when your child is referred. These guidelines (sometimes called procedural safeguards) outline your rights as a parent to control what happens to your child during each step of the process.

The parents' rights also describe how you can proceed if you disagree with any part of the CER or the IEP—mediation and hearings both are options. You can get information about low-cost or free legal representation from the school district or, if your child is in Early Intervention (for kids ages 3 to 5), through that program.

Attorneys and paid advocates familiar with the IEP process will provide representation if you need it. You also may invite anyone who knows or works with your child whose input you feel would be helpful to join the IEP team.

A Final Word

Parents have the right to choose where their kids will be educated. This choice includes public or private elementary schools and secondary schools, including religious schools. It also includes charter schools and home schools.

However, it is important to understand that the rights of children with disabilities who are placed by their parents in private elementary schools and secondary schools are not the same as those of kids with disabilities who are enrolled in public schools or placed by public agencies in private schools when the public school is unable to provide a free appropriate public education (FAPE).

Two major differences that parents, teachers, other school staff, private school representatives, and the kids need to know about are:

1. Children with disabilities who are placed by their parents in private schools may not get the same services they would receive in a public school.

2. Not all kids with disabilities placed by their parents in private schools will receive services.

The IEP process is complex, but it's also an effective way to address how your child learns and functions. If you have concerns, don't hesitate to ask questions about the evaluation findings or the goals recommended by the team. You know your child best and should play a central role in creating a learning plan tailored to his or her specific needs.

Chapter 53

Supports, Modifications, and Accommodations for Students

For many students with disabilities—and for many without—the key to success in the classroom lies in having appropriate adaptations, accommodations, and modifications made to the instruction and other classroom activities.

Some adaptations are as simple as moving a distractible student to the front of the class or away from the pencil sharpener or the window. Other modifications may involve changing the way that material is presented or the way that students respond to show their learning.

Adaptations, accommodations, and modifications need to be individualized for students, based upon their needs and their personal learning styles and interests. It is not always obvious what adaptations, accommodations, or modifications would be beneficial for a particular student, or how changes to the curriculum, its presentation, the classroom setting, or student evaluation might be made. This text is intended to help teachers and others find information that can guide them in making appropriate changes in the classroom based on what their students need.

A Quick Look at Terminology

You might wonder if the terms supports, modifications, and adaptations all mean the same thing. The simple answer is: No, not completely,

"Supports, Modifications, and Accommodations for Students," by the National Dissemination Center for Children with Disabilities (NICHCY, www.nichcy.org), September 2010.

but yes, for the most part. (Don't you love a clear answer?) People tend to use the terms interchangeably, to be sure, and we will do so here, for ease of reading, but distinctions can be made between the terms.

Sometimes people get confused about what it means to have a modification and what it means to have an accommodation. Usually a modification means a change in what is being taught to or expected from the student. Making an assignment easier so the student is not doing the same level of work as other students is an example of a modification.

An accommodation is a change that helps a student overcome or work around the disability. Allowing a student who has trouble writing to give his answers orally is an example of an accommodation. This student is still expected to know the same material and answer the same questions as fully as the other students, but he doesn't have to write his answers to show that he knows the information. What is most important to know about modifications and accommodations is that both are meant to help a child to learn.

Different Types of Supports

Special Education

By definition, special education is "specially designed instruction" (§300.39). And IDEA [Individual with Disabilities Education Act] defines that term as follows: Specially designed instruction means adapting, as appropriate to the needs of an eligible child under this part, the content, methodology, or delivery of instruction:

- to address the unique needs of the child that result from the child's disability; and

- to ensure access of the child to the general curriculum, so that the child can meet the educational standards within the jurisdiction of the public agency that apply to all children.

Thus, special education involves adapting the "content, methodology, or delivery of instruction." In fact, the special education field can take pride in the knowledge base and expertise it's developed in the past 30-plus years of individualizing instruction to meet the needs of students with disabilities.

Adapting Instruction

Sometimes a student may need to have changes made in class work or routines because of his or her disability. Modifications can be made to:

- what a child is taught, and/or
- how a child works at school.

For example: Jack is an 8th-grade student who has learning disabilities in reading and writing. He is in a regular 8th-grade class that is team-taught by a general education teacher and a special education teacher. Modifications and accommodations provided for Jack's daily school routine (and when he takes state or district-wide tests) include the following:

- Jack will have shorter reading and writing assignments.
- Jack's textbooks will be based upon the 8th-grade curriculum but at his independent reading level (4th grade).
- Jack will have test questions read/explained to him, when he asks.
- Jack will give his answers to essay-type questions by speaking, rather than writing them down.

Modifications or accommodations are most often made in the following areas:

- **Scheduling** (for example, giving the student extra time to complete assignments or tests or breaking up testing over several days)
- **Setting** (for example, working in a small group or working one-on-one with the teacher)
- **Materials** (for example, providing audiotaped lectures or books, giving copies of teacher's lecture notes, or using large print books, Braille, or books on CD [digital text])
- **Instruction** (for example, reducing the difficulty of assignments, reducing the reading level, or using a student/peer tutor)
- **Student response** (for example, allowing answers to be given orally or dictated, using a word processor for written work, or using sign language, a communication device, Braille, or native language if it is not English)

Because adapting the content, methodology, and/or delivery of instruction is an essential element in special education and an extremely valuable support for students, it's equally essential to know as much as possible about how instruction can be adapted to address the needs of an individual student with a disability. The special education teacher who serves on the IEP (individualized education program) team can contribute his or her expertise in this area, which is the essence of special education.

Related Services

One look at IDEA's definition of related services and it's clear that these services are supportive in nature, although not in the same way that adapting the curriculum is. Related services support children's special education and are provided when necessary to help students benefit from special education. Thus, related services must be included in the treasure chest of accommodations and supports we're exploring. Related services means transportation and such developmental, corrective, and other supportive services as are required to assist a child with a disability to benefit from special education.

Here's the list of related services in the law.

- Speech-language pathology and audiology services
- Interpreting services
- Psychological services
- Physical and occupational therapy
- Recreation, including therapeutic recreation
- Early identification and assessment of disabilities in children
- Counseling services, including rehabilitation counseling
- Orientation and mobility services
- Medical services for diagnostic or evaluation purposes
- School health services and school nurse services
- Social work services in schools

This is not an exhaustive list of possible related services. There are others (not named here or in the law) that states and schools routinely make available under the umbrella of related services. The IEP team decides which related services a child needs and specifies them in the child's IEP.

Supplementary Aids and Services

One of the most powerful types of supports available to children with disabilities are the other kinds of supports or services (other than special education and related services) that a child needs to be educated with nondisabled children to the maximum extent appropriate. Some examples of these additional services and supports, called supplementary aids and services in IDEA, are the following:

- Adapted equipment: Such as a special seat or a cut-out cup for drinking

- Assistive technology: Such as a word processor, special software, or a communication system

- Training for staff, student, and/or parents

- Peer tutors

- A one-on-one aide

- Adapted materials: Such as books on tape, large print, or highlighted notes

- Collaboration/consultation among staff, parents, and/or other professionals

The IEP team, which includes the parents, is the group that decides which supplementary aids and services a child needs to support his or her access to and participation in the school environment. The IEP team must really work together to make sure that a child gets the supplementary aids and services that he or she needs to be successful. Team members talk about the child's needs, the curriculum, and school routine, and openly explore all options to make sure the right supports for the specific child are included.

Program Modifications or Supports for School Staff

If the IEP team decides that a child needs a particular modification or accommodation, this information must be included in the IEP. Supports are also available for those who work with the child, to help them help that child be successful. Supports for school staff must also be written into the IEP. Some of these supports might include the following:

- Attending a conference or training related to the child's needs

- Getting help from another staff member or administrative person

- Having an aide in the classroom

- Getting special equipment or teaching materials

Accommodations in Large Assessments

IDEA requires that students with disabilities take part in state or district-wide assessments. These are tests that are periodically given to all students to measure achievement. It is one way that schools determine how well and how much students are learning. IDEA now states that students with disabilities should have as much involvement in the general curriculum as possible. This means that, if a child is receiving instruction in the general curriculum, he or she could take the same standardized test that the school district or state gives to nondisabled children. Accordingly, a child's IEP must include all modifications or accommodations that the child needs so that he or she can participate in state or district-wide assessments.

The IEP team can decide that a particular test is not appropriate for a child. In this case, the IEP must include:

- an explanation of why that test is not suitable for the child, and

- how the child will be assessed instead (often called alternate assessment).

Ask your state and/or local school district for a copy of their guidelines on the types of accommodations, modifications, and alternate assessments available to students.

Conclusion

Even a child with many needs is to be involved with nondisabled peers to the maximum extent appropriate. Just because a child has severe disabilities or needs modifications to the general curriculum does not mean that he or she may be removed from the general education class. If a child is removed from the general education class for any part of the school day, the IEP team must include in the IEP an explanation for the child's nonparticipation.

Because accommodations can be so vital to helping children with disabilities access the general curriculum, participate in school (including extracurricular and nonacademic activities), and be educated alongside their peers without disabilities, IDEA reinforces their use again and again, in its requirements, in its definitions, and in its principles. The wealth of experience that the special education field has gained over the years since IDEA was first passed by Congress is the very resource you'll want to tap for more information on what accommodations are appropriate for students, given their disability, and how to make those adaptations to support their learning.

Chapter 54

Transitioning Students with Disabilities to Higher Education and Adulthood

The attitude and self-advocacy skills of students with disabilities may be two of the most important factors in determining their success or failure in postsecondary education. Students with disabilities need to be prepared to work collaboratively with the institution's disability coordinator to enable them to have an equal opportunity to participate in an institution's programs and activities. To ensure that students with disabilities possess the desired levels of self-advocacy to succeed in postsecondary education, high school educators may want to encourage the students to do the following:

Understand their disabilities: Students with disabilities need to know the functional limitations that result from their disabilities and understand their strengths and weaknesses. They should be able to explain their disabilities to an institution's disability coordinators or other appropriate staff. As part of this process, students should be able to explain where they have had difficulty in the past, as well as what has helped them overcome such problems and what specific adjustments might work in specific situations. To assist students in this area, high school educators can encourage high school students to be active participants in their IEP (individualized education program) or Section 504 meetings. High school personnel also can suggest that students practice explaining their disabilities, as well as why they

Excerpted from "Transition of Students With Disabilities To Postsecondary Education: A Guide for High School Educators," by the U.S. Department of Education (ED, www.ed.gov), March 2011.

need certain services, to appropriate secondary staff or through role-playing exercises to prepare them to engage in such conversations with confidence in a postsecondary setting.

Accept responsibility for their own success: All students, including those with disabilities, must take primary responsibility for their success or failure in postsecondary education. Students with disabilities, in particular, are moving from a system where parents and school staff usually advocated on their behalf to a system where they will be expected to advocate for themselves. An institution's staff will likely communicate directly with students when issues arise and are generally not required to interact with students' parents. In general, students with disabilities should expect to complete all course requirements, such as assignments and examinations. Students with disabilities need to identify the essential academic and technical standards that they will be required to meet for admission and continued participation in an institution's program. Students also need to identify any academic adjustments they may need as a result of their disabilities to meet those standards and how to request those adjustments. Students with disabilities need to understand that, while federal disability laws guarantee them an equal opportunity to participate these laws do not guarantee that students will achieve a particular outcome, for example, good grades.

Take an appropriate preparatory curriculum: Because all students will be expected to meet an institution's essential standards, students with disabilities need to take a high school curriculum that will prepare them to meet those standards. If students with disabilities plan to attend a rigorous postsecondary institution, they, like their peers without disabilities, need to make high school curriculum choices that support that goal. High school guidance counselors and state VR (vocational rehabilitation) agency counselors, in particular, can play an important role in students' curriculum planning. For all students, good study skills and the ability to write well are critical factors of success in postsecondary education. High school educators can help students in these areas by offering or identifying opportunities, such as workshops, courses, or tutoring programs, that emphasize the importance of reading, writing, and good study skills. In addition, staff should encourage students to enroll in classes that will focus on writing and study skills in their freshman year of postsecondary education.

Learn time management skills: Although a primary role of high school educators is to provide monitoring, direction, and guidance to students as they approach the end of their high school career, staff also need to prepare students to act independently and to manage their own time with little to no supervision. High school educators can assist students by identifying resources that will help them learn time management and scheduling skills.

Acquire computer skills: Because postsecondary students use computers to complete a multitude of tasks, from registering for classes to accessing course material and obtaining grades, it is essential that students learn to use computers if they are to be prepared for postsecondary education. Ideally, students with disabilities need to start using computers as early as possible in school to increase their familiarity with, and their comfort level in using, computers. Students with visual impairments, hearing impairments, learning disabilities, or mobility impairments may have problems with inputting data or reading a computer monitor. Assistive technology can help certain students with disabilities use computers and access information.

Consider supplemental postsecondary education preparatory programs: A variety of institutions of postsecondary education have summer programs in which students can participate while they are still in high school, or after graduation, to ease their transition to postsecondary education. These programs often expose students to experiences that they are likely to encounter in postsecondary education, such as living in dorms, relating to other students, and eating in dining halls. The programs may also focus on instruction in certain subject areas, such as math or English, or in certain skills, such as computer, writing, or study skills, that can prepare a student to be successful in postsecondary education. High school educators can assist students with disabilities by identifying such program opportunities in their area of residence.

Research postsecondary education programs: Students with disabilities may select any program for which they are qualified but should be advised to review carefully documentation standards and program requirements for their program or institution of interest. For example, students should pay close attention to an institution's program requirements, such as language or math, to avoid making a large financial and time commitment only to realize several years into a program that they cannot, even with academic adjustments, meet an essential requirement for program completion. Campus visits, which include visits to the disability services office, can be helpful in locating an environment that best meets a student's interests and needs. In addition, while all institutions have a legal obligation to provide appropriate services, certain colleges may be able to provide better services than others due to their size or location.

Get involved on campus: To help students avoid the isolation that can occur away from home during the first year of postsecondary education, high school educators should encourage students to live on campus and to become involved in campus activities. Attendance at orientation programs for freshmen is a good first step in discovering ways to get involved in the postsecondary education environment.

Part Six

Legal, Employment, and Financial Concerns for People with Disabilities

Chapter 55

A Guide to Disability Rights Laws

This guide provides an overview of federal civil rights laws that ensure equal opportunity for people with disabilities.

Americans with Disabilities Act (ADA)

The ADA prohibits discrimination on the basis of disability in employment, state and local government, public accommodations, commercial facilities, transportation, and telecommunications. It also applies to the United States Congress.

To be protected by the ADA, one must have a disability or have a relationship or association with an individual with a disability. An individual with a disability is defined by the ADA as a person who has a physical or mental impairment that substantially limits one or more major life activities, a person who has a history or record of such an impairment, or a person who is perceived by others as having such an impairment. The ADA does not specifically name all of the impairments that are covered.

ADA Title I: Employment

Title I requires employers with 15 or more employees to provide qualified individuals with disabilities an equal opportunity to benefit

Excerpted from "A Guide to Disability Rights Laws," U.S. Department of Justice, Civil Rights Division, Disability Rights Section, 2006. Reviewed by David A. Cooke, MD, FACP, July 23, 2011.

from the full range of employment-related opportunities available to others. For example, it prohibits discrimination in recruitment, hiring, promotions, training, pay, social activities, and other privileges of employment. It restricts questions that can be asked about an applicant's disability before a job offer is made, and it requires that employers make reasonable accommodation to the known physical or mental limitations of otherwise qualified individuals with disabilities, unless it results in undue hardship. Religious entities with 15 or more employees are covered under Title I.

Title I complaints must be filed with the U. S. Equal Employment Opportunity Commission (EEOC) within 180 days of the date of discrimination, or 300 days if the charge is filed with a designated state or local fair employment practice agency. Individuals may file a lawsuit in federal court only after they receive a "right-to-sue" letter from the EEOC. Charges of employment discrimination on the basis of disability may be filed at any U.S. Equal Employment Opportunity Commission field office. Field offices are located in 50 cities throughout the United States and are listed in most telephone directories under "U.S. Government."

ADA Title II: State and Local Government Activities

Title II covers all activities of state and local governments regardless of the government entity's size or receipt of federal funding. Title II requires that state and local governments give people with disabilities an equal opportunity to benefit from all of their programs, services, and activities (e.g., public education, employment, transportation, recreation, health care, social services, courts, voting, and town meetings).

State and local governments are required to follow specific architectural standards in the new construction and alteration of their buildings. They also must relocate programs or otherwise provide access in inaccessible older buildings, and communicate effectively with people who have hearing, vision, or speech disabilities. Public entities are not required to take actions that would result in undue financial and administrative burdens. They are required to make reasonable modifications to policies, practices, and procedures where necessary to avoid discrimination, unless they can demonstrate that doing so would fundamentally alter the nature of the service, program, or activity being provided.

Complaints of Title II violations may be filed with the Department of Justice within 180 days of the date of discrimination. In certain situations, cases may be referred to a mediation program sponsored by the Department. The Department may bring a lawsuit where it has investigated a matter and has been unable to resolve violations.

ADA Title II: Public Transportation

The transportation provisions of Title II cover public transportation services, such as city buses and public rail transit (e.g., subways, commuter rails, Amtrak). Public transportation authorities may not discriminate against people with disabilities in the provision of their services. They must comply with requirements for accessibility in newly purchased vehicles, make good faith efforts to purchase or lease accessible used buses, remanufacture buses in an accessible manner, and, unless it would result in an undue burden, provide paratransit where they operate fixed-route bus or rail systems. Paratransit is a service where individuals who are unable to use the regular transit system independently (because of a physical or mental impairment) are picked up and dropped off at their destinations.

ADA Title III: Public Accommodations

Title III covers businesses and nonprofit service providers that are public accommodations, privately operated entities offering certain types of courses and examinations, privately operated transportation, and commercial facilities. Public accommodations are private entities who own, lease, lease to, or operate facilities such as restaurants, retail stores, hotels, movie theaters, private schools, convention centers, doctors' offices, homeless shelters, transportation depots, zoos, funeral homes, day care centers, and recreation facilities including sports stadiums and fitness clubs. Transportation services provided by private entities are also covered by Title III.

Public accommodations must comply with basic nondiscrimination requirements that prohibit exclusion, segregation, and unequal treatment. They also must comply with specific requirements related to architectural standards for new and altered buildings; reasonable modifications to policies, practices, and procedures; effective communication with people with hearing, vision, or speech disabilities; and other access requirements. Additionally, public accommodations must remove barriers in existing buildings where it is easy to do so without much difficulty or expense, given the public accommodation's resources. Courses and examinations related to professional, educational, or trade-related applications, licensing, certifications, or credentialing must be provided in a place and manner accessible to people with disabilities, or alternative accessible arrangements must be offered. Commercial facilities, such as factories and warehouses, must comply with the ADA's architectural standards for new construction and alterations.

Complaints of Title III violations may be filed with the Department of Justice. In certain situations, cases may be referred to a mediation program sponsored by the Department. The Department is authorized to bring a lawsuit where there is a pattern or practice of discrimination in violation of Title III, or where an act of discrimination raises an issue of general public importance. Title III may also be enforced through private lawsuits. It is not necessary to file a complaint with the Department of Justice (or any Federal agency), or to receive a "right-to-sue" letter, before going to court.

ADA Title IV: Telecommunications Relay Services

Title IV addresses telephone and television access for people with hearing and speech disabilities. It requires common carriers (telephone companies) to establish interstate and intrastate telecommunications relay services (TRS) 24 hours a day, 7 days a week.

TRS enables callers with hearing and speech disabilities who use telecommunications devices for the deaf (TDDs), which are also known as teletypewriters (TTYs), and callers who use voice telephones to communicate with each other through a third party communications assistant. The Federal Communications Commission (FCC) has set minimum standards for TRS services. Title IV also requires closed captioning of federally funded public service announcements.

Telecommunications Act

Section 255 and Section 251(a)(2) of the Communications Act of 1934, as amended by the Telecommunications Act of 1996, require manufacturers of telecommunications equipment and providers of telecommunications services to ensure that such equipment and services are accessible to and usable by persons with disabilities, if readily achievable. These amendments ensure that people with disabilities will have access to a broad range of products and services such as telephones, cell phones, pagers, call-waiting, and operator services, which were often inaccessible to many users with disabilities.

Fair Housing Act

The Fair Housing Act, as amended in 1988, prohibits housing discrimination on the basis of race, color, religion, sex, disability, familial status, and national origin. Its coverage includes private housing, housing that receives Federal financial assistance, and State and local government housing. It is unlawful to discriminate in any aspect of selling or renting housing or to deny a dwelling to a buyer or renter because of the disability of that individual, an individual associated with the buyer or renter, or an individual who intends to live in the residence. Other covered activities include, for example, financing, zoning practices, new construction design, and advertising.

The Fair Housing Act requires owners of housing facilities to make reasonable exceptions in their policies and operations to afford people with disabilities equal housing opportunities. For example, a landlord with a "no pets" policy may be required to grant an exception to this rule and allow an individual who is blind to keep a guide dog in the residence. The Fair Housing Act also requires landlords to allow tenants with disabilities to make reasonable access-related modifications to their private living space, as well as to common use spaces. (The landlord is not required to pay for the changes.) The Act further requires that new multifamily housing with four or more units be designed and built to allow access for persons with disabilities. This includes accessible common use areas, doors that are wide enough for wheelchairs, kitchens and bathrooms that allow a person using a wheelchair to maneuver, and other adaptable features within the units.

Air Carrier Access Act

The Air Carrier Access Act prohibits discrimination in air transportation by domestic and foreign air carriers against qualified individuals with physical or mental impairments. It applies only to air carriers that provide regularly scheduled services for hire to the public. Requirements address a wide range of issues including boarding assistance and certain accessibility features in newly built aircraft and new or altered airport facilities. People may enforce rights under the Air Carrier Access Act by filing a complaint with the U.S. Department of Transportation, or by bringing a lawsuit in federal court.

Voting Accessibility for the Elderly and Handicapped Act

The Voting Accessibility for the Elderly and Handicapped Act of 1984 generally requires polling places across the United States to be physically accessible to people with disabilities for federal elections. Where no accessible location is available to serve as a polling place, a political subdivision must provide an alternate means of casting a ballot on the day of the election. This law also requires states to make available registration and voting aids for disabled and elderly voters, including information by telecommunications devices for the deaf (TDDs), which are also known as teletypewriters (TTYs).

National Voter Registration Act

The National Voter Registration Act of 1993, also known as the "Motor Voter Act," makes it easier for all Americans to exercise their fundamental right to vote. One of the basic purposes of the Act is to increase the historically low registration rates of minorities and persons with disabilities that have resulted from discrimination. The Motor Voter Act requires all offices of state-funded programs that are primarily engaged in providing services to persons with disabilities to provide all program applicants with voter registration forms, to assist them in completing the forms, and to transmit completed forms to the appropriate state official.

Civil Rights of Institutionalized Persons Act

The Civil Rights of Institutionalized Persons Act (CRIPA) authorizes the U.S. Attorney General to investigate conditions of confinement at state and local government institutions such as prisons, jails, pretrial detention centers, juvenile correctional facilities, publicly operated nursing homes, and institutions for people with psychiatric or developmental disabilities. Its purpose is to allow the Attorney General to uncover and correct widespread deficiencies that seriously jeopardize the health and safety of residents of institutions. The Attorney General does not have authority under CRIPA to investigate isolated incidents or to represent individual institutionalized persons.

The Attorney General may initiate civil law suits where there is reasonable cause to believe that conditions are "egregious or flagrant," that they are subjecting residents to "grievous harm," and that they are part of a "pattern or practice" of resistance to residents' full enjoyment of constitutional or federal rights, including Title II of the ADA and Section 504 of the Rehabilitation Act.

Individuals with Disabilities Education Act

The Individuals with Disabilities Education Act (IDEA) (formerly called P.L. 94-142 or the Education for all Handicapped Children Act of 1975) requires public schools to make available to all eligible children with disabilities a free appropriate public education in the least restrictive environment appropriate to their individual needs. IDEA requires public school systems to develop appropriate Individualized

Education Programs (IEPs) for each child. The specific special education and related services outlined in each IEP reflect the individualized needs of each student.

IDEA also mandates that particular procedures be followed in the development of the IEP. Each student's IEP must be developed by a team of knowledgeable persons and must be at least reviewed annually. The team includes the child's teacher; the parents, subject to certain limited exceptions; the child, if determined appropriate; an agency representative who is qualified to provide or supervise the provision of special education; and other individuals at the parents' or agency's discretion. If parents disagree with the proposed IEP, they can request a due process hearing and a review from the state educational agency if applicable in that state. They also can appeal the state agency's decision to state or federal court.

Rehabilitation Act

The Rehabilitation Act prohibits discrimination on the basis of disability in programs conducted by federal agencies, in programs receiving federal financial assistance, in federal employment, and in the employment practices of federal contractors. The standards for determining employment discrimination under the Rehabilitation Act are the same as those used in Title I of the Americans with Disabilities Act.

Section 501

Section 501 requires affirmative action and nondiscrimination in employment by federal agencies of the executive branch.

Section 503

Section 503 requires affirmative action and prohibits employment discrimination by federal government contractors and subcontractors with contracts of more than $10,000.

Section 504

Section 504 states that "no qualified individual with a disability in the United States shall be excluded from, denied the benefits of, or be subjected to discrimination under" any program or activity that either receives federal financial assistance or is conducted by any executive agency or the United States Postal Service.

Each federal agency has its own set of Section 504 regulations that apply to its own programs. Agencies that provide federal financial assistance also have Section 504 regulations covering entities that receive federal aid. Requirements common to these regulations include reasonable accommodation for employees with disabilities; program accessibility; effective communication with people who have hearing or vision disabilities; and accessible new construction and alterations. Each agency is responsible for enforcing its own regulations. Section 504 may also be enforced through private lawsuits. It is not necessary to file a complaint with a federal agency or to receive a "right-to-sue" letter before going to court.

Section 508

Section 508 establishes requirements for electronic and information technology developed, maintained, procured, or used by the federal government. Section 508 requires federal electronic and information technology to be accessible to people with disabilities, including employees and members of the public.

An accessible information technology system is one that can be operated in a variety of ways and does not rely on a single sense or ability of the user. For example, a system that provides output only in visual format may not be accessible to people with visual impairments and a system that provides output only in audio format may not be accessible to people who are deaf or hard of hearing. Some individuals with disabilities may need accessibility-related software or peripheral devices in order to use systems that comply with Section 508.

Architectural Barriers Act

The Architectural Barriers Act (ABA) requires that buildings and facilities that are designed, constructed, or altered with federal funds, or leased by a federal agency, comply with federal standards for physical accessibility. ABA requirements are limited to architectural standards in new and altered buildings and in newly leased facilities. They do not address the activities conducted in those buildings and facilities. Facilities of the U.S. Postal Service are covered by the ABA.

Chapter 56

Questions and Answers about the Americans with Disabilities Act

Barriers to employment, transportation, public accommodations, public services, and telecommunications have imposed staggering economic and social costs on American society and have undermined our well-intentioned efforts to educate, rehabilitate, and employ individuals with disabilities. By breaking down these barriers, the Americans with Disabilities Act (ADA) will enable society to benefit from the skills and talents of individuals with disabilities, will allow us all to gain from their increased purchasing power and ability to use it, and will lead to fuller, more productive lives for all Americans.

The Americans with Disabilities Act gives civil rights protections to individuals with disabilities similar to those provided to individuals on the basis of race, color, sex, national origin, age, and religion. It guarantees equal opportunity for individuals with disabilities in public accommodations, employment, transportation, state and local government services, and telecommunications.

Excerpted from "Americans with Disabilities Act: Questions and Answers," by the U.S. Equal Employment Opportunity Commission (EEOC, www.ada.gov), part of the U.S. Department of Justice, October 9, 2008.

What employers are covered by title I of the ADA, and when is the coverage effective?

The title I employment provisions apply to private employers, state and local governments, employment agencies, and labor unions. Employers with 25 or more employees were covered as of July 26, 1992. Employers with 15 or more employees were covered 2 years later, beginning July 26, 1994.

What practices and activities are covered by the employment nondiscrimination requirements?

The ADA prohibits discrimination in all employment practices, including job application procedures, hiring, firing, advancement, compensation, training, and other terms, conditions, and privileges of employment. It applies to recruitment, advertising, tenure, layoff, leave, fringe benefits, and all other employment-related activities.

Who is protected from employment discrimination?

Employment discrimination is prohibited against "qualified individuals with disabilities." This includes applicants for employment and employees. An individual is considered to have a "disability" if s/he has a physical or mental impairment that substantially limits one or more major life activities, has a record of such an impairment, or is regarded as having such an impairment. Persons discriminated against because they have a known association or relationship with an individual with a disability also are protected.

The first part of the definition makes clear that the ADA applies to persons who have impairments and that these must substantially limit major life activities such as seeing, hearing, speaking, walking, breathing, performing manual tasks, learning, caring for oneself, and working. An individual with epilepsy, paralysis, HIV infection, AIDS, a substantial hearing or visual impairment, mental retardation, or a specific learning disability is covered, but an individual with a minor, nonchronic condition of short duration, such as a sprain, broken limb, or the flu, generally would not be covered.

The second part of the definition protecting individuals with a record of a disability would cover, for example, a person who has recovered from cancer or mental illness.

The third part of the definition protects individuals who are regarded as having a substantially limiting impairment, even though they may not have such an impairment. For example, this provision would protect a qualified individual with a severe facial disfigurement from being denied employment because an employer feared the "negative reactions" of customers or coworkers.

Who is a qualified individual with a disability?

A qualified individual with a disability is a person who meets legitimate skill, experience, education, or other requirements of an employment position that he or she holds or seeks, and who can perform the essential functions of the position with or without reasonable accommodation. Requiring the ability to perform "essential" functions assures that an individual with a disability will not be considered unqualified simply because of inability to perform marginal or incidental job functions. If the individual is qualified to perform essential job functions except for limitations caused by a disability, the employer must consider whether the individual could perform these functions with a reasonable accommodation. If a written job description has been prepared in advance of advertising or interviewing applicants for a job, this will be considered as evidence, although not conclusive evidence, of the essential functions of the job.

Does an employer have to give preference to a qualified applicant with a disability over other applicants?

No. An employer is free to select the most qualified applicant available and to make decisions based on reasons unrelated to a disability. For example, suppose two persons apply for a job as a typist and an essential function of the job is to type 75 words per minute accurately. One applicant, an individual with a disability, who is provided with a reasonable accommodation for a typing test, types 50 words per minute; the other applicant who has no disability accurately types 75 words per minute. The employer can hire the applicant with the higher typing speed, if typing speed is needed for successful performance of the job.

What limitations does the ADA impose on medical examinations and inquiries about disability?

An employer may not ask or require a job applicant to take a medical examination before making a job offer. It cannot make any pre-employment inquiry about a disability or the nature or severity of a disability. An employer may, however, ask questions about the ability to perform specific job functions and may, with certain limitations, ask an individual with a disability to describe or demonstrate how he or she would perform these functions.

An employer may condition a job offer on the satisfactory result of a post-offer medical examination or medical inquiry if this is required of all entering employees in the same job category. A post-offer examination or inquiry does not have to be job-related and consistent with business necessity.

However, if an individual is not hired because a post-offer medical examination or inquiry reveals a disability, the reason(s) for not hiring must be job-related and consistent with business necessity. The employer also must show that no reasonable accommodation was available that would enable the individual to perform the essential job functions, or that accommodation would impose an undue hardship. A post-offer medical examination may disqualify an individual if the employer can demonstrate that the individual would pose a "direct threat" in the workplace (i.e., a significant risk of substantial harm to the health or safety of the individual or others) that cannot be eliminated or reduced below the direct threat level through reasonable accommodation.

Such a disqualification is job-related and consistent with business necessity. A post-offer medical examination may not disqualify an individual with a disability who is currently able to perform essential job functions because of speculation that the disability may cause a risk of future injury.

After a person starts work, a medical examination or inquiry of an employee must be job-related and consistent with business necessity. Employers may conduct employee medical examinations where there is evidence of a job performance or safety problem, examinations required by other federal laws, examinations to determine current fitness to perform a particular job, and voluntary examinations that are part of employee health programs.

Information from all medical examinations and inquiries must be kept apart from general personnel files as a separate, confidential medical record, available only under limited conditions.

Tests for illegal use of drugs are not medical examinations under the ADA and are not subject to the restrictions of such examinations.

What is reasonable accommodation?

Reasonable accommodation is any modification or adjustment to a job or the work environment that will enable a qualified applicant or employee with a disability to participate in the application process or to perform essential job functions. Reasonable accommodation also includes adjustments to assure that a qualified individual with a disability has rights and privileges in employment equal to those of employees without disabilities.

What are some of the accommodations applicants and employees may need?

Examples of reasonable accommodation include making existing facilities used by employees readily accessible to and usable by an individual with a disability; restructuring a job; modifying work schedules; acquiring or modifying equipment; providing qualified readers or interpreters; or appropriately modifying examinations, training, or other programs. Reasonable accommodation also may include reassigning a current employee to a vacant position for which the individual is qualified, if the person is unable to do the original job because of a disability even with an accommodation. However, there is no obligation to find a position for an applicant who is not qualified for the position sought. Employers are not required to lower quality or quantity standards as an accommodation; nor are they obligated to provide personal use items such as glasses or hearing aids.

The decision as to the appropriate accommodation must be based on the particular facts of each case. In selecting the particular type of reasonable accommodation to provide, the principal test is that of effectiveness, i.e., whether the accommodation will provide an opportunity for a person with a disability to achieve the same level of performance and to enjoy benefits equal to those of an average, similarly situated person without a disability. However, the accommodation does not have to ensure equal results or provide exactly the same benefits.

When is an employer required to make a reasonable accommodation?

An employer is only required to accommodate a "known" disability of a qualified applicant or employee. The requirement generally will be triggered by a request from an individual with a disability, who frequently will be able to suggest an appropriate accommodation. Accommodations must be made on an individual basis, because the nature and extent of a disabling condition and the requirements of a job will vary in each case. If the individual does not request an accommodation, the employer is not obligated to provide one except where an individual's known disability impairs his or her ability to know of, or effectively communicate a need for, an accommodation that is obvious to the employer. If a person with a disability requests, but cannot suggest, an appropriate accommodation, the employer and the individual should work together to identify one. There are also many public and private resources that can provide assistance without cost.

Chapter 57

Housing and Safety Issues for People with Disabilities

Chapter Contents

Section 57.1—The State of Housing for People
with Disabilities 502

Section 57.2—Disability Rights in Housing 507

Section 57.3—Understanding the Fair Housing
Amendments Act 511

Section 57.4—Homelessness among People with
Disabilities.. 517

Section 57.5—Fire Safety for People with Disabilities
and Their Caregivers 519

Section 57.6—Disaster Preparedness for People with
Disabilities and Special Needs 521

Section 57.1

The State of Housing for People with Disabilities

The state of housing for people with disabilities provides important historical context for some of the major policy barriers in the area of housing and disability. The past history of people with disabilities, currently the largest minority group in the United States, has very much influenced our current state of housing policies and practices in design and government programs.

Legislative history from the turn of the century shows that the disability community has been viewed as everything from "unfit" to "dangerous" to a "detriment to normal society." These views directly led to the establishment of our nation's very long history of government imposed segregation of people with disabilities. This segregation and isolation has occurred in all aspects of community life from education and transportation to recreation and employment and most importantly, housing. The main form of housing under state imposed segregation has been large warehouse-like state operated institutions and smaller institutions such as group homes. People with disabilities were considered sick and in need of treatment to be cured. Our housing options therefore, have resembled that of medical centers, very different from what most people call home. The perception that people with disabilities need to be treated unfortunately continues in our society today.

Institutions were eventually exposed as inhumane, isolated environments spurring the De-Institutionalization movement in the 1960s—people with disabilities were placed in small congregate settings in the community as an alternative.

The 1970s represented a turning point—people with disabilities began to stand up to their history of mistreatment, segregation, overmedicalization, and paternalism. In 1973 one man named Ed Roberts, who used a power wheelchair due to polio, helped give birth to the disability rights movement when he demanded admission to

University of California at Berkeley and refused to be forced to live in an institution.

The 1980s and the 1990s brought a further shift toward integration, inclusion, and recognition that we are a community deserving of human and civil rights with passage of civil rights laws protecting people with disabilities in the areas of housing, transportation, education, recreation, and public accommodations. The amendment of the Fair Housing Act to include people with disabilities, though an important victory, came in 1988, 20 years after the original act was passed.

The protections made it illegal to discriminate against people with disabilities in the rental or sale of housing and mandated accessible design and construction.

Section 504 of the Rehab Act mandates any entity receiving public funds to give access to people with disabilities in all programs, services, or activities. Design and construction requirements under Section 504 state that all buildings of five or more units must have 5% of those units usable for persons with mobility impairments and 2% of the units must be accessible for people with hearing/visual impairments. In addition, landlords must pay for any "reasonable accommodation" or modification which the tenant requests. Section 504 legal requirements are clear but implementation has been weak and not too much has been changed for residents with disabilities in public assisted housing.

Lack of Affordable, Accessible, and Integrated Housing

Too much of our present housing status resembles that of our past. The reality is people with disabilities still don't have the same housing choices the general population has. The choices we have (nursing homes, group homes, segregated apartment complexes) are not what nondisabled people consider housing. The lack of accessible housing in our country has reached crisis levels and people with disabilities have named housing the number-one issue. There are still far too many people living in nursing homes—our long term care system favors providing services to people with disabilities in institutions rather than in their own homes—four out of every five Medicaid dollars go toward providing services to people with disabilities in institutions rather in their own homes.

Also, the state of Illinois is one of the top 10 worst states in the nation for keeping people with disabilities in these institutions. Because of work disincentives, employment discrimination, and the lack of educational opportunities, over 70% of people with disabilities are not working and are on benefits, and people receiving Social Security Insurance (SSI) earn an average of $650 per month. This poverty has resulted in tremendous need for affordable housing which people with disabilities face alongside millions of other Americans. A recent report from the Technical Assistance Collaborative showed that there is not one single housing market in the United States in which a person on SSI (without a subsidy) could afford even a modest efficiency unit. However, if you link the need for affordability with the need for accessibility the search for housing becomes like finding a needle in a haystack.

Access Living, a Center for Independent Living for people with disabilities in metropolitan Chicago, the United States Department of Justice, and the John Marshall Law School in Chicago conducted systemic testing of suburban newly constructed multi-family housing and found 47 of 48 buildings were out of compliance with the federal Fair Housing Act accessibility requirements. The gross lack of accessible apartments in Illinois and throughout the United States forces many people with disabilities to settle for apartments whose only accessible feature is a 32-inch front door entry, even if the kitchen and bathrooms are inaccessible; even worse, many more people are forced into institutional settings because of the lack of accessible housing.

Probably most troubling though, is the fact that we have not yet moved beyond our policies of state-sponsored segregation. Despite the fact that we now have laws and rights protecting people with disabilities and despite the 1988 preamble of the amended Fair Housing Act which declares "a national commitment to end the unnecessary exclusion of people with disabilities from the American mainstream" the United States government still continues to fund, build, and operate housing which segregates people with disabilities on the basis and type of their disabilities. While this would be considered illegal housing practice on the basis of any other protected class, it is still permitted and encouraged by our nation and our government on the basis of disability.

Providers in the private rental market continue to grossly discriminate against people with disabilities; in 2004 the Urban Institute (under contract with the U.S. Department of Housing and Urban Development [HUD]), worked in partnership with Access Living of Metropolitan Chicago to design, and conduct the study "Discrimination Against Persons With Disabilities: Barriers At Every Step." The study (released in 2005) focused on the Chicago area private rental housing market, and its treatment of people with physical disabilities and people with hearing impairments. The findings were based on more than 200 tests where people with and without disabilities posed as applicants for rental units. The findings showed that people with disabilities face discrimination more than any other protected class, and that more than 30% of the Chicago housing stock was not even visitable by people with physical disabilities.

Housing Design

Housing Design is one of the basic elements that impacts our segregation, our housing choices, as well as our ability to be a part of the American mainstream.

Whether or not a home is accessible can literally determine where a person lives, and whether a person is truly a part of his or her community. If a wheelchair user cannot visit friends and neighbors, participate in block club meetings, or go to dinner parties because there are stairs, that person cannot participate in his or her community fully. But accessibility's impact on community life doesn't rest solely on the wheelchair user, it impacts the wheelchair user's friends, neighbors, and families who live in those inaccessible houses and cannot invite their disabled friends and relatives to their homes.

Further, it is important to consider that as we all get older and can no longer function as we once did, we will likely prefer to remain in our homes. It is the design of the homes we live in that will determine whether we are displaced as we get older.

Public Housing and Design

With the national transformation of public housing in the United States, the disability community is thinking deeply about design issues. Because public housing is the disability community's number one source of housing, the local and national trends demolishing public housing high rises are troubling. While these buildings are often blighted and in disrepair, they are also a symbol of accessibility for people who are blind, visually impaired, hard of hearing, deaf, and to those using wheelchairs. The demolition of public housing is giving way to inaccessible, walk-up townhouses which are exempt from the Fair Housing Act accessibility requirements and are unusable by persons with mobility impairments. This new housing style may address issues of economic and racial segregation but they leave behind and further segregate people with disabilities from the new public housing.

Housing for All

Efforts to work with our local and our national policy makers to rethink how we design housing in ways that it can be both attractive and livable for all—with and without disabilities—have met with little success, and there is still much work to be done. We challenge architects and designers to think outside of the box. Advocates in the disability rights movement have worked hard to create housing whose accessible features are undetectable, yet usable by everyone. We must think outside of the box—be creative and innovative and inclusive. The disability community does not think of a wide 32-inch clear doorway or a 12:1 ramp, or a 15-inch outlet as merely building codes, but as civil rights—as those elements which will allow people with disabilities to have shelter while becoming truly active members of our community.

It is important to remember that in every country, disability is one of the largest and fastest growing segments of the population. Disability cuts across all racial, ethnic, economic, social, age, gender, and geographic boundaries.

Whether disability is acquired from birth, from illness or from traumatic injury, it is part of the human condition—a condition that will impact virtually all of us in this society or someone we love, at some point in our lives.

This is why the international disability community feels such urgency to have our policy makers, architects, designers, and developers be thoughtful and inclusive not just to the needs of our citizens living with disabilities now, but to all of us who will acquire disabilities in the future. In 2008 the United Nations entered into force the first human rights treaty of the twenty-first century, The Conference for the Rights of People with Disabilities. One hundred twenty-seven countries have signed the U.N. treaty; the United States shamefully has not.

Our traditional views that disability issues or accessible design is something impacting only a small portion of our society must be cast away. Accessibility is not a special needs issue—it is an issue of civil rights, a matter of independence, and a matter of importance to our entire population—it is everybody's issue; it is a human issue.

Access Living

Access Living is a not-for-profit, non-residential center for independent living which is consumer controlled. We provide services and advocacy to people with all types of disabilities in Chicago. Our goal is to ensure full integration and participation of people with disabilities into the mainstream of society. Access Living's advocacy and service programs include housing, education, health care, economic development, deinstitutionalization, civil rights enforcement, and peer support as they relate to disability.

Section 57.2

Disability Rights in Housing

From "Disability Rights in Housing," by the U.S. Department of Housing and Urban Development (HUD, www.hud.gov), May 25, 2006. Reviewed by David A. Cooke, MD, FACP, July 23, 2011.

Definition of Disability

Federal laws define a person with a disability as "Any person who has a physical or mental impairment that substantially limits one or more major life activities; has a record of such impairment; or is regarded as having such an impairment."

In general, a physical or mental impairment includes hearing, mobility and visual impairments, chronic alcoholism, chronic mental illness, AIDS [acquired immunodeficiency syndrome], AIDS-related complex, and mental retardation that substantially limits one or more major life activities. Major life activities include walking, talking, hearing, seeing, breathing, learning, performing manual tasks, and caring for oneself.

Disability Rights in Private and Public Housing

Regardless of whether you live in private or public housing, federal laws provide the following rights to persons with disabilities:

- **Prohibits discrimination against persons with disabilities:** It is unlawful for a housing provider to refuse to rent or sell to a person simply because of a disability. A housing provider may not impose different application or qualification criteria, rental fees or sales prices, and rental or sales terms or conditions than those required of or provided to persons who are not disabled.

507

Example: A housing provider may not refuse to rent to an otherwise qualified individual with a mental disability because he or she is uncomfortable with the individual's disability. Such an act would violate the Fair Housing Act because it denies a person housing solely on the basis of their disability.

- **Requires housing providers to make reasonable accommodations for persons with disabilities:** A reasonable accommodation is a change in rules, policies, practices, or services so that a person with a disability will have an equal opportunity to use and enjoy a dwelling unit or common space. A housing provider should do everything he or she can to assist, but he or she is not required to make changes that would fundamentally alter the program or create an undue financial and administrative burden. Reasonable accommodations may be necessary at all stages of the housing process, including application, tenancy, or to prevent eviction. Example: A housing provider would make a reasonable accommodation for a tenant with mobility impairment by fulfilling the tenant's request for a reserved parking space in front of the entrance to their unit, even though all parking is unreserved.

- **Requires housing providers to allow persons with disabilities to make reasonable modifications:** A reasonable modification is a structural modification that is made to allow persons with disabilities the full enjoyment of the housing and related facilities. Examples of a reasonable modification would include allowing a person with a disability to install a ramp into a building, lower the entry threshold of a unit, or install grab bars in a bathroom.

- **Reasonable modifications are usually made at the resident's expense:** However, there are resources available for helping fund building modifications. Additionally, if you live in federally assisted housing the housing provider may be required to pay for the modification if it does not amount to an undue financial and administrative burden.

- **Requires that new covered multifamily housing be designed and constructed to be accessible:** In covered multifamily housing consisting of four or more units with an elevator built for first occupancy after March 13, 1991, all units must comply with the following seven design and construction requirements of the Fair Housing Act:

- Accessible entrance on an accessible route

- Accessible public and common-use areas

- Usable doors

- Accessible route into and through the dwelling unit

- Accessible light switches, electrical outlets, thermostats, and environmental controls

- Reinforced walls in bathrooms

- Usable kitchens and bathrooms

In covered multifamily housing without an elevator that consists of four or more units built for first occupancy after March 13, 1991, all ground floor units must comply with the Fair Housing Act seven design and construction requirements.

These requirements apply to most public and private housing. However, there are limited exemptions for owner-occupied buildings with no more than four units, single-family housing sold or rented without the use of a broker, and housing operated by organizations and private clubs that limit occupancy to members.

If you live in federally assisted multifamily housing consisting of five or more units, 5 percent of these units (or at least one unit whichever is greater) must meet more stringent physical accessibility requirements. Additionally, 2 percent of units (or at least one unit whichever is greater) must be accessible for persons with visual or hearing disabilities.

People with Disabilities in Federally Assisted Housing

Federal law makes it illegal for an otherwise qualified individual with a disability to be excluded, solely because of his or her disability, from programs receiving federal financial assistance.

Zoning and Land Use

It is unlawful for local governments to utilize land use and zoning policies to keep persons with disabilities from locating to their area.

State and Local Laws

Many states and localities have fair housing laws that are substantially equivalent to the Federal Fair Housing Act. Some of these laws prohibit discrimination on additional bases, such as source of income or marital status. Some of these laws may impose more stringent design and construction standards for new multifamily housing.

The Americans with Disabilities Act (ADA)

In most cases, the ADA does not apply to residential housing. Rather, the ADA applies to places of public accommodation such as restaurants, retail stores, libraries, and hospitals as well as commercial facilities such as office buildings, warehouses, and factories. However, Title III of the ADA covers public and common use areas at housing developments when these public areas are, by their nature, open to the general public. For example, it covers the rental office since the rental office is open to the general public.

Title II of the ADA applies to all programs, services, and activities provided or made available by public entities. This includes housing when the housing is provided or made available by a public entity. For example, housing covered by Title II of the ADA includes public housing authorities that meet the ADA definition of "public entity," and housing operated by states or units of local government, such as housing on a state university campus.

Section 57.3

Understanding the Fair Housing Amendments Act

Excerpted from "Understanding the Fair Housing Amendments Act," © 2004 United Spinal Association. Reprinted with permission. Additional information, including the complete text of this document, is available at www .unitedspinal.org. The United Spinal Association states that the text is current and up-to-date.

Introduction

The Fair Housing Amendments Act (FHAA) was signed into law on September 13, 1988, and became effective on March 12, 1989. The Act amends Title VIII of the Civil Rights Act of 1968, which prohibits discrimination on the basis of race, color, religion, sex, or national origin in housing sales, rentals, or financing. The FHAA extends this protection to persons with a disability and families with children.

This law is intended to increase housing opportunities for people with disabilities. However, individual citizens must come forward with concerns, file complaints, or sue if they believe their rights have been violated. The government has no other way of detecting discrimination as it occurs. As a result, it is important to understand this legislation and how to make it work for you.

Understanding the Fair Housing Amendments Act will help both persons with disabilities and advocates better understand the FHAA. This text will explain the law.

Who Is Protected?

The FHAA added persons with a "handicapping condition," along with families with children, as protected classes under the Civil Rights Act. The legislation adopts the definition of handicapping condition found in Section 504 of the Rehabilitation Act of 1973, as amended. This definition includes any person who actually has a physical or mental impairment, has a record of having such an impairment, or is regarded as having such an impairment that substantially limits one or more major life activity such as hearing, seeing, speaking, breathing, performing manual tasks, walking, and caring for one's self.

Types of Housing Facilities Covered

This law pertains to all types of housing, whether privately or publicly funded. Some examples of types of facilities include, but are not limited to, condominiums, cooperatives, mobile homes, trailer parks, time shares, and any unit that is designed or used as a residence. It also includes any land or vacant property, which is sold or leased as residential property.

Prohibited Actions

The FHAA prohibits a wide array of activities that discriminate against persons with disabilities and families with children in the sale or rental of housing. The following specifically outlines illegal actions:

- Refusal to sell or rent a dwelling unit when a bona fide offer has been made, where the refusal is based on race, color, religion, sex, disability, familial status, or national origin.

- Imposing different terms and conditions or treating people differently with the provision of service because of race, color, religion, sex, disability, familial status, or national origin.

- Discouraging an individual from living in a community or neighborhood, if the restriction is based on race, color, religion, sex, disability, familial status, or national origin. This activity is frequently referred to as steering.

- Advertising, posting notices, or making statements in such a way as to deny access to an individual if that denial is based on race, color, religion, sex, disability, familial status, or national origin.

- Misrepresenting the availability of a dwelling because of the applicant's race, color, religion, sex, disability, familial status, or national origin.

- Blockbusting by encouraging the sale or rental of a dwelling by implying that people of a certain race, color, religion, sex, disability, familial status, or origin are entering the community in large numbers.

The FHAA expands the traditional list of prohibited activities to actions, which relate directly to discrimination based on disability. The following are examples of such activities:

- It is illegal for a landlord to refuse to allow a tenant with a disability to make modifications, at the tenant's expense, which would permit the tenant to fully enjoy the premises. The landlord can, where reasonable, require the tenant to restore the interior of the premises to the condition it was in prior to the modification. Premises are defined to include interior and exterior parts. Therefore, refusing to permit a tenant to make modifications to a lobby, entryway, parking lot, or laundry room, is also discriminatory. This is discussed in greater detail in the "reasonable accommodations" section.

- Asking a question designed to determine whether an applicant or anyone associated with that applicant has a disability is unlawful under FHAA. However, the Act does provide for certain inquiries, provided they are asked of all applicants whether or not they have a disability.

A housing provider may ask:

- if an applicant can meet the financial requirements of ownership or tenancy;

- if an applicant is eligible for housing that is available only to persons with a disability or a specific disability;

- if a person is eligible for a priority available only to persons with a disability or a specific disability;

- if a person is a current substance abuser;

- if an applicant has ever been convicted of the illegal manufacture or distribution of a controlled substance.

Reasonable Accommodations

FHAA requires two types of reasonable accommodations to make existing housing more accessible to persons with disabilities. These accommodations consist of structural modifications and policy changes.

Structural Modifications

Housing providers must permit reasonable modifications of existing premises if such modifications are necessary for a person with a disability to be able to live in and use the premises.

- The cost of the modification is to be paid by the resident with a disability.

513

- Modifications may be made to the interior of the individual's unit as well as any public and common use areas of a building, including lobbies, hallways, and laundry rooms.

- Modifications may be requested in any type of dwelling; however, in a rental situation, the landlord may reasonably condition permission for modification on the following:

  - the renter agreeing to restore the interior of the premises to the condition that existed before the modification, ordinary wear and tear excepted;

  - the renter providing a reasonable description of the proposed modifications; and

  - the renter providing reasonable assurance that the work will be done in a workmanlike manner with all applicable building permits being obtained.

A renter should be aware that a landlord must not increase any customarily required security deposit. However, where it is necessary to ensure with reasonable certainty that funds will be available for any necessary restoration at the end of the tenancy, the landlord may require that the tenant pay a reasonable amount of money not to exceed the cost of the restorations, into an interest bearing escrow account, over a reasonable period of time. The interest earned on the account accrues to the benefit of the tenant. This means that when the tenant with a disability moves and the unit is restored to its original condition, any money left in the account is given to the tenant.

As a result of these rules, FHAA has, in effect, created three classifications of modifications:

- modifications that do not have to be restored;

- modifications that need to be restored to the original condition but do not require establishment of an escrow account; and

- modifications that need to be restored and are relatively expensive; therefore, an escrow account may be required.

An example of the first modification category would be widening a bathroom door, which does not affect the usability of any other space, such as a closet. Here, a wider door would not affect the next tenant's use of the apartment.

A modification, which may fall in the second category, would be the removal of a base cabinet under the kitchen sink. In this situation, the next tenant would want the storage space under the sink, therefore the tenant with a disability would be required to restore the cabinet. The cost to replace one cabinet would not be tremendous, so an escrow account would probably not be required. If all the cabinets in the kitchen were replaced and the counter lowered, which is obviously more expensive, an escrow account may be required. The traditional example of a situation where an escrow account may be needed is when a tenant removes the bathtub and replaces it with a roll-in shower.

Remember, although a landlord may condition permission, he/she cannot deny permission for modifications needed so that the tenant with a disability can use and enjoy his/her home.

Policy Changes

FHAA requires that the housing provider make reasonable modifications in rules, policies, practices, or services necessary to give persons with disabilities equal opportunity to use and enjoy the dwelling. Examples of modifications that would be required include:

- Allowing a tenant who is blind to have a guide dog even though the building has a no pet policy. This same rule would apply to individuals who need a service animal, emotional support animal, or a therapy animal.

- Reserving a parking space for a tenant with a mobility impairment that is accessible and close to an accessible route when other tenants must park on a first come, first served basis.

- Waiving a rule that allows only tenants to use laundry facilities in order to accommodate a tenant with a disability who cannot gain access to the laundry facilities by allowing his/her friend or aide to do the laundry.

In short, any policy or rule that denies people with disabilities access to a facility or service may be a violation of FHAA.

Accessibility Requirements in New Construction

Newly constructed multi-family dwellings with four or more units must provide basic accessibility to people with disabilities, if the building was ready for first occupancy on or after March 13, 1991. The design features mentioned here apply to all units in buildings with elevators and to ground floor units in multi-level buildings without elevators.

Multi-story townhouses are exempt from these requirements. The following are the FHAA's required accessible design features:

- At least one building entrance must be on an accessible route.

- All public and common use areas must be readily accessible.

- All doors into and within all premises must be wide enough to allow passage by persons in wheelchairs.

- All premises must contain an accessible route into and through the dwelling unit.

- All light switches, electrical outlets, thermostats, and environmental controls must be placed in an accessible location.

- Reinforcements in the bathroom walls for later installation of grab bars around toilet, tub, and shower must be provided.

- Usable kitchens and bathrooms must be provided so that a person who uses a wheelchair can maneuver about the space.

Although FHAA does not include any exceptions to these requirements, the Department of Housing and Urban Development (HUD) has determined that the provision requiring at least one building entrance be on an accessible route may be exempted if it is impractical to do so because of terrain or unusual site characteristics. For example, an accessible route to a building constructed on stilts would be impractical. The burden of proving impracticality is on the designer or builder of the housing facility. HUD has indicated that only infrequent cases will qualify for this exception.

Section 57.4

Homelessness among People with Disabilities

Excerpted from "Questions and Answers on Special Education
and Homelessness," by the U.S. Department of Education
(ED, www.ed.gov), February 2008.

What are the evaluation and placement requirements under Section 504 for homeless children?

A process of evaluation and reevaluation in accordance with Section 504 is required to determine whether a child has or continues to have a disability under Section 504. A recipient that operates a public elementary or secondary education program or activity must conduct an evaluation of any individual who, because of disability, is believed to need special education or related services. The evaluation must use established standards and procedures, including tests and other evaluation materials that have been properly validated for the specific purpose and must be administered by trained personnel. In interpreting evaluation data and in making placement decisions, the recipient must draw upon information from a variety of sources, including aptitude and achievement tests, teacher recommendations, physical condition, social or cultural background, and adaptive behavior, and must ensure that information obtained from these sources is documented and carefully considered. If the student is found to have a disability under Section 504, then an appropriate placement decision is made by a group of persons who are knowledgeable about the student, the meaning of the evaluation data, and the placement options. School districts also may create a plan or other document describing the evaluation and placement decisions they make pursuant to Section 504. A recipient also is required to establish procedures for the periodic reevaluation of students who have been provided special education and related services. The Section 504 regulations specify that evaluation procedures established under IDEA (Individuals with Disabilities Education Act) would satisfy this requirement.

If a public agency determines that a homeless child has a disability following the homeless child's initial evaluation, what steps must be taken before the child can receive special education and related services for the first time?

After completion of administration of assessments and other evaluation measures, a group of qualified professionals, including the parents of the child, must determine whether the child is a "child with a disability" and the educational needs of the child. The public agency must provide the parent with a copy of the evaluation report and documentation of the eligibility determination at no cost. If the homeless child is an unaccompanied homeless youth, the requirements for appointment of surrogate parents would be applicable, and the requirements for eligibility determinations that are applicable to parents would apply to the surrogate parent appointed to represent the child in special education matters.

In interpreting evaluation data for purposes of determining whether the child is a child with a disability, and the educational needs of the child, each public agency must draw upon information from a variety of sources, including aptitude and achievement tests, parent input, teacher recommendations, as well as information about the child's physical condition, social or cultural background, and adaptive behavior. Each public agency also must ensure that information obtained from all of these sources is documented and carefully. If a determination is made that the child has a disability and needs special education and related services, an IEP (individualized education program) that meets the requirements must be developed for the child.

Section 57.5

Fire Safety for People with Disabilities and Their Caregivers

From "People with Disabilities and Their Caregivers," by the U.S. Fire Administration (USFA, www.usfa.dhs.gov), January 27, 2011.

Approximately 3,500 Americans die and 18,300 are injured in fires each year. The risk of death or injury from fire is even greater for people with physical, mental, or sensory disabilities. The good news is deaths resulting from failed emergency escapes are preventable through preparation.

The United States Fire Administration (USFA) and the Disabled American Veterans (DAV) want people with disabilities, their caregivers, and all Americans to know that there are special precautions you can take to protect yourself and your home from fire.

Why Are People with Disabilities at Risk?

People with disabilities should be more cautious because of physical limitations and a decreased ability to react in an emergency.

People with disabilities are typically fiercely independent and do not wish to alter their lives from those of the general public. However, this can lead them to ignore their special fire safety needs. In some cases people with disabilities may need the help of a caregiver to practice proper fire safety precautions.

Fire Safety Precautions

Install and Maintain Smoke Alarms

People with disabilities should be aware of the special fire warning devices that are available.

- Smoke alarms with a vibrating pad or flashing light are available for the deaf or hard of hearing. Additionally, smoke alarms with a strobe light outside the house to catch the attention of neighbors and emergency call systems for summoning help are also available.

519

- Ask the manager of your building, or a friend or relative to install at least one smoke alarm on each level of your home.

- Make sure your smoke alarms are tested monthly and change the batteries at least once a year.

Live near an Exit

Although you have the legal right to live where you choose, you'll be safest on the ground floor if you live in an apartment building.

- If you live in a multi-story home, arrange to sleep on the first floor.

- Being on the ground floor and near an exit will make your escape easier.

Plan Your Escape

Plan your escape around your capabilities.

- Know at least two exits from every room.

- If you use a walker or wheelchair, check all exits to be sure you get through the doorways.

- Make any necessary accommodations, such as providing exit ramps and widening doorways, to facilitate an emergency escape.

Don't Isolate Yourself

People with disabilities have often been excluded from the development and practicing of escape plans and fire safety drills. As a result, their vital input is omitted and their fire safety needs remain unfulfilled. Speak up to ensure that all parties receive the fire safety information that everyone deserves.

- Speak to your family members, building manager, or neighbors about your fire safety plan and practice it with them.

- Contact your local fire department's non-emergency line and explain your special needs. They will probably suggest escape plan ideas, and may perform a home fire safety inspection and offer suggestions about smoke alarm placement and maintenance.

- Ask emergency providers to keep your special needs information on file.

- Keep a phone near your bed and be ready to call 911 or your local emergency number if a fire occurs.

Section 57.6

Disaster Preparedness for People with Disabilities and Special Needs

Excerpted from "Preparing Makes Sense for People
with Disabilities and Special Needs," by the Department of
Homeland Security (www.ready.gov), November 10, 2010.

The likelihood that you and your family will recover from an emergency tomorrow often depends on the planning and preparation done today. Although each person's abilities and needs are unique, every individual can take steps to prepare for all kinds of emergencies from fires and floods to potential terrorist attacks. By evaluating your own personal needs and making an emergency plan that fits those needs, you and your loved ones can be better prepared.

This text outlines commonsense measures individuals with disabilities, special needs, and their caregivers can take to start preparing for emergencies before they happen.

Get a Kit of Emergency Supplies

The first step is to consider how an emergency might affect your individual needs. Plan to make it on your own, for at least 3, days. It's possible that you will not have access to a medical facility or even a drugstore. It is crucial that you and your family think about what kinds of resources you use on a daily basis and what you might do if those resources are limited or not available.

Basic Supplies

Think first about the basics for survival—food, water, clean air and any life-sustaining items you require. Consider two kits. In one kit put everything you will need to stay where you are and make it on your own for a period of time. The other kit should be a lightweight, smaller version you can take with you if you have to leave your home.

Recommended basic emergency supplies include the following:

- Water, 1 gallon of water per person per day for at least 3 days, for drinking and sanitation

- Food, at least a 3-day supply of non-perishable food and a can opener if the kit contains canned food

- Battery-powered or hand crank radio and an NOAA Weather Radio with tone alert and extra batteries for both

- Flashlight and extra batteries

- First aid kit

- Whistle to signal for help

- Dust mask to help filter contaminated air and plastic sheeting and duct tape to shelter-in-place

- Moist towelettes, garbage bags, and plastic ties for personal sanitation

- Wrench or pliers to turn off utilities

- Local maps

- Pet food, extra water, and supplies for your pet or service animal

Include Medications and Medical Supplies

If you take medicine or use a medical treatment on a daily basis, be sure you have what you need on hand to make it on your own for at least a week. You should also keep a copy of your prescriptions as well as dosage or treatment information. If it is not possible to have a week-long supply of medicines and supplies, keep as much as possible on hand and talk to your pharmacist or doctor about what else you should do to prepare.

If you undergo routine treatments administered by a clinic or hospital or if you receive regular services such as home health care, treatment, or transportation, talk to your service provider about their emergency plans. Work with them to identify back-up service providers within your area and the areas you might evacuate to. If you use medical equipment in your home that requires electricity to operate, talk to your health care provider about what you can do to prepare for its use during a power outage.

Additional Items

In addition, there may be other things specific to your personal needs that you should also have on hand. If you use eyeglasses, hearing aids and hearing aid batteries, wheelchair batteries, and oxygen, be sure you always have extras in your home. Also have copies of your medical insurance, Medicare, and Medicaid cards readily available. If you have a service animal, be sure to include food, water, collar with ID tag, medical records, and other emergency pet supplies.

Include Emergency Documents

Include copies of important documents in your emergency supply kits such as family records, medical records, wills, deeds, social security number, charge and bank account information, and tax records. It is best to keep these documents in a waterproof container. If there is any information related to operating equipment or life-saving devices that you rely on, include those in your emergency kit as well, and also make sure that a trusted friend or family member has copies of these documents. Include the names and numbers of everyone in your personal support network, as well as your medical providers. If you have a communication disability, make sure your emergency information list notes the best way to communicate with you. Also be sure you have cash or travelers' checks in your kits in case you need to purchase supplies.

Make a Plan for What You Will Do in an Emergency

The reality of a disaster situation is that you will likely not have access to everyday conveniences. To plan in advance, think through the details of your everyday life. If there are people who assist you on a daily basis, list who they are and how you will contact them in an emergency. Create your own personal support network by identifying others who will help you in an emergency. Think about what modes of transportation you use and what alternative modes could serve as back-ups. If you require handicap accessible transportation be sure your alternatives are also accessible. If you have tools or aids specific to your disability, plan how you would cope without them. For example, if you use a communication device, mobility aid, or rely on a service animal, what will you do if these are not available? If you are dependent on life-sustaining equipment or treatment such as a dialysis machine, find out the location and availability of more than one facility. For every aspect of your daily routine, plan an alternative procedure. Make a plan and write it down. Keep a copy of your plan in your emergency supply kits and a list of important information and contacts in your wallet. Share your plan with your family, friends, care providers, and others in your personal support network.

Create a Personal Support Network

If you anticipate needing assistance during a disaster, make a list of family, friends, and others who will be part of your plan. Talk to these people and ask them to be part of your support network. Share each aspect of your emergency plan with everyone in your group, including a friend or relative in another area who would not be impacted by the same emergency who can help if necessary. Make sure everyone knows how you plan to evacuate your home, school, or workplace and where you will go in case of a disaster. Make sure that someone in your personal support network has an extra key to your home and knows where you keep your emergency supplies. Teach them how to use any lifesaving equipment or administer medicine in case of an emergency. If you use a wheelchair, oxygen, or other medical equipment show friends how to use these devices so they can move you if necessary or help you evacuate. Practice your plan with those who have agreed to be part of your personal support network.

Inform your employer and coworkers about your disability and let them know specifically what assistance you will need in an emergency. This is particularly important if you need to be lifted or carried. Talk about communication difficulties, physical limitations, equipment instructions, and medication procedures. If you are hearing impaired, discuss the best ways to alert you in an emergency. If you have a cognitive disability, be sure to work with your employer to determine how to best notify you of an emergency and what instruction methods are easiest for you to follow. Always participate in exercises, trainings, and emergency drills offered by your employer.

Develop a Family Communications Plan

Your family may not be together when disaster strikes, so plan how you will contact one another and review what you will do in different situations. Consider a plan where each family member calls or e-mails the same friend or relative in the event of an emergency. It may be easier to make a long-distance phone call than to call across town, so an out-of-town contact, not in the impacted area, may be in a better position to communicate among separated family members. You may have trouble getting through, or the phone system may be down altogether, but be patient. For more information on how to develop a family communications plan, visit www.ready.gov.

Chapter 58

Employees with Disabilities

Chapter Contents

Section 58.1—Why Work Matters to People with
            Disabilities... 526

Section 58.2—In the Workplace: Reasonable
            Accommodations for Employees with
            Disabilities... 528

Section 58.3—Job Accommodation Situations and
            Solutions 529

Section 58.4—Accommodations for Employees with
            Psychiatric Disabilities 532

Section 58.1

Why Work Matters to People with Disabilities

Excerpted from "Why Work Matters for People with Disabilities," by Dan O'Brien, Acting Associate Commissioner, Office of Employment Support Programs, Social Security Administration, Disability.gov, July 21, 2010.

While working in the mental health field, I discovered that supporting people to work could facilitate and help sustain recovery. As the director of an employment program at a large, urban mental health center, I had unique opportunities to assist people every day. One woman's story, while typical, stands out in my memory.

Beth (a pseudonym) would check into the center every day, and we wouldn't see her again until she checked out at the end of the day. So one day, I looked all over for her and found her—hiding in the closet. From that day forward, I visited her in the closet and invited her to engage in the real work of running the clubhouse at the center. Slowly, Beth increased her activity and confidence level.

After several months, we got her a part-time job in the community where she thrived with the short-term help of a job coach. She later moved on to a regular full-time job. We didn't hear from her for a year or so, but one day she entered the center, and we had a great visit. I took her to see the staff members that had helped her—Beth was looking good and strutting her stuff.

After she left, a staff person asked me who she was. I had to remind her about the woman I talked out of the closet. The staff person could not believe it was the same person. Beth had reclaimed herself. Being employed enabled her to completely transform her appearance, her energy level, and her demeanor. She had literally come out of the closet and become an extraordinary example that recovery through work is possible.

All people with disabilities should be given the help they need to find work, whether they are Social Security disability beneficiaries or other Americans who seek to enhance their autonomy and purpose through employment. Today, with the celebrations of the Americans with Disabilities Act (ADA), we find more pathways and support for employment opportunities for people with disabilities. We all must do more to give people a chance to work, to ensure they are able to retain their employment, and to develop real and sustaining careers.

This reminds me of another person I met in Oklahoma many years ago. A young man had been shuffled through about 20 foster homes while growing up. He had schizophrenia and fetal alcohol syndrome. Due to his disabilities, he couldn't follow more than two-step instructions. In spite of these limitations, we found a good job match for him, and he succeeded with short-term help from a job coach.

Months later, I visited him at his work site. I will never forget how he looked me in the eye with confidence as he shook my hand and said, "Thanks for helping me get this job. This is the first time in my life that I ever felt real." He meant that work gave his life meaning, that people depended on him, and he was an essential part of the work team—he felt important for the first time.

We need to enable millions more Americans with disabilities to succeed by helping them to choose and retain work. Like the people I've mentioned, every individual with a disability has the potential to be a work success story.

Section 58.2

In the Workplace: Reasonable Accommodations for Employees with Disabilities

Excerpted from "Support Employees with Disabilities," by the Centers for Disease Control and Prevention (CDC, www.cdc.gov), December 6, 2010.

Defining a Disability

Title I of the American with Disabilities Act (ADA) protects qualified individuals with disabilities from employment discrimination. Under the ADA, a person has a disability if he has a physical or mental impairment that substantially limits a major life activity. The ADA also protects individuals who have a record of a substantially limiting impairment, and people who are regarded as having a substantially limiting impairment.

Today, about 50 million Americans, or one in five people, are living with at least one disability, and most Americans will experience a disability some time during the course of their lives.

Disabilities Should Not Limit Employee Performance

Anyone can have a disability; however, it should not limit that person's ability to do his or her job. The Americans with Disabilities Act requires employers to provide an employee identified as having a disability with reasonable accommodations. A reasonable accommodation (RA) is any change or adjustment to a job or work environment that permits a qualified applicant or employee with a disability to participate in the job application process, to perform the essential functions of a job, or to enjoy benefits and privileges of employment equal to those enjoyed by employees without disabilities.

Reasonable accommodation may include acquiring or modifying equipment or devices; job restructuring; part-time or modified work schedules; reassignment to a vacant position; adjusting or modifying examinations, training materials, or policies; providing readers and interpreters, and making the workplace readily accessible to and usable by people with disabilities.

In addition to changes to a workspace or workplace materials and policies, reasonable accommodation may involve altering a building or external facility to make it accessible to those with disabilities. Examples of accessibility reasonable accommodation may include the following:

- Building ramps that are easily accessible

- Raised lettering and Braille are used on signs, such as those on elevators, near bathrooms, and exits

- Parking spaces close to entrances

- Removal of obstructions in hallways

- Evacuation plans for those with disabilities

- Widening of interior doorways and entryways

Section 58.3

Job Accommodation Situations and Solutions

From "Investing in People: Job Accommodation Situations and Solutions," by the Office of Disability Employment Policy (ODEP, www.dol.gov/odep), U.S. Department of Labor, August 2005. Reviewed by David A. Cooke, MD, FACP, July 23, 2011.

All employees need the right tools and work environment to effectively perform their jobs. Similarly, individuals with disabilities may need workplace adjustments—or accommodations—to maximize the value they can add to their employer.

An accommodation can be simple, such as putting blocks under a table's legs so that a person who uses a wheelchair can roll up to it. It might involve advanced technology, such as installing a screen reader on a computer so that a person who is blind can manage documents. It may be procedural, such as altering a work schedule or job assignments.

When thinking about accommodations, the focus should not be on the person's disability but rather on essential job tasks and the physical functions necessary to complete them. Consider a receptionist who cannot answer the phone because he or she cannot grasp the receiver. A handle could be attached to the receiver to enable him or her to balance it on the hand. Or, the receptionist could use a headset, eliminating the need for grasping altogether. The reason the person can't grasp the receiver is immaterial. With a simple accommodation, the employee can answer the phone.

Because accommodations are for individuals, they are individual in nature. But by requiring employers and employees to think creatively about how tasks are accomplished, an accommodation can benefit more than a single employee—it can benefit business. Devising accommodations can uncover strategies that help others, regardless of whether they have disabilities. For instance, headsets may help other receptionists better perform their duties and reduce neck strain. Similarly, magnifying glasses at work stations help people with visual disabilities read documents and may reduce eyestrain for others. When an accommodation has widespread benefit, it is referred to as universal design. Perhaps the most ubiquitous example of universal design is curb cuts. These were designed to enable people who use wheelchairs to get on and off sidewalks, but they are routinely used by people for other purposes, such as pushing strollers or carts.

Thus, an accommodation is an investment that promises an immediate return—an investment in a qualified worker who happens to have a disability and is, or could become, a valuable asset to a business. Moreover, accommodations usually are not expensive. According to the Job Accommodation Network (JAN), a free and confidential service from the U.S. Department of Labor's Office of Disability Employment Policy that provides individualized accommodation solutions, two thirds of accommodations cost less than $500, with nearly a quarter costing nothing at all. Yet, more than half of the employers surveyed said that each accommodation benefited their organization an average of $5,000.

In the following text are real-life examples of successful accommodations that were implemented by employers after consulting JAN.

Situation: A woman with a severe developmental disability worked in an envelope manufacturing facility operating a machine that stacked boxes. She needed to stack 20 boxes at a time, but could not keep a mental count past 10.

Solution: The employer installed a punch counter and trained the woman to include punching in her routine—tape, stack, punch; tape, stack, punch. As the woman's productivity soared, the employer realized that keeping count is difficult for many people and decided to install counters at other machines. Cost: $10.

Situation: A person who is blind was a switchboard operator for a large building. As such, she needed to know which telephone lines were on hold, in use, or ringing.

Solution: The employer installed a light probe that emitted a noise signaling which console buttons were blinking and which ones were steadily lit. The console was also modified to audibly differentiate incoming calls from internal calls. Cost of light probe: $45. Console modifications were made at no cost to the employer.

Situation: A student with cerebral palsy obtained a work-study position with the landscape crew of his university. His supervisor was concerned that he could not safely operate a push mower because of his motor impairment. The individual agreed that his gait and balance were a concern in safely operating a push mower.

Solution: His supervisor assigned him other tasks, such as mulching, weeding, and picking up litter. Cost: None.

Situation: A college chemistry teacher who used a wheelchair needed to work in a lab designed to accommodate students at a standing height.

Solution: The college provided the teacher with an elevating wheelchair. Cost: $7,000.

Situation: A warehouse worker whose job involved maintaining and delivering supplies had difficulty with the job's physical demands due to fatigue from cancer treatment.

Solution: The individual was provided a three-wheeled scooter at work to reduce the amount of walking required, and the warehouse was rearranged to reduce the amount of climbing and reaching. Cost: $1,500.

Section 58.4

Accommodations for Employees with Psychiatric Disabilities

From "Maximizing Productivity: Accommodations for Employees with Psychiatric Disabilities," by the Office of Disability Employment Policy (ODEP, www.dol.gov/odep), U.S. Department of Labor, March 2006. Reviewed by David A. Cooke, MD, FACP, July 23, 2011.

A psychiatric disability can impact various aspects of an individual's life, including the ability to achieve maximum productivity in the workplace. The National Institute of Mental Health estimates that one in five people will experience a psychiatric disability in their lifetime, and one in four Americans currently knows someone who has a psychiatric disability. It is likely that most employers have at least one employee with a psychiatric disability.

Under the Americans with Disabilities Act (ADA) and other nondiscrimination laws, most employers must provide "reasonable accommodations" to qualified employees with disabilities. Many employers are aware of different types of accommodations for people with physical and communication disabilities, but they may be less familiar with accommodations for employees with disabilities that are not visible, such as psychiatric disabilities. Over the last few years, increasing numbers of employers have expressed a desire and need for information and ideas on accommodations for employees with psychiatric disabilities.

In the following text are examples of accommodations that have helped employees with psychiatric disabilities to more effectively perform their jobs. The list does not include all possible accommodations, but it is a good starting point and provides some of the most effective and frequently used workplace accommodations.

- **Flexible workplace:** Telecommuting and/or working from home

- **Scheduling:** Part-time work hours, job sharing, adjustments in the start or end of work hours, compensation time, and/or "make up" of missed time

- **Leave:** Sick leave for reasons related to mental health, flexible use of vacation time, additional unpaid or administrative leave for treatment or recovery, leaves of absence, and/or use of occasional leave (a few hours at a time) for therapy and other related appointments

- **Breaks:** Breaks according to individual needs rather than a fixed schedule, more frequent breaks and/or greater flexibility in scheduling breaks, provision of backup coverage during breaks, and telephone breaks during work hours to call professionals and others needed for support

- **Other policies:** Beverages and/or food permitted at workstations, if necessary, to mitigate the side effects of medications, on-site job coaches

Modifications

- Reduction and/or removal of distractions in the work area
- Addition of room dividers, partitions, or other soundproofing or visual barriers between workspaces to reduce noise or visual distractions
- Private offices or private space enclosures
- Office/work space location away from noisy machinery
- Reduction of workplace noise that can be adjusted (such as telephone volume)
- Increased natural lighting or full spectrum lighting
- Music (with headset) to block out distractions

Equipment/Technology

- Tape recorders for recording/reviewing meetings and training sessions
- "White noise" or environmental sound machines
- Handheld electronic organizers, software calendars, and organizer programs
- Remote job coaching, laptop computers, personal digital assistants, and office computer access via remote locations
- Software that minimizes computerized distractions such as pop-up screens

Job Duties

- Modification or removal of non-essential job duties or restructuring of the job to include only the essential job functions

- Division of large assignments into smaller tasks and goals

- Additional assistance and/or time for orientation activities, training, and learning job tasks and new responsibilities

- Additional training or modified training materials

Management/Supervision

- Implementation of flexible and supportive supervision style; positive reinforcement and feedback; adjustments in level of supervision or structure, such as more frequent meetings to help prioritize tasks; and open communication with supervisors regarding performance and work expectations

- Additional forms of communication and/or written and visual tools, including communication of assignments and instructions in the employee's preferred learning style (written, verbal, e-mail, demonstration); creation and implementation of written tools such as daily "to-do" lists, step-by-step checklists, written (in addition to verbal) instructions, and typed minutes of meetings

- Regularly scheduled meetings (weekly or monthly) with employees to discuss workplace issues and productivity, including annual discussions as part of performance appraisals to assess abilities and discuss promotional opportunities

- Development of strategies to deal with problems before they arise

- Written work agreements that include any agreed-upon accommodations, long-term and short-term goals, expectations of responsibilities, and consequences of not meeting performance standards

- Education of all employees about their right to accommodations

- Relevant training for all employees, including coworkers and supervisory staff

Chapter 59

Social Security Disability Benefits

Disability is something most people do not like to think about. But the chances that you will become disabled probably are greater than you realize. Studies show that a 20-year-old worker has a three in 10 chance of becoming disabled before reaching full retirement age.

This text provides basic information on Social Security disability benefits and is not intended to answer all questions. For specific information about your situation, you should talk with a Social Security representative.

Disability benefits are paid through two programs—the Social Security disability insurance program and the Supplemental Security Income (SSI) program. This text is about the Social Security disability program.

Who can get Social Security disability benefits?

Social Security pays benefits to people who cannot work because they have a medical condition that is expected to last at least 1 year or result in death. Federal law requires this very strict definition of disability. While some programs give money to people with partial disability or short-term disability, Social Security does not.

Certain family members of disabled workers also can receive money from Social Security.

Excerpted from "Disability Benefits," by the Social Security Administration (SSA, www.ssa.gov), July 2011.

How do I meet the earnings requirement for disability benefits?

In general, to get disability benefits, you must meet two different earnings tests:

1. A "recent work" test based on your age at the time you became disabled

2. A "duration of work" test to show that you worked long enough under Social Security

Certain blind workers have to meet only the "duration of work" test. Table 59.1 shows the rules for how much work you need for the "recent work" test based on your age when your disability began. The rules in this table are based on the calendar quarter in which you turned or will turn a certain age.

The calendar quarters are the following:

• First quarter: January 1 through March 31

• Second quarter: April 1 through June 30

• Third quarter: July 1 through September 30

• Fourth quarter: October 1 through December 31

Table 59.2 shows examples of how much work you need to meet the "duration of work test" if you become disabled at various selected ages. For the "duration of work" test, your work does not have to fall within a certain period of time. This table does not cover all situations.

Table 59.1. Rules for Work Needed for the Recent Work Test

If you become disabled	Then you generally need:
In or before the quarter you turn age 24	1.5 years of work during the 3-year period ending with the quarter your disability began.
In the quarter after you turn age 24 but before the quarter you turn age 31	Work during half the time for the period beginning with the quarter after you turned 21 and ending with the quarter you became disabled. Example: If you become disabled in the quarter you turned age 27, then you would need 3 years of work out of the 6-year period ending with the quarter you became disabled.
In the quarter you turn age 31 or later	Work during 5 years out of the 10-year period ending with the quarter your disability began.

Table 59.2. Examples of Work Needed for the Duration of Work Test

If you become disabled	Then you generally need:
Before age 28	1.5 years of work
Age 30	2 years
Age 34	3 years
Age 38	4 years
Age 42	5 years
Age 44	5.5 years
Age 46	6 years
Age 48	6.5 years
Age 50	7 years
Age 52	7.5 years
Age 54	8 years
Age 56	8.5 years
Age 58	9 years
Age 60	9.5 years

How do I apply for disability benefits?

There are two ways that you can apply for disability benefits. You can do the following:

1. Apply at www.socialsecurity.gov/disabilityonline.

2. Call the toll-free number, 800-772-1213, to make an appointment to file a disability claim at your local Social Security office or to set up an appointment for someone to take your claim over the telephone. The disability claims interview lasts about 1 hour. If you are deaf or hard of hearing, you may call the toll-free TTY number, 800-325-0778, between 7 a.m. and 7 p.m. on business days. If you schedule an appointment, the SSA will send you a Disability Starter Kit to help you get ready for your disability claims interview. The Disability Starter Kit also is available online at www.socialsecurity.gov/disability.

When should I apply and what information do I need?

You should apply for disability benefits as soon as you become disabled. It can take a long time to process an application for disability benefits (3 to 5 months). To apply for disability benefits, you will need to complete an application for Social Security benefits and the Adult Disability Report.

You can complete the Adult Disability Report online at www.social-security.gov/disabilityreport. You also can print the Adult Disability Report, complete it and return it to your local Social Security office. We may be able to process your application faster if you help us by getting any other information we need.

The information we need includes the following:

- Your Social Security number

- Your birth or baptismal certificate

- Names, addresses, and phone numbers of the doctors, caseworkers, hospitals, and clinics that took care of you and dates of your visits

- Names and dosage of all the medicine you take

- Medical records from your doctors, therapists, hospitals, clinics, and caseworkers that you already have in your possession

- Laboratory and test results

- A summary of where you worked and the kind of work you did

- A copy of your most recent W-2 Form (Wage and Tax Statement) or, if you are self-employed, your federal tax return for the past year

In addition to the basic application for disability benefits, there are other forms you will need to fill out. One form collects information about your medical condition and how it affects your ability to work. Other forms give doctors, hospitals, and other health care professionals who have treated you permission to send us information about your medical condition.

Do not delay applying for benefits if you cannot get all of this information together quickly. We will help you get it.

Chapter 60

Tax Benefits and Credits for People with Disabilities

Income

All income is taxable unless it is specifically excluded by law. The following discussions highlight some income items (both taxable and nontaxable) that are of particular interest to people with disabilities and those who care for people with disabilities.

Dependent Care Benefits

Dependent care benefits include the following:

1. Amounts your employer paid directly to either you or your care provider for the care of your qualifying person(s) while you work

2. The fair market value of care in a daycare facility provided or sponsored by your employer

3. Pretax contributions you made under a dependent care flexible spending arrangement

Exclusion or deduction: If your employer provides dependent care benefits under a qualified plan, you may be able to exclude these benefits from your income. Your employer can tell you whether your benefit plan qualifies. To claim the exclusion, you must complete Part III of Form 2441, Child and Dependent Care Expenses. You cannot use Form 1040EZ.

Excerpted from "Tax Highlights for Persons with Disabilities," by the Internal Revenue Service (IRS, www.irs.gov), February 3, 2010.

If you are self-employed and receive benefits from a qualified dependent care benefit plan, you are treated as both employer and employee. Therefore, you would not get an exclusion from wages. Instead, you would get a deduction for the dependent care benefits. To claim the deduction, you must use Form 2441.

The amount you can exclude or deduct is limited to the smallest of:

- the total amount of dependent care benefits you received during the year;

- the total amount of qualified expenses you incurred during the year;

- your earned income;

- your spouse's earned income; or

- $5,000 ($2,500 if married filing separately).

Statement for employee: Your employer must give you a Form W-2 (or similar statement), showing in box 10 the total amount of dependent care benefits provided to you during the year under a qualified plan. Your employer will also include any dependent care benefits over $5,000 in your wages shown on your Form W-2 in box 1.

Qualifying person(s): A qualifying person is:

- a qualifying child who is under age 13 whom you can claim as a dependent (if the child turned 13 during the year, the child is a qualifying person for the part of the year he or she was under age 13);

- your disabled spouse who is not physically or mentally able to care for himself or herself;

- any disabled person who was not physically or mentally able to care for himself or herself whom you can claim as a dependent (or could claim as a dependent except that the person had gross income of $3,650 or more or filed a joint return);

- any disabled person who was not physically or mentally able to care for himself or herself whom you could claim as a dependent except that you (or your spouse if filing jointly) could be claimed as a dependent on another taxpayer's 2010 return.

For information about excluding benefits on Form 1040, Form 1040NR, or Form 1040A, see Form 2441 and its instructions.

Social Security and Railroad Retirement Benefits

If you received social security or equivalent tier 1 railroad retirement benefits during the year, part of the amount you received may be taxable.

Are any of your benefits taxable? If the only income you received during the year was your social security or equivalent tier 1 railroad retirement benefits, your benefits generally are not taxable and you probably do not have to file a return.

If you received income during the year in addition to social security or equivalent tier 1 railroad retirement benefits, part of your benefits may be taxable if all of your other income, including tax-exempt interest, plus half of your benefits are more than:

- $25,000 if you are single, head of household, or qualifying widow(er);

- $25,000 if you are married filing separately and lived apart from your spouse for all of 2010;

- $32,000 if you are married filing jointly; or

- $0 if you are married filing separately and lived with your spouse at any time during 2010.

For more information, see the instructions for Form 1040, lines 20a and 20b, or Form 1040A, lines 14a and 14b.

Supplemental security income (SSI) payments: Social security benefits do not include SSI payments, which are not taxable. Do not include these payments in your income.

Disability Pensions

If you retired on disability, you must include in income any disability pension you receive under a plan that is paid for by your employer. You must report your taxable disability payments as wages on line 7 of Form 1040 or Form 1040A until you reach minimum retirement age. Minimum retirement age generally is the age at which you can first receive a pension or annuity if you are not disabled.

You may be entitled to a tax credit if you were permanently and totally disabled when you retired.

Beginning on the day after you reach minimum retirement age, payments you receive are taxable as a pension or annuity. Report the payments on lines 16a and 16b of Form 1040 or on lines 12a and 12b of Form 1040A.

Retirement and profit-sharing plans: If you receive payments from a retirement or profit-sharing plan that does not provide for disability retirement, do not treat the payments as a disability pension. The payments must be reported as a pension or annuity.

Accrued leave payment: If you retire on disability, any lump-sum payment you receive for accrued annual leave is a salary payment. The payment is not a disability payment. Include it in your income in the tax year you receive it.

Military and Government Disability Pensions

Generally, you must report disability pensions as income, but do not include certain military and government disability pensions.

VA disability benefits: Do not include disability benefits you receive from the Department of Veterans Affairs (VA) in your gross income.

Do not include in your income any veterans' benefits paid under any law, regulation, or administrative practice administered by the VA. These include the following:

- Education, training, and subsistence allowances
- Disability compensation and pension payments for disabilities paid either to veterans or their families
- Grants for homes designed for wheelchair living
- Grants for motor vehicles for veterans who lost their sight or the use of their limbs
- Veterans' insurance proceeds and dividends paid either to veterans or their beneficiaries, including the proceeds of a veteran's endowment policy paid before death
- Interest on insurance dividends left on deposit with the VA
- Benefits under a dependent-care assistance program
- The death gratuity paid to a survivor of a member of the Armed Forces who died after September 10, 2001
- VA payments to hospital patients and resident veterans for their services under the VA's therapeutic or rehabilitative programs

Other Payments

You may receive other payments that are related to your disability. The following payments are not taxable.

- Benefit payments from a public welfare fund, such as payments due to blindness

- Workers' compensation for an occupational sickness or injury if paid under a workers' compensation act or similar law

- Compensatory (but not punitive) damages for physical injury or physical sickness

- Disability benefits under a "no-fault" car insurance policy for loss of income or earning capacity as a result of injuries

- Compensation for permanent loss or loss of use of a part or function of your body, or for your permanent disfigurement

Itemized Deductions

If you file Form 1040, you generally can either claim the standard deduction or itemize your deductions. You must use Schedule A (Form 1040) to itemize your deductions.

See your form instructions for information on the standard deduction and the deductions you can itemize. The following discussions highlight some itemized deductions that are of particular interest to persons with disabilities.

Medical Expenses

When figuring your deduction for medical expenses, you can generally include medical and dental expenses you pay for yourself, your spouse, and your dependents. Medical expenses are the cost of diagnosis, cure, mitigation, treatment, or prevention of disease and the costs for treatments affecting any part or function of the body. They include the costs of equipment, supplies, diagnostic devices, and transportation for needed medical care and payments for medical insurance.

You can deduct only the amount of your medical and dental expenses that is more than 7.5% of your adjusted gross income shown on Form 1040, line 38.

The following list highlights some of the medical expenses you can include in figuring your medical expense deduction.

- Artificial limbs, contact lenses, eyeglasses, and hearing aids

- The part of the cost of Braille books and magazines that is more than the price of regular printed editions

- Cost and repair of special telephone equipment for hearing-impaired persons

- Cost and maintenance of a wheelchair or a three-wheel motor vehicle commercially known as an autoette

- Cost and care of a guide dog or other animal aiding a person with a physical disability

- Costs for a school that furnishes special education if a principal reason for using the school is its resources for relieving a mental or physical disability (This includes the cost of teaching Braille and lip reading and the cost of remedial language training to correct a condition caused by a birth defect.)

- Premiums for qualified long-term care insurance, up to certain amounts

- Improvements to a home that do not increase its value if the main purpose is medical care (An example is constructing entrance or exit ramps)

- Improvements that increase a home's value, if the main purpose is medical care, may be partly included as a medical expense.

Impairment-Related Work Expenses

If you are disabled, you can take a business deduction for expenses that are necessary for you to be able to work. If you take a business deduction for these impairment- related work expenses, they are not subject to the 7.5% limit that applies to medical expenses.

You are disabled if you have:

- a physical or mental disability (for example, blindness or deafness) that functionally limits your being employed; or

- a physical or mental impairment (including, but not limited to, a sight or hearing impairment) that substantially limits one or more of your major life activities, such as performing manual tasks, walking, speaking, breathing, learning, or working.

Impairment-related expenses defined: Impairment-related expenses are those ordinary and necessary business expenses that are:

- necessary for you to do your work satisfactorily;

- for goods and services not required or used, other than incidentally, in your personal activities; and

- not specifically covered under other income tax laws.

Chapter 61

Preparing for the Future: End-of-Life Planning

Chapter Contents

Section 61.1—Frequently Asked Questions about
    End-of-Life Care.. 546

Section 61.2—Wills, Advance Directives, and Other
    Documents Associated with End-of-Life
    Planning 548

Section 61.1

Frequently Asked Questions about End-of-Life Care

"End-of-Life Care: Questions and Answers," by the National Cancer Institute (NCI, www.cancer.gov), part of the National Institutes of Health, October 30, 2002. Reviewed by David A. Cooke, MD, FACP, July 23, 2011.

When a patient's health care team determines that a disease (like cancer) can no longer be controlled, medical testing and treatment often stop. But the patient's care continues. The care focuses on making the patient comfortable. The patient receives medications and treatments to control pain and other symptoms, such as constipation, nausea, and shortness of breath. Some patients remain at home during this time, whereas others enter a hospital or other facility. Either way, services are available to help patients and their families with the medical, psychological, and spiritual issues surrounding dying. A hospice often provides such services.

The time at the end of life is different for each person. Each individual has unique needs for information and support. The patient's and family's questions and concerns about the end of life should be discussed with the health care team as they arise.

The following information can help answer some of the questions that many patients, their family members, and caregivers have about the end of life.

How long is the patient expected to live?

Patients and their family members often want to know how long a person is expected to live. This is a hard question to answer. Although doctors may be able to make an estimate based on what they know about the patient, they might be hesitant to do so. Doctors may be concerned about over- or under-estimating the patient's life span. They also might be fearful of instilling false hope or destroying a person's hope.

When caring for the patient at home, when should the caregiver call for professional help?

When caring for a patient at home, there may be times when the caregiver needs assistance from the patient's health care team. A caregiver can contact the patient's doctor or nurse for help in any of the following situations:

- The patient is in pain that is not relieved by the prescribed dose of pain medication.
- The patient shows discomfort, such as grimacing or moaning.
- The patient is having trouble breathing and seems upset.
- The patient is unable to urinate or empty the bowels.
- The patient has fallen.
- The patient is very depressed or talking about committing suicide.
- The caregiver has difficulty giving medication to the patient.
- The caregiver is overwhelmed by caring for the patient, or is too grieved or afraid to be with the patient.
- At any time the caregiver does not know how to handle a situation.

What are some ways that caregivers can provide emotional comfort to the patient?

Everyone has different needs, but some emotions are common to most dying patients. These include fear of abandonment and fear of being a burden. They also have concerns about loss of dignity and loss of control. Some ways caregivers can provide comfort are as follows:

- Keep the person company—talk, watch movies, read, or just be with the person.
- Allow the person to express fears and concerns about dying, such as leaving family and friends behind. Be prepared to listen.
- Be willing to reminisce about the person's life.
- Avoid withholding difficult information. Most patients prefer to be included in discussions about issues that concern them.
- Reassure the patient that you will honor advance directives, such as living wills.
- Ask if there is anything you can do.
- Respect the person's need for privacy.

Section 61.2

Wills, Advance Directives, and Other Documents Associated with End-of-Life Planning

Advance Care Planning

What is an advance directive? Advance directive is a general term that describes two types of legal documents:

- Living will

- Healthcare power of attorney

These documents allow you to instruct others about your future healthcare wishes and appoint a person to make healthcare decisions if you are not able to speak for yourself. Each state regulates the use of advance directives differently.

What is a living will?

A living will allows you to put in writing your wishes about medical treatments for the end of your life in the event that you cannot communicate these wishes directly. Different states name this document differently. For example, it may be called a directive to physicians, healthcare declaration, or medical directive. Regardless of what it is called, its purpose is to guide your family and doctors in deciding about the use of medical treatments for you at the end of life.

Your legal right to accept or refuse treatment is protected by the Constitutions and case law. However, your state law may define when the living will goes into effect, and may limit the treatments to which the living will applies. You should read your state's document carefully to ensure that it reflects your wishes. You can add further instructions or write your own living will to cover situations that the state suggested document might not address. Even if your state does not have a living will law, it is wise to put your wishes about the use of life-sustaining medical treatments in writing as a guide to healthcare providers and loved ones.

What is the difference between a will, a living trust, and a living will?

A will (last will and testament) and living trusts are both financial documents; they allow you to plan who receives your financial assets and property. A living will deals with medical issues while you are alive. It allows you to express your preferences about your medical care at the end of life.

Wills and living trusts are complex legal instruments, for which you will need and want legal advice to complete them. Although a living will is a legal document, you do not need a lawyer to complete it.

Healthcare Power of Attorney

What is a healthcare power of attorney?

This can also be called a healthcare proxy, appointment of a healthcare agent, or durable power of attorney for healthcare. The person you appoint may be called your healthcare agent, surrogate, attorney-in-fact, or healthcare proxy. The person you appoint usually is authorized to deal with all medical situations when you cannot speak for yourself. Thus, he or she can speak for you if you become temporarily incapacitated—after an accident, for example—as well as if you become permanently incapacitated because of illness or injury.

What is the difference between financial power of attorney, a financial durable power of attorney, and a healthcare power of attorney?

A financial power of attorney and a financial durable power of attorney are both legal documents that let you appoint someone to make financial decisions for you. A power of attorney is effective only while you still handle your own finances, where as a durable power of attorney remains valid even after you have lost the ability to make financial decisions due to illness and injury.

A healthcare power of attorney (which in some states is called a durable power of attorney for medical or healthcare) only permits the appointed person to make medical decisions for you if you cannot make those decisions yourself. It does not authorize the person to handle your financial affairs, and normally does not empower him or her to make decisions while you can still make them.

Generally, the law requires your agent to make the same medical decisions that you would have made, if possible. To help your agent do this, it is essential that you discuss your values about the quality of life that is important to you and the kinds of decisions you would make in various situations. These discussions along with a living will will help your agent to form a picture of your views regarding the use of medical treatments.

Why bother with an advance directive if I want my family to make the necessary decisions for me?

Depending on your state's laws, your family might not be allowed to make decisions about life-sustaining treatment for you without a living will stating your wishes. Some states laws do permit family members to make all medical decisions for their incapacitated loved ones. However, other states require clear evidence of the person's own wishes or a legally designated decision maker.

Even in states that do permit family decision-making, you should still prepare advance directives for three reasons:

- You can name the person with whom you are most comfortable (this person does not need to be a family member) to make sure your wishes are honored.

- Your living will makes your specific wishes known.

- It is a gift to loved ones faced with making decisions about your care.

Should I prepare a living will and also use a medical power of attorney to appoint an agent?

Yes, each document offers something the other does not. Together they provide the best insurance that your wishes will be honored.

Benefits of appointing a healthcare agent: The person who you appoint as your agent can respond as your care needs and conditions changes in a way that no document can. In addition, you are legally authorizing that person to make decisions based not only on what you expressed in writing or verbally, but also on the knowledge of you as a person.

Benefits of having a living will: If your agent must decide whether or not to begin, continue, or discontinue medical treatment, your living will can reassure your agent that he or she is following your wishes. Further, if the person you appointed as an agent is unavailable or unwilling to speak for you, or if other people challenge a decision about medical treatments, your living will can guide your caregivers.

What if I do not have anyone to appoint as my agent?

If you do not have anyone to appoint as your agent, it is especially important that you complete a clear living will and that you talk about it with anyone who might be involved with your healthcare. This might include family members, even if you do not want them to be your agent.

It also could include social workers, spiritual caregivers, visiting nurses, or aids who are helping you in some way. You should discuss it with any physicians that you see regularly and give them a copy to put in your medical record. If you are admitted to a hospital or long-term care facility, you should have a copy of your living will made a part of your medical record.

When will my advance directive go into effect?

Your advance directive becomes legally valid as soon as you sign them in front of the required witnesses. However, they normally do not go into effect unless you are unable to make your own decisions. Each state establishes its own guidelines for when an advance directive becomes active. The rules may differ for living wills and healthcare power of attorney, as described in the following text.

Living will: In most states, before your living will can guide medical decision making, two physicians must certify that you are unable to make medical decisions and that you are in the medical conditions specified in the state's living will law (such as terminal illness or permanent unconsciousness). Other requirements may also apply, depending upon the state.

Healthcare power of attorney: Most healthcare powers of attorneys go into effect when your physician concludes that you are unable to make your own decisions. If you regain the ability to make decisions, your agent cannot continue to act for you. Many states have additional requirements that apply only to decisions about life-sustaining medical treatments.

Will my advance directive be honored if I am in an accident or experience a medical crisis at home and emergency technicians are called?

In these emergency situations, unless you are able to speak for yourself emergency personnel are obligated to do what is necessary to stabilize a person for transfer to a hospital, both from accident sites and from a home or other facility. After a physician fully evaluates the person's condition and determines the underlying conditions, an advance directive can be implemented.

Emergency medical technicians cannot honor living wills or healthcare power of attorneys. However, in many localities, the specific crisis of cardiac arrest/respiratory arrest is addressed by a document called a non-hospital Do-Not-Resuscitate Order. These non-hospital DNR orders instruct emergency personnel not to perform cardiopulmonary resuscitation (CPR).

These are physician orders that apply to situations in which the person's heart has stopped beating or breathing has stopped. For all other conditions, emergency medical technicians are still required to treat and transport the person to the nearest hospital for evaluation by a physician. If you wish to find out whether non-hospital DNR orders are available in your locality, contact your local emergency medical services or department of health.

Will my advance directive be honored in another state?

The answer to this question varies from state to state. Some states do honor an advance directive from another state; others will honor out-of-state documents to the extent they match the state's own law; and some states do not address the issue.

If you spend a significant amount of time in more than one state, it is recommended that you complete an advance directive for all the states involved. It will be easier to have your advance directive honored if they are the ones with which the medical facility is familiar.

How can I change what is in my advance directive?

If you want to change anything in an advance directive once you have completed it, you should complete a new document. For this reason you should review your advance directive periodically to endure that the forms still reflect your wishes.

Must my advance directive be witnessed?

Yes, every state has some type of witnessing requirement. Most require two adult witnesses; some also require a notary. Some states give you the option of having two witnesses or a notary alone as a witness. The purpose of witnessing is to confirm that you really are the person who signed the document, you were not forced to sign it, and you appeared to understand what you were doing. The witnesses do not need to know the content of the document.

Generally, a person you appoint as your agent or alternative agent cannot be a witness. In some states your witnesses cannot be any relatives by blood or marriage, or anyone who would benefit from your estate. Some states prohibit your doctor and employees of a healthcare institution in which you are a resident from acting as a witness. To ensure it is done correctly read the instructions carefully to see who can and cannot be a witness on your state-specific form.

What should I do with my completed advance directive?

Make several photocopies of the completed documents. Keep the original documents in a safe but easily accessible place, and tell others where you put them; you can note on the photocopies the locations where the originals are kept. Do not keep your advance directive in a safe deposit box. Other people may need access to them.

Give photocopies to your agent and alternate agent. Be sure your doctors have copies of your advance directives and give copies to everyone who might be involved with your healthcare, such as your family, clergy, or friends. Your local hospital might also be willing to file your advance directive in case you are admitted in the future. If you have surgery or are being admitted to a hospital, bring a copy with you and ask for it to be placed in your medical record.

Do healthcare providers run any legal risk by honoring advance directive?

No. Most advance directives statutes state explicitly that providers run no legal risk for honoring valid advance directives.

What if my healthcare provider will not honor my advance directive?

In many states, healthcare providers can refuse to honor an advance directive for ethical, moral, or religious reasons. For this reason, it is important to ask in advance if a healthcare provider has personal views or if an institution has any policy that would prevent them from honoring a person's treatment choices. If you know that your personal doctor is unable or unwilling to carry out your wishes, it would be wise to change to a physician who will respect them.

Who would make decisions about my medical care if I did not complete an advance directive?

There is not a simple answer to this question. In general, physicians consult with families when the person cannot make decisions. A number of states have passed surrogate decision making statutes. These laws create a decision-making process by identifying the individuals who may make decisions for a person who has no advance directive.

Is there a federal law about advance directives?

Yes, the Patient Self-Determination Act (PSDA) is a federal law regarding advance directives. It requires medical facilities that receive Medicaid and Medicare funds to have procedures for handling a person's advance directive, and to tell individuals upon admission about their rights under state law to use advance directives. The PSDA does not set standards for what an advance directive must say; it does not require facilities to provide advance directive forms; and it does not require people to have an advance directive. Rather PSDA's purpose is to make people aware of their rights.

Can I state my wishes about organ donation, cremation, or burial in my advance directive?

Several states permit you to indicate your wishes regarding organ donation. In those states that do not specifically address the issues of organ donation you may state your wishes in your advance directive. However, you should consider expressing your wishes through a form designed for that purpose. You should also make your family aware of your wishes. Since your advance directive and the authority of your agent technically ceases upon your death, you should tell your wishes about cremation or burial to your family or the executor of your estate.

Healthcare Agent—Appointing One

Whom can I appoint to be my healthcare agent?

Your agent can be almost any adult whom you trust to make healthcare decisions for you. However, most states do not permit you to appoint your attending physician (unless the individual resigns as your physician) or employees of the facility in which you are a resident (unless they are related to you by blood or marriage).

The most important considerations are that the agent be someone:

- you trust;
- who knows you well;
- who will honor your wishes.

Ideally, it should be someone who is not afraid to ask questions of doctors in order to get information needed to make decisions. Your agent may need to be forceful and not everyone is comfortable accepting this sort of responsibility, which is why it is very important to have a discussion with the person you plan to name as your healthcare agent before you select him or her.

Often people assume that their closest relatives know what they would want, so they think it is unnecessary to discuss wishes with them. However, people sometimes find that when they actually talk with their loved ones about end-of-life issues, they have very different views. Talking openly about your preferences is key to assuring that your agent knows what you want.

Everyone's situation is unique. Your decision about whom to appoint must be guided by your own relationships.

Can I appoint more than one person to be my healthcare agent?

In many states only one person can act as your agent at one time. Doctors can communicate more effectively if they know that there is one person who can receive information and make decisions. You can and should appoint an alternative agent in case the primary agent is unavailable or unable to serve.

What should I tell my agent?

Your agent needs to:

- know when and how you would want life-sustaining treatments provided to you;
- understand personal and spiritual values that guide your thinking about death and dying;
- have a copy of your living will.

To achieve a clearer understanding between you and your agent you might discuss some concrete situations. The following are some examples:

1. If you should suffer a massive stroke or had a head injury from which you were unlikely to regain consciousness, how you want to be treated?

2. Would you want life-sustaining treatments that might prolong your life if you suffered from a progressive debilitating disease such as Alzheimer's disease, Parkinson's, or a similar disease and could no longer make decisions? If you want treatments, which ones? For how long? Indefinitely?

3. If you were in any of these situations, would you want to receive artificial nutrition and fluids?

4. If you were seriously ill and your heart stopped beating or you stopped breathing, would you want resuscitation attempts? Would you want to have a ventilator breathe for you? If so for how long?

Although you cannot review every specific situation that might arise, discussions like this can help your agent understand how you think about the use of medical treatments at the end of life. Sometimes sharing your personal concerns and values, your spiritual beliefs, or your views about what makes life worth living can be as helpful to your agent as talking about specific treatments and circumstances. For example:

*   How important is it to be physically independent and to stay in your own home?

*   How do your religious or spiritual beliefs affect your attitudes toward dying and death? And medical care?

*   What aspects of your life give it the most meaning?

*   What are your particular concerns about dying? About death?

*   Would you want your agent to take into account the effect of your illness on any other people?

*   Should financial concerns enter into decisions about your treatment?

These are not simple questions and your views may change over time. It is important that you review these issues with your agent from time to time.

How does my agent make decisions?

Under most states' laws your agent is expected to make decisions based on specific knowledge of your wishes. If your agent does not know what you would want in a particular situation, he or she should try to infer your wishes based on their knowledge of you as a person and on your values related to quality of life in general. If your agent lacks this knowledge, decisions must be in your best interest. Generally, the more confident the agent is about the decisions will accurately reflect your wishes; the easier it will be to make them.

In a few states, the law limits the agent's power to refuse some treatments in circumstances. State law, for example, may limit decisions to what the person has specifically stated in the living will. You should carefully review your state's documents.

What if I know members of my family will disagree with my wishes?

To ensure that your wishes are followed, be certain that the person you appoint to be your agent understands your wishes and will abide by them. Your agent has the legal right to make decisions for you even if close family members disagree. However, should close family members express strong disagreement, your agent and your healthcare professional may find it extremely difficult to carry out the decisions you would want. If you foresee that your agent may encounter serious resistance, the following steps can help:

- Communicate with family members you anticipate may object to your decisions.

- Tell them in writing whom you have appointed to be your healthcare agent and explain why you have done so, and send a copy to your agent.

- Let them know that you do not wish for them to be involved with decisions about your medical care and give a copy of these communications to your agent as well.

- Give your primary care physician, if you have one, copies of written communications you have made.

- Prepare a specific, written living will.

- Make it clear in your documents that you want your agent to resolve any uncertainties that could arise with interpreting the living will. A way to say this is: "My agent should make any decisions about how to interpret or when to apply my living will."

Healthcare Agent—Being One

Why would I want to be a healthcare agent?

Accepting the appointment to be a healthcare agent is a way of affirming the importance of your relationship to the person appointing you. However, accepting an appointment requires thoughtful consideration about whether you can fulfill the role appropriately. Acting as a healthcare agent brings significant responsibilities.

What are my responsibilities as a healthcare agent?

As the healthcare agent you have the power to make medical decisions if the person loses the capacity to make them. Unless your authority to act is limited by the person or the state law, you normally can make all medical decisions for the person, not only end-of-life decisions.

Generally, you may speak for the person only as long as they are unable to make decisions. You need to read the state forms and the instructions carefully to find out if there are any limitations to your decision making.

One of an agent's most important functions is as an advocate for the person. Advocacy can involve asking to see medical records, meeting with the physician to get information about the person's diagnosis (the person's illness) and prognosis (what is the likely outcome of the illness, with treatment and without treatment), and getting other information that is needed to make decisions about treatment.

As the agent you may need to be assertive and persistent in seeking information and in speaking up on your loved one's behalf. It is important for you to remember that you have the legal authority to speak for your loved one, not the physician, nurses, or other healthcare professionals.

How do I make decisions as a healthcare agent?

Generally, you will be required, as far as possible, to make the same medical decisions that the individual you are speaking for would have made. To do this you might need to examine any specific statements that the person made (either orally or in writing, such as in a living will), as well as consider the person's beliefs and values. If you have no information about what they would want, you must act in what you believe would be in the person's best interest, using your own judgment. To arrive at that decision, you might ask the person's doctors what kind of benefits and burdens might result from the treatment; and you can draw on knowledge that others have about the person and on their opinions. However, the more you and the person have talked the less likely you will be in the dark about what they would want.

What do I need to know to make decisions?

You can ask the physician to describe how the illness is likely to progress and what decisions are likely to be necessary at some point. If you need information from the doctors, ask for an appointment to meet and come prepared with specific questions. Write your questions down so that you do not forget any of them and you can make good use of the time. You can get information and other support from nurses, social workers, patient representatives, member of the ethics committee, and chaplains.

Medical decision-making is a process. You can make provisional decisions and change them later. For example, you can authorize a trial treatment, and later if the treatment is not having the intended benefit, direct that it be stopped.

Take the time you need to get the information that you feel is necessary to make a thoughtful decision. There may be no "right" decision. You can only make the best decision that you can under the circumstances.

If I withdraw as the agent, can anyone else make decisions for the person?

If the person has appointed an alternative agent, you can withdraw and the alternate agent will become the legal decision maker. If there is not appointed alternate agent, the outcome varies among the states.

In some states, law sets forth a procedure for making decisions for persons who do not have designated decision makers. However, in some states there is no provision for decision making in the absence of an appointed agent unless the person's own wishes are clearly known. If the person's wishes are not known, care decisions are likely left to the physician and healthcare team.

How should I handle my personal feelings with acting as a healthcare agent?

It is very important that you stay in touch with your own feelings while you are acting as an agent. Otherwise, you may not realize that they can affect your behavior and even your decisions.

You may fear that you will not do the right thing or that you are not being assertive enough. You may worry that you are making decisions that make you feel better rather than those that are best for the person you are advocating for. You may also be struggling with grief, particularly if the illness has taken away the person you knew or if you anticipate that the person will soon die.

It is hard to listen and to hear what healthcare professionals are saying when you are under emotional stress. It is difficult to be objective when you are afraid of losing someone you love.

End-of-life decisions can be particularly difficult even when you know the person's wishes very clearly. Try to accept your feelings and be patient with yourself. You can usually defer making a decision until you have a chance to think about it. Do not blame yourself if you forget to ask something or if you are afraid you made the wrong decision. If, after thinking things over, you want to change your mind, you generally can do so. As a rule, you can find another opportunity to ask questions.

It is perfectly appropriate to seek help. People without medical experience cannot be expected to understand the healthcare systems and the medical issues that are involved. You should expect to need guidance in dealing with them. Some physicians can be quite sympathetic to the issues you are dealing with and, if asked, will try to help. If you feel particularly comfortable with a nurse, talk with him or her. Chaplains often have a great deal of experience dealing with individuals and families struggling with difficult decisions and can be very helpful, even if you do not share a common religious outlook. Patient representatives and social workers also may be resources. Look to your own friends and communities. Sometimes people you do not know well, but who have gone through similar situations, can be a wealth of support and information.

Life-Sustaining Treatments

Life-sustaining treatments are medical procedures that replace or support a failing essential bodily function (one that is necessary to keep you alive). They are also sometimes called life support or life prolonging treatments.

Why would I not want life-sustaining treatments?

If a good chance exists that a life-sustaining treatment will improve your condition (e.g., temporary use of a ventilator to support breathing until you are able to breathe on your own), you might accept the treatment. However, if your condition is complicated by many problems (e.g., serious brain damage, kidney failure) and continues to deteriorate with no likelihood of recovery, you might not want life-sustaining treatment.

If I refuse life support, will I still receive treatment for any pain I might have?

Yes. Many people mistakenly think that by refusing life-sustaining medical treatments they could be refusing all medical care. An individual is not refusing pain management and supportive care when they are refusing life support. This kind of care is often called "palliative care." It is not just pain medication, although pain management is an important part of palliative care. Palliative care is care for the whole person and includes spiritual and social supports as well as support for those caring for the person.

Artificial Nutrition and Hydration

What is artificial nutrition and hydration?

Artificial nutrition and hydration is a medical treatment that allows a person to receive nutrition (food) and hydration (fluids) when they are no longer able to take them by mouth. It is a chemically balanced mix of nutrients and fluids, provided by placing a tube directly into the stomach, the intestine, or a vein.

When is it used?

Artificial nutrition and hydration is given to a person who for some reason cannot eat or drink enough to sustain life or health. Doctors can provide nutrition and hydration through intravenous (IV) administration or by putting a tube in the stomach.

Is artificial nutrition and hydration different from ordinary eating and drinking?

Yes, an obvious difference is that providing artificial nutrition and hydration requires technical skill. Professional skill and training are necessary to insert the tube and to make decisions about how much and what type of feed to give the person.

Can I refuse artificial nutrition and hydration?

Yes. Artificial nutrition and hydration are life-sustaining treatments and your refusal is protected under the law.

Is it appropriate to give artificial nutrition and hydration to people who are at the end of life?

Yes. As with any medical treatment, artificial nutrition and hydration should be given if they contribute to the overall treatment goals for the person. These treatment goals should always focus on the person's wishes and interests.

What does the law say about artificial nutrition and hydration?

Every state law allows individuals to refuse artificial nutrition and hydration through the use of an advance directive such as a living will or durable power of attorney for healthcare. However, state laws vary as to what must be done to make wishes known. In many states nutrition and hydration is considered a medical treatment that may be refused in an advance directive. But in some states individuals are required to state specifically whether or not they would want artificial nutrition and hydration at the end of life. When there is uncertainty or conflict about whether or not a person would want the treatment, treatment usually will be continued.

Can artificial nutrition and hydration be stopped once it has been started?

Yes. As with any other medical treatment, stopping treatment is both legally and ethically appropriate if treatment is of no benefit to the person or it is unwanted. In fact, the law requires that treatment be stopped if the person does not want it.

Conflicts about stopping artificial nutrition and hydration often arise because the person's wishes are not clearly known or the person has not designated an agent to make decisions for him or her. In situations of uncertainty, the usual fallback option is to continue treatment. It is important that individuals talk to their doctors and loved ones about their wishes regarding the use of artificial nutrition and hydration at the end of life so they will be honored.

Can anything be done if the doctor insists on providing artificial nutrition and hydration?

Yes. If individuals have made their wishes know, the doctor must honor those wishes or transfer their care to another doctor who will honor them. To keep this kind of conflict from developing, it is wise for people to talk with their physicians before a medical crisis arises, if possible, so they know their physician will honor their end-of-life choices.

Is it considered suicide to refuse artificial nutrition and hydration?

No. When a person is refusing life-sustaining treatment at the end of life, including artificial nutrition and hydration, it is not considered an act of suicide. A person at the end of life is dying, not by choice, but because of a particular condition or disease. Continuing treatment may delay the moment of death but cannot change the underlying condition.

Are life insurance policies affected if life-sustaining treatments are refused?

No. Because death is not the result of suicide, life insurance policies are not affected when medical treatments are stopped.

Some points to think about when making decisions about the use of artificial nutrition and hydration:

1. What are your wishes?

2. What quality of life is important to you?

3. What is the goal or purpose for providing artificial nutrition and hydration?

4. Will it prolong life? Will it bring about a cure?

5. Will it contribute to the level of comfort?

6. Are there religious, cultural, or personal values that would affect a decision to continue or stop treatment?

7. Are there any benefits that artificial nutrition and hydration would offer?

Cardiopulmonary Resuscitation

Whether to resuscitate someone who has a cardiac or respiratory arrest is one of the most common end-of-life medical decisions that individuals and their families must make. Yet many people lack the necessary information to make an informed decision about cardiopulmonary resuscitation (CPR).

What is cardiopulmonary resuscitation?

Cardiopulmonary resuscitation (CPR) refers to a group of procedures that may include artificial respiration and intubation to support or restore breathing, and chest compressions or the use of electrical stimulation or medication to support or restore heart function. Intubation refers to endotracheal incubation which is the insertion of a tube through the mouth or nose into the tracheal (windpipe) to create and maintain an open airway to assist breathing. These procedures can either replace the normal work of the heart and lungs or stimulate the person's own heart and lungs to begin working again.

When is CPR used?

CPR is when a person stops breathing (respiratory arrest) and the heart stops beating (cardiac arrest). During cardiac arrest all body functions stop, including breathing and the blood stops going to the brain. Sometimes, however, a person may stop breathing while the heart continues to beat. This respiratory arrest may result from choking, or serious lung or neurological disease. If untreated, respiratory arrest will rapidly lead to cardiac arrest.

Why would someone want to refuse CPR?

CPR's success rate depends heavily upon how quickly it is started and the person's underlying medical condition. When a person is seriously ill or dying, cardiac arrest marks the moment of a disease when the body is shutting down. If CPR is initiated, it disrupts the body's natural dying process.

Do-Not-Resuscitate (DNR) Order

What is a Do-Not-Resuscitate (DNR) Order?

A DNR order is a physician's written order instructing healthcare providers not to attempt CPR in case of cardiac or respiratory arrest. A person with a valid DNR order will not be given CPR. Unlike a living will or a medical power of attorney, a person cannot prepare a DNR order. Although it is a written request of an individual, his or her family or healthcare agent, it must be signed by a physician to be valid.

Why is a DNR order needed to refuse CPR?

Without a physician's order not to resuscitate, the healthcare team must initiate CPR because in an emergency there is no time to call the attending physician, determine the person's wishes, or consult the family or healthcare agent. If a person wishes to refuse CPR, that wish must be communicated to the healthcare team by a DNR order signed by the attending physician.

Does a DNR order mean a person won't receive any treatment?

No. "Do not resuscitate" does not mean, "do not treat." A DNR order covers only one type of medical treatment—CPR. Other types of treatment, including intravenous fluids, artificial nutrition and hydration, and antibiotics must be discussed with the physician separately. In addition, although CPR will not be given to a person who has a DNR order, all measures can and should be used to keep a person comfortable.

Who can consent to a DNR order?

An individual, his or her healthcare agent, or a family member (as provided by state law), can agree to a DNR order. Although policies may differ, in general a DNR order must first be discussed with a person if he or she has the capacity to make medical decisions. If the person is incapacitated and is unable to make this decision, a physician can then consult instructions in a living will or speak with an appointed healthcare agent. If there are no written advance directives, a physician might consult a family member or a close friend of the individual.

When should a DNR order be discussed with a physician?

If a person is seriously ill or dying, discuss a DNR order with the physician as soon as possible. Ideally, a decision about a DNR order should be made while a person is alert and able to think clearly. However, if a person does not have the capacity to make a decision about a DNR order, it is important that this discussion be initiated as soon as possible. Ideally the physician would raise the issue, but the family or healthcare agent should not hesitate to approach the physician with their concerns. A discussion initiated sooner rather than later gives individuals and their families' time to reflect on the decision.

What questions should be asked when discussing a DNR order with a physician?

Before making a decision about CPR, individuals and their loved ones need to understand both the burdens and benefits of CPR. These can vary depending on individual's underlying condition. The physician should be prepared to:

- describe the procedures;

- address the probability for successful resuscitation based upon the person's medical condition;

- define what is meant by successful resuscitation—does successful mean the person will be able to leave the hospital? In what condition? If it is unlikely that the person will be able to leave the hospital, what can the resuscitation attempt accomplish?

If the physician does not think resuscitation would be successful, he or she should be willing to discuss the reasons why.

What if an individual, healthcare agent, or family member disagrees with the physician's recommendation?

First, the person or appropriate family member should approach the physician to clear up any misunderstandings about the person's wishes, prognosis, and treatment options. They can also request that a meeting be arranged with the physician, nurse, and other members of the healthcare team to discuss possible reasons why an agreement cannot be reached. Often, conflicts arise because of a lack of communication. However, if differences cannot be resolved, it is important that the person, agent, or family learn what resources the facility has to mediate and resolve conflict.

Healthcare facilities are required to have a process in place for resolving conflicts over decisions about CPR. A social worker or patient representative may be a good source of information about what to do. The family should also ask to see a copy of the facility's policy on DNR orders. The policy should describe the facility's process for resolving conflict. For example, many facilities give individuals and their families the opportunity to bring disputes before an ethics committee that can provide a neutral environment in which to mediate and resolve conflict.

Can a physician write a DNR order without consulting the individual?

Yes, in limited circumstances. In special circumstances, if a person is incapacitated and an authorized decision maker is not available, a physician may, depending upon the facility's policy, write a DNR order if he or she believes that CPR would not be successful appropriate treatment given the person's underlying illness. In general, however, physicians are obligated to discuss a DNR order with an individual or his or her authorized decision maker, and must obtain consent before treatment can be withheld or withdrawn. Informed consent is a basic right that must be respected by a facility's policy on DNR orders.

Will a DNR order remain effective when a person is transferred between healthcare facilities, for example, from a nursing home to a hospital?

Yes. A person's DNR order should accompany him or her on every transfer. Once the person arrives at the new facility, a new DNR order may need to be written based on that facility's policy. It is important that family and friends monitor the transfer to ensure that the DNR order accompanies the person and is properly documented in the medical record at the new facility. A DNR order or other important documents like a living will and medical power of attorney can be misplaced or overlooked during a transfer.

Will a DNR order be honored during surgery?

Usually not. DNR orders often are suspended during surgery. Cardiac or respiratory arrest during surgery may be due to the circumstances of surgery and not the underlying illness, and the chances of a successful resuscitation may be better. It is important that the individual or decision-maker talk to the surgeon in advance to make sure all parties understand what should happen in the event of an arrest during or shortly after surgery. The surgeon should also discuss how soon after surgery a DNR order will be reinstated.

Can a DNR order be revoked?

Yes. The individual or authorized surrogate can cancel a DNR order at any time by notifying the attending physician, who must then remove the order from the medical record.

What is a non-hospital DNR order?

Unlike medical facility DNR orders, non-hospital DNR orders are written for people who want to refuse CPR and are outside a healthcare facility, either at home or in a residential care setting. Also referred to as a pre-hospital DNR order, a non-hospital DNR order directs emergency medical care providers, including emergency medical technicians, paramedics, and emergency department physicians, to withhold CPR. These orders must be signed by a physician and generally are written on an official form but, depending upon the state, they also may be issued on a bracelet, necklace, or wallet card. Although honored by emergency medical providers, non-hospital DNR orders are not binding upon bystanders who may initiate resuscitative measures in an emergency.

Why are non-hospital DNR orders needed?

Emergencies demand an immediate response. Emergency medical service (EMS) personnel are trained to act quickly and to save lives. Once called to a scene, they must do all they can to stabilize and transport a person to the nearest hospital, including administering CPR if necessary. If a person wishes to refuse CPR in the home, he or she must have a non-hospital DNR order. Without a non-hospital DNR order, EMS will initiate CPR if a person is in cardiac or respiratory arrest. It is important to remember, however, that as long as a person has decision-making capacity, he or she can refuse any form of medical treatment, including emergency care.

Are non-hospital DNR orders governed by state law?

Yes. Many states have laws in place governing non-hospital DNR orders. With the growth of hospice care and the increasing desire of dying persons to spend their last days at home, has come the need to protect people from unwanted emergency care. Non-hospital DNR laws allow qualified persons to refuse emergency resuscitative measures under certain conditions. Check with the State Department of Health and county EMS agency to determine if a statewide policy or any local protocols governing non-hospital DNR orders exist.

Who should consider a non-hospital DNR order and when?

Non-hospital DNR orders generally are intended for seriously ill persons who have chosen to die at home. Depending upon state law or policy, there may be restrictions on who can qualify for a non-hospital DNR order. Remember, these orders must be signed by a physician to be valid.

Can a non-hospital DNR order be revoked?

Yes. The person or the person's authorized surrogate can cancel a non-hospital DNR order at any time by notifying the physician who signed the order and by destroying the form and/or bracelet, wallet card, etc.

What happens to a non-hospital DNR order when someone is taken to a hospital?

If a person is admitted to the hospital for any reason, it is important that the non-hospital DNR order goes with the person. If EMS personnel are involved, they should take the order with them in the ambulance, but it is still advisable for family members to bring a copy of the order with them. Although the admitting physician should write a new DNR order at the hospital, it is important that family members make sure that a facility DNR order is in place. Hospital personnel are sometimes unfamiliar with DNR laws or policies, and in an emergency, important papers can be overlooked.

Do-Not-Intubate (DNI) Order

What is a Do-Not-Intubate (DNI) Order?

When a DNR order is discussed the doctor might ask if a do-not-intubate order is also wanted. Intubation may be considered separately from resuscitation because a person can have trouble breathing or might not be getting enough oxygen before the heart actually stops beating or breathing stops (a cardiac or respiratory arrest).

If this condition continues a full arrest will occur. If the person is intubated, cardiac or respiratory arrest might be averted. During intubation a tube is inserted through the mouth or nose into the trachea (windpipe) in order to assist breathing; a machine (ventilator) may be connected to that tube to push oxygen into the lungs.

Refusal of resuscitation is not necessarily the same as refusal of intubation. It is important that all concerned understand the decisions being made since some institutional DNR policies include intubation, while others treat it separately.

If a person does not want life mechanically sustained it is important to be sure that intubation is addressed as part of the discussion of DNR.

Part Seven

Additional Help and Information

Chapter 62

Glossary of Terms Related to Disabilities

access: An individual's ability to obtain appropriate health care services. Barriers to access can be financial, geographic, organizational, and sociological. Efforts to improve access often focus on providing/improving health coverage.

accessibility: Removal of barriers that would hinder a person with a disability from entering, functioning, and working within a facility. Required restructuring of the facility cannot cause undue hardship for the employer.

activities of daily living (ADLs): Basic personal activities that include bathing, eating, dressing, mobility, transferring from bed to chair, and using the toilet. ADLs are used to measure how dependent a person may be on requiring assistance in performing any or all of these activities.

adult day care: A daytime community-based program for functionally impaired adults that provides a variety of health, social, and related support services in a protective setting.

advance health care directive: Also called advance directive. A written instructional health care directive and/or appointment of an agency, or a written refusal to appoint an agent or execute a directive.

Definitions in this chapter were compiled from documents published by the U.S. Department of Health and Human Services (HHS, www.hhs.gov).

assistive devices: Tools that enable individuals with disabilities to perform essential job functions, e.g., telephone headsets, adapted computer keyboards, enhanced computer monitors.

birth defect: Conditions that cause structural changes in one or more parts of the body; are present at birth; and have an adverse effect on health, development, or functional ability.

caregiver: Person who provides support and assistance with various activities to a family member, friend, or neighbor. May provide emotional or financial support, as well as hands-on help with different tasks. Caregiving may also be done from long distance.

cognitive impairment: Deterioration or loss of intellectual capacity that requires continual supervision to protect the person or others, as measured by clinical evidence and standardized tests that reliably measure impairment in the area of (1) short or long-term memory, (2) orientation as to person, place and time, or (3) deductive or abstract reasoning. Such loss in intellectual capacity can result from Alzheimer disease or similar forms of dementia.

comorbidity: Condition that exists at the same time as the primary condition in the same patient (e.g., hypertension is a comorbidity of many conditions such as diabetes, ischemic heart disease, end-stage renal disease, etc.).

developmental disability: A disability that originates before age 18, can be expected to continue indefinitely, and constitutes a substantial handicap to the disabled's ability to function normally.

disability: The limitation of normal physical, mental, social activity of an individual. There are varying types (functional, occupational, learning), degrees (partial, total), and durations (temporary, permanent) of disability.

group home: Also called adult care home or board and care home. Residence that offers housing and personal care services for three to 16 residents. Services (such as meals, supervision, and transportation) are usually provided by the owner or manager. May be single family home.

guardian: A judicially appointed guardian or conservator having authority to make a health care decision for an individual.

home health care: Includes a wide range of health-related services such as assistance with medications, wound care, intravenous (IV) therapy, and help with basic needs such as bathing, dressing, mobility, etc., which are delivered at a person's home.

home medical equipment: Also called durable medical equipment. Equipment such as hospital beds, wheelchairs, and prosthetics used at home. May be covered by Medicaid and in part by Medicare or private insurance.

impairment: Any loss or abnormality of psychological, physiological, or anatomical function.

individualized education program (IEP): A written statement of the educational program designed to meet a child's individual needs. Every child who receives special education services must have an IEP.

independent living facility: A facility (house, apartment, etc.) in which a child/youth is permitted to live or reside independently without a paid caretaker.

learning disability: A disorder in one or more of the basic psychological processes involved in understanding or in using language, spoken or written, which may manifest itself in an imperfect ability to listen, think, speak, read, write, spell, or to do mathematical calculation. The term includes such conditions as perceptual handicaps, brain injury, and minimal brain dysfunction.

life-sustaining treatment: Medical procedures that replace or support an essential bodily function. Life-sustaining treatments include cardiopulmonary resuscitation (CPR), mechanical ventilation, artificial nutrition and hydration, dialysis, and certain other treatments.

long-term care: Range of medical and/or social services designed to help people who have disabilities or chronic care needs. Services may be short- or long-term and may be provided in a person's home, in the community, or in residential facilities (e.g., nursing homes or assisted living facilities).

mental illness/impairment: A deficiency in the ability to think, perceive, reason, or remember, resulting in loss of the ability to take care of one's daily living needs.

nursing home: Facility licensed by the state to offer residents personal care as well as skilled nursing care on a 24-hour-a-day basis. Provides nursing care, personal care, room and board, supervision, medication, therapies, and rehabilitation. Rooms are often shared, and communal dining is common.

occupational health services: Health services concerned with the physical, mental, and social well-being of an individual in relation to his or her working environment and with the adjustment of individuals to their work. The term applies to more than the safety of the workplace and includes health and job satisfaction.

occupational therapy: Designed to help patients improve their independence with activities of daily living through rehabilitation, exercises, and the use of assistive devices. May be covered in part by Medicare.

physical therapy: Designed to restore/improve movement and strength in people whose mobility has been impaired by injury and disease. May include exercise, massage, water therapy, and assistive devices. May be covered in part by Medicare.

rehabilitation: The combined and coordinated use of medical, social, educational, and vocational measures for training or retaining individuals disabled by disease or injury to the highest possible level of functional ability. Several different types of rehabilitation are distinguished—vocational, social, psychological, medical, and educational.

residential care: The provision of room, board, and personal care. Residential care falls between the nursing care delivered in skilled and intermediate care facilities and the assistance provided through social services. It can be broadly defined as the provision of 24-hour supervision of individuals who, because of old age or impairments, necessarily need assistance with the activities of daily living.

respite care: Service in which trained professionals or volunteers come into the home to provide short-term care (from a few hours to a few days) for a disabled person to allow caregivers some time away from their caregiving role.

special education: A type of education some children with disabilities receive. Special education may include specially designed instruction in classrooms, at home, or in private or public institutions, and may be accompanied by related services such as speech therapy, occupational and physical therapy, psychological counseling, and medical diagnostic services necessary to the child's education.

speech therapy: Designed to help restore speech through exercises. May be covered by Medicare.

support groups: Groups of people who share a common bond (e.g., caregivers) who come together on a regular basis to share problems and experiences. May be sponsored by social service agencies, senior centers, religious organizations, as well as organizations such as the Alzheimer's Association.

Chapter 63

Directory of Organizations That Help People with Disabilities

Government Agencies That Provide Information about Disabilities

Administration on Aging (AOA)

One Massachusetts Avenue, NW
Washington, DC 20001
Phone: 202-619-0724
Fax: 202-357-3555
Website: www.aoa.gov
E-mail: aoainfo@aoa.hhs.gov

Administration on Developmental Disabilities (ADD)

Administration for Children and Families
U.S. Department of Health and Human Services
Mail Stop: HHH 405-D
370 L'Enfant Promenade, SW
Washington, DC 20447
Phone: 202-690-6590
Fax: 202-690-6904
or 202-205-8037
Website: www.acf.hhs.gov/programs/add

Resources in this chapter were compiled from several sources deemed reliable; all contact information was verified and updated in July 2011. The information under the heading "Americans with Disabilities Act National Network Centers" is from "ADA Home," by the Americans with Disabilities Act National Network (www.adata.org), an undated document. The information under the heading "Summer Camps for Children with Disabilities" is from "Summer Camps 2008," by the National Dissemination Center for Children with Disabilities (NICHCY), www.nichcy.org, 2008.

Agency for Healthcare Research and Quality (AHRQ)
Office of Communications and Knowledge Transfer
540 Gaither Road, Suite 2000
Rockville, MD 20850
Phone: 301-427-1104
Website: www.ahrq.gov

Centers for Disease Control and Prevention (CDC)
1600 Clifton Road
Atlanta, GA 30333
Toll-Free: 800-CDC-INFO
(232-4636)
Toll-Free TTY: 888-232-6348
Phone: 404-639-3311
Website: www.cdc.gov
E-mail: cdcinfo@cdc.gov

Disability.gov
Website: www.disability.gov

Eldercare Locator
Toll-Free: 800-677-1116
Website: www.eldercare.gov
E-mail: eldercarelocator@n4a.org

Federal Communications Commission (FCC)
445 12th Street, SW
Washington, DC 20554
Toll-Free: 888-225-5322
Toll-Free TTY: 888-835-5322
Toll-Free Fax: 866-418-0232
Website: www.fcc.gov
E-mail: fccinfo@fcc.gov

Healthfinder®
National Health Information Center
P.O. Box 1133
Washington, DC 20013-1133
Toll-Free: 800-336-4797
Phone: 301-565-4167
Fax: 301-984-4256
Website: www.healthfinder.gov
E-mail: healthfinder@nhic.org

Library of Congress (LOC)
101 Independence Avenue, SE
Washington, DC 20540
Phone: 202-707-5000
Website: www.loc.gov

Maternal and Child Health Bureau (MCHB)
Human Resources and Services Administration
5600 Fishers Lane
Rockville, MD 20857
Website: www.mchb.hrsa.gov

National Cancer Institute (NCI)
NCI Office of Communications and Education
Public Inquiries Office
6116 Executive Boulevard
Suite 300
Bethesda, MD 20892-8322
Toll-Free: 800-4-CANCER
(422-6237)
Toll-Free TTY: 800-332-8615
Website: www.cancer.gov
E-mail:
cancergovstaff@mail.nih.gov

National Center for Complementary and Alternative Medicine (NCCAM)

National Institutes of Health
NCCAM Clearinghouse
P.O. 7923
Gaithersburg, MD 20898-7923
Toll-Free: 888-644-6226
Toll-Free TTY: 866-464-3615
Toll-Free Fax: 866-464-3616
Website: www.nccam.nih.gov
E-mail: info@nccam.nih.gov

National Center for Health Statistics (NCHS)

3311 Toledo Road
Hyattsville, MD 20782
Toll-Free: 800-232-4636
Website: www.cdc.gov/nchs
E-mail: cdcinfo@cdc.gov

National Council on Disability (NCD)

1331 F Street, NW, Suite 850
Washington, DC 20004
Phone: 202-272-2004
TTY: 202-272-2074
Fax: 202-272-2022
Website: www.ncd.gov
E-mail: ncd@ncd.gov

National Heart, Lung and Blood Institute (NHLBI)

NHLBI Health Information Center
Attention: Website
P.O. Box 30105
Bethesda, MD 20824-0105
Phone: 301-592-8573
TTY: 240-629-3255
Fax: 240-629-3246
Website: www.nhlbi.nih.gov
E-mail: nhlbiinfo@nhlbi.nih.gov

National Institute of Arthritis and Musculoskeletal and Skin Diseases (NIAMS)

Information Clearinghouse
National Institutes of Health
1 AMS Circle
Bethesda, MD 20892-3675
Toll-Free: 877-22-NIAMS
(226-4267)
Phone: 301-495-4484
TTY: 301-565-2966
Fax: 301-718-6366
Website: www.niams.nih.gov
E-mail: NIAMSInfo@mail.nih.gov

National Institute of Child Health and Human Development (NICHD)

P.O. Box 3006
Rockville, MD 20847
Toll-Free: 800-370-2943
Toll-Free TTY: 888-320-6942
Toll-Free Fax: 866-760-5947
Website: www.nichd.nih.gov
E-mail: NICHDInformation
ResourceCenter@mail.nih.gov

National Institute of Dental and Craniofacial Research (NIDCR)

National Institutes of Health
Bethesda, MD 20892-2190
Toll-Free: 866-232-4528
Phone: 301-496-4261
Fax: 301-480-4098
Website: www.nidcr.nih.gov
E-mail: nidcrinfo@mail.nih.gov

National Institute of Mental Health (NIMH)
Science Writing, Press, and Dissemination Branch
6001 Executive Boulevard
Room 8184, MSC 9663
Bethesda, MD 20892-9663
Toll-Free: 866-615-6464
Toll-Free TTY: 866-415-8051
Phone: 301-443-4513
TTY: 301-443-8431
Fax: 301-443-4279
Website: www.nimh.nih.gov
E-mail: nimhinfo@nih.gov

National Institute of Neurological Disorders and Stroke (NINDS)
NIH Neurological Institute
P.O. Box 5801
Bethesda, MD 20824
Toll-Free: 800-352-9424
Phone: 301-496-5751
TTY: 301-468-5981
Website: www.ninds.nih.gov
E-mail: braininfo@ninds.nih.gov

National Institute on Aging (NIA)
Building 31, Room 5C27
31 Center Drive, MSC 2292
Bethesda, MD 20892
Phone: 301-496-1752
Toll-Free TTY: 800-222-4225
Fax: 301-496-1072
Website: www.nia.nih.gov

National Institute on Deafness and Other Communication Disorders (NIDCD)
National Institutes of Health
31 Center Drive, MSC 2320
Bethesda, MD 20892-2320
Toll-Free: 800-241-1044
Toll-Free TTY: 800-241-1055
Phone: 301-496-7243
Fax: 301-402-0018
Website: www.nidcd.nih.gov
E-mail: nidcdinfo@nidcd.nih.gov

National Institute on Disability and Rehabilitation Research (NIDRR)
U.S. Department of Education
400 Maryland Avenue, SW
Mailstop PCP-6038
Washington, DC 20202
Phone: 202-245-7640 (Voice and TTY)
Fax: 202-245-7323 or 202-245-7643
Website: www.ed.gov/about/offices/list/osers/nidrr

National Technical Information Service (NTIS)
5301 Shawnee Road
Alexandria, VA 22312
Toll-Free: 800-553-NTIS (553-6847)
Phone: 703-605-6000
Website: www.ntis.gov
E-mail: info@ntis.gov

National Women's Health Information Center (NWHIC)
Office on Women's Health
200 Independence Avenue, SW
Room 712E
Washington DC 20201
Toll-Free: 800-994-9662
Toll-Free TDD: 888-220-5446
Phone:202-690-7650
Fax: 202-205-2631
Website: www.womenshealth.gov

Office of Disability Employment Policy (ODEP)
U.S. Department of Labor
200 Constitution Avenue, NW
Washington, DC 20210
Toll-Free: 866-4-USA-DOL
(487-2365)
Toll-Free TTY: 877-889-5627
Website: www.dol.gov/odep

U.S. Department of Education (ED)
400 Maryland Avenue, SW
Washington, DC 20202
Toll-Free: 800-USA-LEARN
(872-5327)
Toll-Free TTY: 800-437-0833
Website: www2.ed.gov

U.S. Department of Housing and Urban Development (HUD)
451 7th Street, SW
Washington, DC 20410
Phone: 202-708-1112
TTY: 202-708-1455
Website: www.hud.gov

U.S. Department of Justice
950 Pennsylvania Avenue, NW
Civil Rights Division
Disability Rights Section–NYA
Washington, DC 20530
Toll-Free: 800-514-0301
Toll-Free TTY: 800-514-0383
Fax: 202-307-1197
Website: www.ada.gov

U.S. Department of Transportation (DOT)
1200 New Jersey Avenue, SE
Washington, DC 20590
Toll-Free: 866-377-8642
Toll-Free TTY: 800-877-8339
Phone: 202-366-4000
Website: www.dot.gov

U.S. Department of Veterans Affairs (VA)
810 Vermont Avenue, NW
Washington, DC 20420
Toll-Free: 800-827-1000
Website: www.va.gov

U.S. Equal Employment Opportunity Commission (EEOC)
131 M Street, NE
Washington, DC 20507
Toll-Free: 800-669-4000
Toll-Free TTY: 800-669-6820
Phone: 202-663-4900
Website: www.eeoc.gov
E-mail: info@eeoc.gov

U.S. Food and Drug Administration (FDA)
10903 New Hampshire Avenue
Silver Spring, MD 20993
Toll-Free: 888-INFO-FDA
(463-6332)
Website: www.fda.gov

U.S. Government Printing Office (GPO)
732 North Capitol Street, NW
Washington, DC 20401-0001
Toll-Free: 866-512-1800
Phone: 202-512-1800
Fax: 202-512-2104
Website: www.gpo.gov
E-mail: ContactCenter@gpo.gov

U.S. National Library of Medicine (NLM)
8600 Rockville Pike
Bethesda, MD 20894
Toll-Free: 888-FIND-NLM
(346-3656)
Toll-Free TDD: 800-735-2258
Phone: 301-594-5983
Fax: 301-402-1384
Website: www.nlm.nih.gov
E-mail: custserv@nlm.nih.gov

U.S. Social Security Administration (SSA)
Office of Public Inquiries
Windsor Park Building
6401 Security Boulevard
Baltimore, MD 21235
Toll-Free: 800-772-1213
Toll-Free TTY: 800-325-0778
Website: www.ssa.gov

Private Agencies That Provide Information about Disabilities

AARP
601 E Street, NW
Washington DC 20049
Toll-Free: 888-OUR-AARP
(687-2277)
Toll-Free TTY: 877-434-7598
Website: www.aarp.org
E-mail: member@aarp.org

AbilityJobs
ABILITY Mail Center
P.O. Box 10878
Costa Mesa, CA 92627
Website: www.abilityjobs.com
E-mail: custserv@jobtarget.com

Adaptive Environments Center
200 Portland Street
Boston, MA 02114
Phone: 617-695-1225
Fax: 617-482-8099
Website: www.adaptenv.org
E-mail: info@
HumanCenteredDesign.org

Alzheimer's Association
225 North Michigan Avenue
Floor 17
Chicago, IL 60601-7633
Toll-Free: 800-272-3900
Phone: 312-335-8700
TDD: 312-335-5886
Toll-Free Fax: 866-699-1246
Website: www.alz.org
E-mail: info@alz.org

Alzheimer's Foundation of America
322 Eighth Avenue, 7th Floor
New York, NY 10001
Toll-Free: 866-232-8484
Fax: 646-638-1546
Website: www.alzfdn.org
E-mail: info@alzfdn.org

American Academy of Family Physicians
P.O. Box 11210
Shawnee Mission, KS 66207-1210
Toll-Free: 800-274-2237
Phone: 913-906-6000
Fax: 913-906-6075
Website: www.aafp.org
E-mail: contactcenter@aafp.org

American Academy of Physical Medicine and Rehabilitation
9700 West Bryn Mawr Avenue
Suite 200
Rosemont, IL 60018-5701
Phone: 847-737-6000
Fax: 847-737-6001
Website: www.aapmr.org
E-mail: info@aapmr.org

American Council of the Blind
2200 Wilson Boulevard
Suite 650
Arlington, VA 22201
Toll-Free: 800-424-8666
Phone: 202-467-5081
Fax: 703-465-5085
Website: www.acb.org
E-mail: info@acb.org

American Foundation for the Blind
2 Penn Plaza, Suite 1102
New York, NY 10121
Toll-Free: 800-AFB-LINE (232-5463)
Phone: 212-502-7600
Toll-Free Fax: 888-545-8331
Website: www.afb.org
E-mail: afbinfo@afb.net

American Geriatrics Society Foundation for Health in Aging
The Empire State Building
350 Fifth Avenue, Suite 801
New York, NY 10118
Toll-Free: 800-563-4916
Phone: 212-755-6810
Fax: 212-832-8646
Website: www.healthinaging.org

American Health Assistance Foundation
22512 Gateway Center Drive
Clarksburg, MD 20871
Toll-Free: 800-437-2423
Phone: 301-948-3244
Fax: 301-258-9454
Website: www.ahaf.org/alzheimers
E-mail: info@ahaf.org

American Heart Association
National Center
7272 Greenville Avenue
Dallas, TX 75231
Toll-Free: 800-AHA-USA-1 (242-8721)
Website: www.heart.org

American Medical Association
515 North State Street
Chicago, IL 60654
Toll-Free: 800-621-8335
Website: www.ama-assn.org

American Parkinson Disease Association
135 Parkinson Avenue
Staten Island, NY 10305
Toll-Free: 800-223-2732
Phone: 718-981-8001
Fax: 718-981-4399
Website: www.apdaparkinson.org
E-mail: apda@apdaparkinson.org

American Printing House for the Blind
1839 Frankfort Avenue
P.O. Box 6085
Louisville, KY 40206-0085
Toll-Free: 800-223-1839
Phone: 502-895-2405
Fax: 502-899-2284
Website: www.aph.org
E-mail: info@aph.org

American Psychiatric Association
1000 Wilson Boulevard
Suite 1825
Arlington, VA 22209
Toll-Free: 888-35-PSYCH
(357-7924)
Website: www.psych.org
E-mail: apa@psych.org

American Psychological Association
750 First Street, NE
Washington, DC 20002-4242
Toll-Free: 800-374-2721
Phone: 202-336-5500
TDD/TTY: 202-336-6123
Website: www.apa.org

American Society on Aging
71 Stevenson Street, Suite 1450
San Francisco, CA 94105-2938
Toll-Free: 800-537-9728
Phone: 415-974-9600
Fax: 415-974-0300
Website: www.asaging.org
E-mail: info@asaging.org

American Speech-Language-Hearing Association
2200 Research Boulevard
Rockville, MD 20850-3289
Toll-Free: 800-638-8255
TTY: 301-296-5650
Phone: 301-296-5700
Fax: 301-296-8580
Website: www.asha.org
E-mail: actioncenter@asha.org

Amputee Coalition of America
900 East Hill Avenue, Suite 205
Knoxville, TN 37915-2566
Toll-Free: 888-AMP-KNOW
(888-267-5669)
Phone: 865-524-8772
TTY: 865-525-4512
Fax: 865-525-7917
Website:
www.amputee-coalition.org

Amyotrophic Lateral Sclerosis Association

1275 K Street, NW, Suite 1050
Washington, DC 20005
Toll-Free: 800-782-4747
Phone: 202-407-8580
Fax: 202-289-6801
Website: www.alsa.org
E-mail: alsinfo@alsa-national.org

The Arc

1660 L Street, NW, Suite 301
Washington, DC 20036
Toll-Free: 800-433-5255
Phone: 202-534-3700
Fax: 202-534-3731
Website: www.thearc.org
E-mail: info@thearc.org

Arthritis Foundation

P.O. Box 7669
Atlanta, GA 30357-0669
Toll-Free: 800-283-7800
Website: www.arthritis.org

Assisted Living Federation of America

1650 King Street, Suite 602
Alexandria, VA 22314
Phone: 703-894-1805
Website: www.alfa.org
E-mail: info@ALFA.org

Associated Services for the Blind and Visually Impaired

919 Walnut Street
Philadelphia, PA 19107
Phone: 215-627-0600
Fax: 215-922-0692
Website: www.asb.org
E-mail: asbinfo@asb.org

Association of University Centers on Disabilities

1010 Wayne Avenue, Suite 920
Silver Spring, MD 20910
Phone: 301-588-8252
Fax: 301-588-2842
Website: www.aucd.org
E-mail: aucdinfo@aucd.org

Autism Society

4340 East-West Highway
Suite 350
Bethesda, MD 20814
Toll-Free: 800-3AUTISM
(328-8476)
Phone: 301-657-0881
Website: www.autism-society.org

Birth Defect Research for Children, Inc.

976 Lake Baldwin Lane
Suite 104
Orlando, FL 32814
Phone: 407-895-0802
Website: www.birthdefects.org
E-mail: staff@birthdefects.org

Brain Injury Association of America

1608 Spring Hill Road
Suite 110
Vienna, VA 22182
Toll-Free: 800-444-6443
Phone: 703-761-0750
Fax: 703-761-0755
Website: www.biausa.org
E-mail:
braininjuryinfo@biausa.org

Brain Trauma Foundation
7 World Trade Center
250 Greenwich Street
34th Floor
New York, NY 10017
Phone: 212-772-0608
Fax: 212-772-0357
Website: www.braintrauma.org
E-mail:
education@braintrauma.org

Cleveland Clinic
9500 Euclid Avenue
Cleveland, OH 44195
Toll-Free: 800-223-2273
TTY: 216-444-0261
Website: my.clevelandclinic.org

Cystic Fibrosis Foundation
6931 Arlington Road, 2nd Floor
Bethesda, MD 20814
Toll-Free: 800-FIGHT CF
(344-4823)
Phone: 301-951-4422
Fax: 301-951-6378
Website: www.cff.org
E-mail: info@cff.org

Easter Seals
233 South Wacker Drive
Suite 2400
Chicago, IL 60606
Toll-Free: 800-221-6827
Phone: 312-726-6200
Fax: 312-726-1494
Website: www.easterseals.com

Epilepsy Foundation
8301 Professional Place
Landover, MD 20785
Toll-Free: 800-332-1000
Fax: 301-577-2684
Website:
www.epilepsyfoundation.org
E-mail: info@efa.org

Family Caregiver Alliance
180 Montgomery Street
Suite 900
San Francisco, CA 94104
Toll-Free: 800-445-8106
Phone: 415-434-3388
Website: www.caregiver.org
E-mail: info@caregiver.org

Goodwill Industries
15810 Indianola Drive
Rockville, MD 20855
Toll-Free: 800-741-0186
Website: www.goodwill.org
E-mail: contactus@goodwill.org

International Dyslexia Association
40 York Road, 4th Floor
Baltimore, MD 21204
Phone: 410-296-0232
Fax: 410-321-5069
Website: www.interdys.org

Job Accommodation Network
Toll-Free: 800-526-7234
Toll-Free TTY: 877-781-9403
Website: www.askjan.org
E-mail: jan@askjan.org

March of Dimes

1275 Mamaroneck Avenue
White Plains, NY 10605
Phone: 914-997-4488
Website: www.marchofdimes.com

Meals-on-Wheels Association of America

203 South Union Street
Alexandria, VA 22314
Phone: 703-548-5558
Fax: 703-548-8024
Website: www.mowaa.org
E-mail: mowaa@mowaa.org

Muscular Dystrophy Association

National Headquarters
3300 East Sunrise Drive
Tucson, AZ 85718
Toll-Free: 800-572-1717
Website: www.mdausa.org
E-mail: mda@mdausa.org

National Adult Day Services Association

1421 East Broad Street
Suite 425
Fuquay Varina, NC 27526
Toll-Free: 877-745-1440
Fax: 919-552-0254
Website: www.nadsa.org
E-mail: NADSAnews@gmail.com

National Alliance for Caregiving

4720 Montgomery Lane
2nd Floor
Bethesda, MD 20814
Website: www.caregiving.org
E-mail: info@caregiving.com

National Association of the Deaf

8630 Fenton Street, Suite 820
Silver Spring, MD 20910
Phone: 301-587-1788
TTY: 301-587-1789
Fax: 301-587-1791
Website: www.nad.org

National Center for Learning Disabilities

381 Park Avenue South
Suite 1401
New York, NY 10016
Toll-Free: 888-575-7373
Phone: 212-545-7510
Fax: 212-545-9665
Website: www.ncld.org
E-mail: ncld@ncld.org

National Center of Physical Activity and Disability

1640 West Roosevelt Road
Chicago, IL 60608-6904
Toll-Free: 800-900-8086
Fax: 312-355-4058
Website: www.ncpad.org
E-mail: ncpad@uic.edu

National Consortium on Deaf-Blindness

345 North Monmouth Avenue
Monmouth, OR 97361
Toll-Free: 800-438-9376
Toll-Free TTY: 800-854-7013
Fax: 503-838-8150
Website: www.nationaldb.org
E-mail: info@nationaldb.org

National Dissemination Center for Children with Disabilities
1825 Connecticut Avenue, NW
Suite 700
Washington, DC 20009
Toll-Free: 800-695-0285
Phone: 202-884-8200
Fax: 202-884-8441
Website: www.nichcy.org
E-mail: nichcy@aed.org

National Down Syndrome Society
666 Broadway, 8th Floor
New York, NY 10012
Toll-Free: 800-221-4602
Fax: 212-979-2873
Website: www.ndss.org
E-mail: info@ndss.org

National Family Caregivers Association
10400 Connecticut Avenue
Suite 500
Kensington, MD 20895-3944
Toll-Free: 800-896-3650
Phone: 301-942-6430
Fax: 301-942-2302
Website: www.nfcacares.org
E-mail:
info@thefamilycaregiver.org

National Federation of the Blind
200 East Wells Street
Baltimore, MD 21230
Phone: 410-659-9314
Fax: 410-685-5653
Website: www.nfb.org
E-mail: pmaurer@nfb.org

National Hospice and Palliative Care Organization/National Hospice Foundation
1731 King Street, Suite 100
Alexandria, VA 22314
Toll-Free: 800-658-8898
Phone: 703-837-1500
Fax: 703-837-1233
Website: www.nhpco.org
E-mail: nhpco_info@nhpco.org

National Multiple Sclerosis Society
733 Third Avenue, 3rd Floor
New York, NY 10017
Toll-Free: 800-344-4867
Website:
www.nationalmssociety.org

National Organization for Rare Disorders
55 Kenosia Avenue
P.O. Box 1968
Danbury, CT 06813-1968
Toll-Free: 800-999-6673
Phone: 203-744-0100
TDD: 203-797-9590
Fax: 203-798-2291
Website: www.rarediseases.org
E-mail: orphan@rarediseases.org

*National Parkinson
Foundation, Inc.*
1501 NW 9th Avenue
Bob Hope Road
Miami, FL 33136-1494
Toll-Free: 800-4PD-Info
(473-4636) (Helpline)
Toll-Free: 800-327-4545
(National Headquarters)
Phone: 305-243-6666
Fax: 305-243-6073
Website: www.parkinson.org
E-mail: contact@parkinson.org

*National Rehabilitation
Information Center*
8201 Corporate Drive, Suite 600
Landover, MD 20785
Toll-Free: 800-346-2742
Phone: 301-459-5900
TTY: 301-459-5984
Fax: 301-459-4263
Website: www.naric.com
E-mail: naricinfo@
heitechservices.com

*National Respite Network
and Resource Center*
Website: www.archrespite.org
Respite Locator: www.
archrespite.org/respitelocator

*National Spinal Cord
Injury Association*
75-20 Astoria Boulevard
Suite 120
Jackson Heights, NY 11370
Toll-Free: 800-962-9629
Phone: 718-512-0010
Fax: 866-387-2196
Website: www.spinalcord.org
E-mail: info@spinalcord.org

National Stroke Association
9707 East Easter Lane, Suite B
Centennial, CO 80112-3747
Toll-Free: 800-787-6537
Phone: 303-649-9299
Fax: 303-649-1328
Website: www.stroke.org
E-mail: info@stroke.org

*Nemours Foundation Center
for Children's Health Media*
1600 Rockland Road
Wilmington, DE 19803
Phone: 302-651-4000
Website: www.kidshealth.org
E-mail: info@kidshealth.org

*Parkinson's Disease
Foundation*
1359 Broadway, Suite 1509
New York, NY 10018
Toll-Free: 800-457-6676
Phone: 212-923-4700
Fax: 212-923-4778
Website: www.pdf.org
E-mail: info@pdf.org

PsychCentral
55 Pleasant Street, Suite 207
Newburyport, MA 01950
Phone: 978-992-0008
Website: www.psychcentral.com
E-mail:
talkback@psychcentral.com

*Regional Resource Center
Program*
Website: www.rrcprogram.org

Rehabilitation Institute of Chicago

345 East Superior Street
Chicago, IL 60611
Toll-Free: 800-354-REHAB
(354-7342)
Phone: 312-238-1000
Website: www.ric.org

Spina Bifida Association

4590 MacArthur Boulevard, NW
Suite 250
Washington, DC 20007
Toll-Free: 800-621-3141
Phone: 202-944-3285
Fax: 202-944-3295
Website: www.
spinabifidaassociation.org
E-mail: sbaa@sbaa.org

United Cerebral Palsy

1660 L Street, NW, Suite 700
Washington, DC 20036
Toll-Free: 800-872-5827
Phone: 202-776-0406
Fax: 202-776-0414
Website: www.ucp.org

United Spinal Association

75-20 Astoria Boulevard
Suite 120
Jackson Heights, NY 11370
Toll-Free: 800-404-2898
Phone: 718-803-3782
Fax: 718-803-0414
Website: www.unitedspinal.org
E-mail: info@unitedspinal.org

Very Special Arts

818 Connecticut Avenue, NW
Suite 600
Washington, DC 20006
Toll-Free: 800-933-8721
Phone: 202-628-2800
TDD: 202-737-0645
Fax: 202-429-0868
Website: www.vsarts.org
E-mail: info@vsarts.org

Visiting Nurses Associations of America

900 19th Street, NW, Suite 200
Washington, DC 20006
Phone: 202-384-1420
Fax: 202-384-1444
Website: www.vnaa.org
E-mail: vnaa@vnaa.org

WE MOVE

5731 Mosholu Avenue
Bronx, NY 10471
Phone: 347-843-6132
Fax: 718-601-5112
Website: www.wemove.org
E-mail: wemove@wemove.org

Web Accessibility Initiative

MIT/CSAIL, Building 32-G530
32 Vassar Street
Cambridge, MA 02139
Phone: 617-253-2613
Website: www.w3.org/WAI
E-mail: site-comments@w3.org

Americans with Disabilities Act National Network Centers

The ADA National Network provides information, guidance, and training on the Americans with Disabilities Act (ADA), tailored to meet the needs of business, government, and individuals at local, regional, and national levels. The ADA National Network consists of 10 regional ADA National Network Centers located throughout the United States that provide personalized, local assistance to ensure that the ADA is implemented wherever possible. The ADA National Network is not an enforcement or regulatory agency, but a helpful resource supporting the ADA's mission to "make it possible for everyone with a disability to live a life of freedom and equality."

New England ADA Center
Serves Region 1 (Connecticut, Maine, Massachusetts, New Hampshire, Rhode Island, and Vermont)
Institute for Human Centered Design
180-200 Portland Street
First Floor
Boston, MA 02114
Phone: 617-695-0085
Fax: 617-482-8099
Website:
www.NewEnglandADA.org

Northeast ADA Center
Serves Region 2 (New Jersey, New York, Puerto Rico, and the U.S. Virgin Islands)
Cornell University
201 Dolgen Hall
Ithaca, NY 14853-3901
Phone: 607-225-6686
Fax: 607-255-2763
Website:
www.dbtacnortheast.org

Mid-Atlantic ADA Center
Serves Region 3 (Delaware, District of Columbia, Maryland, Pennsylvania, Virginia, and West Virginia)
TransCen, Inc.
451 Hungerford Drive
Suite 700
Rockville, MD 20850
Phone: 301-217-0124
Fax: 301-217-0754
Website: www.adainfo.org

Southeast ADA Center
Serves Region 4 (Alabama, Florida, Georgia, Kentucky, Mississippi, North Carolina, South Carolina, and Tennessee)
Project of the Burton Blatt Institute-Syracuse University
1419 Mayson Street
Atlanta, GA 30324
Phone: 404-541-9001
Fax: 404-541-9002
Website: www.sedbtac.org

Great Lakes ADA Center

Serves Region 5 (Illinois,
Indiana, Michigan, Minnesota,
Ohio, and Wisconsin)
University of Illinois/Chicago
Department on Disability and
Human Development
1640 West Roosevelt Road
Room 405
Chicago, IL 60608
Phone: 312-413-1407
Fax: 312-413-1856
Website: www.adagreatlakes.org

Southwest ADA Center

Serves Region 6 (Arkansas,
Louisiana, New Mexico,
Oklahoma, and Texas)
Independent Living Research
Utilization
2323 South Shepherd Boulevard
Suite 1000
Houston, TX 77019
Phone: 713-520-0232
Fax: 713-520-5785
Website: www.dlrp.org

Great Plains ADA Center

Serves Region 7 (Iowa, Kansas,
Missouri, and Nebraska)
University of Missouri/Columbia
100 Corporate Lake Drive
Columbia, MO 65203
Phone: 573-882-3600
Fax: 573-884-4925
Website: www.adaproject.org

Rocky Mountain ADA Center

Serves Region 8 (Colorado,
Montana, North Dakota, South
Dakota, Utah, and Wyoming)
Meeting the Challenge, Inc.
3630 Sinton Road, Suite 103
Colorado Springs, CO 80907
Phone: 719-444-0268
Fax: 719-444-0269
Website:
www.adainformation.org

Pacific ADA Center

Serves Region 9 (Arizona,
California, Hawaii, Nevada,
and the Pacific Basin)
555 12th Street, Suite 1030
Oakland, CA 94607-4046
Phone: 510-285-5600
Fax: 510-285-5614
Website: www.adapacific.org

Northwest ADA Center

Serves Region 10 (Alaska, Idaho,
Oregon, and Washington)
University of Washington
6912 220th Street SW, #105
Mountlake Terrace, WA 98043
Phone: 425-248-2480
Fax: 425-774-9303
Website:
www.dbtacnorthwest.org

Summer Camps for Children with Disabilities

Here are some resources for finding a summer camp. Some of these identify camps available to all children, and some are especially for children who have disabilities. It is also very likely that your community has summer camps or recreational opportunities available, that you won't find listed here. To find out what's available in your community, consult these local sources of information—your child's teachers, parks and/or recreation departments, area private schools, religious organizations, other community groups, parent centers, and fellow parents.

Camp List for Children with Cancer:

Candlelighters Childhood Cancer Foundation
American Childhood Cancer Organization
National Office
P.O. Box 498
Kensington, MD 20895-0498
Toll-Free: 800-366-2223
Phone: 301-962-3520
Website: www.candlelighters.org
E-mail: staff@candlelighters.org

Camps 2011–2012: A Directory of Camps and Summer Programs for Children and Youth with Disabilities and Special Needs in the Metro New York Area:

Resources for Children with Special Needs
Publications/Department B
116 East 16th Street, 5th Floor
New York, NY 10003
Phone: 212-677-4650
Website: http://www.resourcesnyc
.org/sites/default/files/Camps%20
2011-2012%20_English%20
Version_%20FINAL.pdf
E-mail: info@resourcesnyc.org

Discover Camp: Considerations for Sending Your Child with a Disability to Camp for the First Time:

National Center on Physical Activity and Disability
1640 West Roosevelt Road
Chicago, IL 60608-6904
Toll-Free: 800-900-8086 (Voice and TTY)
Website: www.ncpad.org/get/
discover/resources.html
E-mail: ncpad@uic.edu

Easter Seals Nationwide Directory of Day and Residential Camps:

Easter Seals, Inc.
National Office
223 South Wacker Drive
Suite 2400
Chicago, IL 60606
Toll-Free: 800-221-6827
Phone: 312-726-6200
TTY: 312-726-4258
Website: www.easterseals.com/
site/PageServer?pagename=ntl_
directory_camprec
E-mail: info@easterseals.com

593

Guide to Summer Camps and Summer Schools, 2010–2011 (32nd Edition):

Porter Sargent Handbooks
2 LAN Drive, Suite 100
Westford, MA 01886
Phone: 978-692-9708
Website: www.portersargent
.com/gsc.php
E-mail: info@portersargent.com

CampQuest:

National Camp Association, Inc.
610 Fifth Avenue
P.O. Box 5371
New York, NY 10185
Toll-Free: 800-966-CAMP
(966-2267)
Phone: 212-645-0653
Website: www.summercamp.org
E-mail: info@summercamp.org

Peterson's Summer Programs for Kids & Teenagers, 2009:

Available from local bookstores and Amazon: www.amazon.com / Summer-Programs-Kids-Teenagers-Lifetime / dp / 0768925525 / ref =sr_1_1?s=books&ie=UTF8&qid =1308839056&sr=1-1

Websites

American Camp Association
www.campparents.org

Association of Independent Camps
www.aiccamps.org

Brave Kids: Camps and Resources for Children with Chronic, Life-Threatening Illnesses or Disabilities
www.bravekids.org/bkpopular
-campus.aspx

Camp Channel
www.campchannel.com/campers/
search

Camps for Children with Diabetes
www.childrenwithdiabetes.com/
camps

The CampPage Summer Camps Guide
www.camppage.com

CampResource.com: Special Needs Camps
www.campresource.com/summer
-camps/special-needs-camps.cfm

Children's Hemiplegia and Stroke Association (CHASA)
www.chasa.org/summercamps.htm

Children's Oncology Camping Association International
www.cocai.org

Diabetes Education & Camping Association
www.diabetescamps.org

Grown-Up Camps
www.grownupcamps.com

Kids' Camps
www.kidscamps.com

My Summer Camps
www.mysummercamps.com/
camps/Special_Needs_Camps/
index.html

National Center on Physical Activity & Disability (NCPAD) Fun & Leisure: Camp Resources
www.ncpad.org/fun/fact_sheet
.php?sheet=88&view=all

Summer Camps for Amputees and Children with Limb Differences
www.amputee-coalition.org/fact_
sheets/Kidscamps.html

Summer Camps for Deaf and Hard of Hearing Children and Teens
www.gallaudet.edu/clerc_center/
information_and_resources/
info_to_go/resources/summer_
camps_for_deaf_and_hard_of_
hearing_children.html

Summer Camp Search
http://summercamps.com/cgi-bin/
summercamps/search.cgi

Chapter 64

Directory of Organizations for Athletes with Disabilities

Organizations That Provide Information on Multiple Sports

Adaptive Sports Center
Toll-Free: 866-349-2296
Phone: 970-349-5075
Website: www.adaptivesports.org
E-mail: info@adaptivesports.org

Disabled Sports USA
Phone: 301-217-0960
Website: www.dsusa.org
E-mail: programs@dsusa.org

National Sports Center for the Disabled (NSCD)
Phone: 970-726-1540
or 303-316-1540
Website: www.nscd.org
E-mail: info@nscd.org

Partners for Access to the Woods (PAW)
Phone: 970-887-3435
Website: www.outdoors4all.org
E-mail: Partners4all@earthlink.net

Special Olympics
Toll-Free: 800-700-8585
Phone: 202-628-3630
Website: www.specialolympics.org
E-mail: info@specialolympics.org

SPLORE (Special Populations Learning Outdoor Recreation and Education)
Phone: 801-484-4128
Website: www.splore.org
E-mail: info@splore.org

Resources in this chapter were adapted from "Directory of Athletes with Disabilities Organizations," by the American Academy of Physical Medicine and Rehabilitation (AAPMR, www.aapmr.org), 2011. All contact information was verified and updated in July 2011.

United States Association of Blind Athletes (USABA)
Phone: 719-630-0422
Website: www.usaba.org

United States Paralympic Team
Phone: 719-866-2030
Website: www.usparalympics.org
E-mail: paralympicinfo@usoc.org

USA Deaf Sports Federation (USADSF)
Phone: 605-367-5760
TTY: 605-367-5761
Website: www.usdeafsports.org
E-mail:
homeoffice@usdeafsports.org

Wheelchair & Ambulatory Sports, USA
Phone: 732-266-2634
Website: www.wsusa.org
E-mail: Office@wsusa.org

Wilderness Inquiry
Toll-Free: 800-728-0719
Phone: 612-676-9400
TTY: 612-676-9475
Website: www.wildernessinquiry
.org
E-mail: info@wildernessinquiry.org

World T.E.A.M. Sports
Phone: 855-987-8326
Website: www.worldteamsports.org
E-mail: info@worldteamsports.org

Organizations for Blind and Deaf Athletes

American Blind Bowling Association (ABBA)
Website: www.abba1951.org
E-mail: president@abba1951.org

American Blind Skiing Foundation (ABSF)
Website: www.absf.org
E-mail: absf@absf.org

National Softball Association for the Deaf
Phone: 512-444-8847
Website: www.nsad.org
E-mail: commissioner@nsad.org

Skating Athletes Bold at Heart (SABAH)
Phone: 716-362-9600
Website: www.sabahinc.org
E-mail: sabah@sabahinc.org

Ski for Light, Inc.
Phone: 612-827-3232
Website: www.sfl.org
E-mail: info@sfl.org

United States Association of Blind Athletes (USABA)
Phone: 719-630-0422
Website: www.usaba.org

United States Blind Golf Association (USBGA)
Website: www.blindgolf.com
E-mail: usbga@bellsouth.net

United States Deaf Cycling Association (USDCA)
Website: www.usdeafcycling.org

United States Deaf Ski and Snowboard Association (USDSSA)
Website: www.usdssa.org
E-mail: president@usdssa.org

United States Flag Football for the Deaf (USFFD)
Website: www.usffd.org

USA Deaf Soccer Association
Website: www.usdeafsoccer.com

USA Deaf Sports Federation (USADSF)
Phone: 605-367-5760
TTY: 605-367-5761
Website: www.usdeafsports.org
E-mail: homeoffice@usdeafsports.org

USA Deaf Track and Field
Website: www.usadtf.org
E-mail: usadtf@msn.com

Organizations That Provide Information on Specific Sports

Access to Sailing
Phone: 310-874-8629
Website: www.accesstosailing.org
E-mail: info@accesstosailing.org

Achilles International
Phone: 212-354-0300
Website: www.achillesinternational.org
E-mail: info@achillesinternational.org

American Amputee Hockey Association (AAHA)
Phone: 781-297-1393
Website: www.amputeehockey.org

American Amputee Soccer Association
Website: www.ampsoccer.org

American Wheelchair Bowling Association (AWBA)
Website: www.awba.org
E-mail: info@awba.org

Dancing Wheels
Toll-Free: 800-901-8485
Phone: 440-266-1732
Website: www.gggreg.com/DW/pages/dancingwheels.htm
E-mail: gggregagy@aol.com

Fishing Has No Boundaries, Inc.
Toll-Free: 800-243-3462
Phone: 715-634-3185
Website: www.fhnbinc.org

Freedom's Wings International (FWI)
Toll-Free: 800-382-1197
Website: www.freedomswings.org
E-mail: rrfucci@earthlink.net

Handicapped Hunting Resource Guide
Website: www.disabledhunting.net

International Wheelchair Aviators
Phone: 530-258-6709
Website:
www.wheelchairaviators.org
E-mail: dwight_leiss@yahoo.com

International Wheelchair Basketball Federation (IWBF)
Website: www.iwbf.org

National Alliance for Accessible Golf
Phone: 703-299-4296
Website: www.resourcecenter
.usga.org
E-mail: info@accessgolf.org

National Amputee Golf Association (NAGA)
Toll-Free: 800-633-6242
Website: www.nagagolf.org
E-mail: info@nagagolf.org

National Rifle Association (NRA)
Disabled Shooting Services
Phone: 703-267-1450
Website: www.nrahq.org/compete/
disabled.asp
E-mail: competitions@nrahq.org

National Shooting Sports Foundation (NSSF)
Phone: 203-426-1320
Website: www.nssf.org
E-mail: info@nssf.org

National Wheelchair Basketball Association (NWBA)
Phone: 719-266-4082
Website: www.nwba.org

National Wheelchair Poolplayers Association (NWPA)
Phone: 702-437-6792
Website: www.nwpainc.org

Professional Association of Therapeutic Horsemanship (PATH) International
Toll-Free: 800-369-RIDE
(369-7433)
Phone: 303-452-1212
Website: www.pathintl.org
E-mail: pathintl@pathintl.org

Physically Challenged Bowhunters of America, Inc. (PCBA)
Toll-Free: 855-247-7222
Website: www.pcba-inc.org

United Foundation for Disabled Archers (UFFDA)
Phone: 320-634-3660
Website: www.uffdaclub.com
E-mail: info@uffdaclub.com

United States Electric Wheelchair Hockey Association (U.S.EWHA)
Phone: 763-535-4736
Website: www.powerhockey.com
E-mail: info@powerhockey.com

United States Handcycling
Phone: 303-459-4159
Website: www.ushandcycling.org
E-mail: info@ushandcycling.org

United States Rowing
Toll-Free: 800-314-4ROW
(314-4769)
Website: www.usrowing.org
E-mail: members@usrowing.org

United States Sailing: Sailors with Special Needs
Website: www.racing.ussailing
.org/Disabled_Sailing.htm

United States Tennis Wheelchair
Website: www.usta.com

USA Swimming
Phone: 719-866-4578
Website: www.usa-swimming.org

USA Water Ski
Phone: 863-324-4341
Website: www.usawaterski.org
E-mail:
usawaterski@usawaterski.org

Chapter 65

Finding Financial Help for Assistive Devices

Some of the questions most frequently asked by amputees who contact the National Limb Loss Information Center relate to the payment coverage for costs related to prosthetic fitting and associated services, and durable medical equipment (DME) such as wheelchairs, ramps, and other adaptive equipment. The prosthetic fitting process can be very costly depending on the difficulty of the case, pathology, and analogous components used—foot, ankle, knee, hip, hand, elbow, etc. Many durable medical devices such as sophisticated electronic wheelchairs are also very costly, and many people can experience financial hardship when trying to obtain these and other equipment needed to maintain their independence. Before attempting to find a funding source, two basic steps should be taken to lay the groundwork:

1. **Determine what assistive device(s) you need:** Those seeking to replace old or outdated equipment such as wheelchairs or crutches need to determine the specific item needed (make, model, manufacturer, etc.) and from where it will be purchased, and then get a prescription for the device. If there

are changes in disability or ability levels, consult a therapist, physician, or rehabilitation professional to determine necessary features to accommodate them. For those who are newly disabled or in need of new prostheses, consulting with medical and rehabilitation professionals is the essential first step in the process.

2. **Gather information:** No matter where you seek assistance, organized information is important. Keeping the following documentation handy will help avoid frustration and unnecessary delays:

   - Primary disability (time of onset and cause of disability)
   - Secondary disability (time of onset and cause of secondary disability)
   - Employment history
   - Family gross income
   - Monthly expenses (rent or mortgage payments, utilities, outstanding loans and bills, medical expenses, etc.)
   - Health insurance information
   - Name, age, and relationship of dependents

Preparing a Justification Statement

Some funding sources, particularly government programs, require the applicant to prepare a justification statement before funds are actually appropriated. Public or private insurance companies usually require the expected beneficiary, a physician, or a therapist to submit a statement of medical necessity for the purchase. State vocational rehabilitation agencies normally require that applicants demonstrate that the service or technology will enhance their ability to prepare for, get, or keep a job. If employment is not an expected outcome, then the justification statement must show that the device will enhance the individual's independence.

Other funding sources will have their own specific requirements. Success in securing funding frequently depends on the applicant's ability to address each agency's unique requirements. Sources of financial assistance range from Medicare and other insurance to national and local nonprofit organizations. The following is an overview of some of the available resources.

Government Programs

Medicare

In the United States, Medicare is the largest financial resource for prosthetic care. In addition to prostheses, Medicare commonly covers wheelchairs (both manual and power), walkers, and crutches. Ramps, adaptive driving devices, and other nonmedical devices are not covered.

In general, those eligible for Medicare include:

- people 65 years of age and older who are eligible to receive retirement benefits from Social Security or the Railroad Retirement Board or their spouses;

- people under 65 years of age who have received Social Security or Railroad Retirement Board disability benefits for 24 months;

- people with end-stage renal disease (permanent kidney failure requiring dialysis or a transplant).

Medicare has two parts. Part A, for which most people do not have to pay, covers inpatient and outpatient hospitalization, home healthcare, some nursing home care, and hospice care. If you receive a prosthesis through one of these providers, the facility will often bill and receive payment directly from Medicare. Part B pays for professional services (physicians and other healthcare personnel), suppliers of medical devices and equipment (including artificial limbs), and certain outpatient services. If you receive prosthetic care outside of a facility setting, your prosthetist will bill Medicare Part B for you. Most people pay monthly for Part B. Note that if you do not have a Medicare supplement policy, you will be responsible for any copay (usually 20 percent) and deductible amounts. In addition, you may be responsible for the difference between the prosthetist's charge and the amount allowed by Medicare.

Obtaining SSD (Social Security Disability) Medicare Coverage

For those under age 65, the first major obstacle to obtaining Medicare coverage for assistive devices may be getting approval for Social Security Disability (SSD) benefits. Approximately 70 to 75 percent of SSD applicants are denied the first time they apply. Persistence, detailed documentation of your medical history, and the help of an attorney are often the keys to receiving the benefits to which you are entitled.

In addition, most United States Congressional representatives and senators have staff caseworkers whose job is to provide assistance to their constituents who have problems with federal agencies and programs. However, these offices receive thousands of pieces of mail each week. To ensure that your correspondence receives the attention it deserves:

- consult the Blue Pages of your local telephone book or go to house.gov/writerep to determine your Congressional district by ZIP code;

- call the local office of your federal representatives to determine whether the caseworkers are located in the state or in Washington, DC;

- place an initial phone call to the caseworker to establish a relationship and develop a personal contact. However, a written letter is typically required before an office is allowed to pursue action on your behalf.

Contacting one representative's office is usually sufficient. However, if you do not receive the assistance you need from one office, try another.

When disability benefits are awarded, payment is typically made retroactive to the beginning date of either the disability itself or the medical condition that caused the disability. This retroactive date will also apply to the "waiting period" for Medicare eligibility.

L-Codes and Level II Modifiers

The L-Code system is the current method of billing Medicare for orthotic and prosthetic services. This is a unique medical billing "add-on" system, in which a base code identifies, and descriptive language explains, the basic approach taken. Various add-on codes describing multiple options in feet, knees, ankles, and other technology combines with the base code to fully describe the total services the patient is receiving and what is covered by Medicare.

Additionally, Level II, or "K-Modifiers," help organize components and amputees' access to them based on the patient's rehabilitation potential as determined by the prosthetist and ordering physician. Criteria considered for assessing the functional level include the patient's history, current condition including the status of the residual limb and the nature of other medical problems, and the patient's desire to ambulate. Classification levels are [the following]:

- K0 (Level 0): Does not have the ability or potential to ambulate or transfer safely with or without assistance, and a prosthesis does not enhance the quality of life or mobility

- K1 (Level 1): Has the ability or potential to use a prosthesis for transfers or ambulation on level surfaces at fixed cadence—typical of the limited and unlimited household walker

- K2 (Level 2): Has the ability or potential for ambulation with the ability to traverse low-level environmental barriers such as curbs, stairs, or uneven surfaces—typical of the limited community walker

- K3 (Level 3): Has the ability or potential for walking with variable cadence—typical of the community walker who is able to traverse most environmental barriers and may have vocational, therapeutic, or exercise activity that demands prosthetic use beyond simple walking

- K4 (Level 4): Has the ability or potential for prosthetic use that exceeds basic walking skills, exhibiting high impact, stress, or energy levels—typical of the prosthetic demands of the child, active adult, or athlete.

The following determination of coverage for selected prostheses and components with respect to potential functional levels represents the usual case. Exceptions are considered in individual cases if additional documentation is included that justifies the medical necessity. Prostheses are denied as not medically necessary if the patient's potential functional level is "0."

Feet

- Basic lower-limb prostheses include a solid-ankle-cushion-heel (SACH) foot.

- External keel, SACH foot, or single-axis ankle/foot are covered for patients with a functional Level 1 or above.

- Flexible-keel foot and multiaxial ankle/foot candidates are expected to demonstrate a functional Level 2 or greater functional needs.

- Flex-foot system, energy-storing foot, multiaxial ankle/foot, dynamic response, or flex-walk system or equal are covered for patients with a functional Level 3 or above.

Knees

- Basic lower-limb prostheses include a single-axis, constant friction knee.

- Fluid and pneumatic knees are covered for patients with a functional Level 3 or above.

- Other knee systems are covered for patients with a functional Level 1 or above.

Ankles

- Axial rotation units are covered for patients with a functional Level 2 or above.

The following are general policies regarding coverage of prosthetic sockets:

- Test (diagnostic) sockets for "immediate prostheses" are not medically necessary.

- No more than two test sockets for an individual prosthesis are medically necessary without additional documentation.

- No more than two of the same socket inserts are allowed per individual prosthesis at the same time.

- Socket replacements are considered medically necessary if there is adequate documentation of functional or physiological need. The Durable Medical Equipment Regional Carrier (DMERC) recognizes that there are situations where the explanation includes but is not limited to changes in the residual limb, functional need changes, or irreparable damage or wear/tear due to excessive patient weight or prosthetic demands of very active amputees.

When Your Claim Is Denied

If your Medicare claim is denied, it is important to understand why and what options you have. Reasons for denial of claims for durable medical equipment (DME) and prosthetic devices usually fall into five categories:

1. **Lack of medical necessity:** If your claim was denied for this reason, you should appeal the denial. The appeals process must be initiated within 6 months of the processing date of Remittance Advice. There are five levels of appeal:

a. Review: The appeals process is begun by submitting a HCFA [Health Care Financing Administration] 1964 form or a written letter of request. Any additional information, along with all the originals, will be examined by a reviewer who did not participate in the initial decision.

b. Fair Hearing: If the original decision is upheld and your case is valued at $100 or more, you may submit, in writing, a request for a Fair Hearing within 120 days of the Review decision. You can request that the hearing be conducted in person or by phone. A date and hearing officer is assigned to the claim. Before the hearing date, the officer will conduct an "on the record" review of the case and any supporting documentation. The officer has the authority to conclude the case at this point or, if the review is not favorable, the scheduled hearing will be conducted.

c. Administrative Law Judge: Claims denied in the Fair Hearing and valued over $500 can proceed to this level. The request must be submitted in writing within 60 days of the Fair Hearing decision.

d. Appeals Council and Judicial Review: Claims must be valued over $1000 to be eligible for these levels, and each requires filing within 60 days of the previous decision. Claims that are denied in review and do not meet the dollar limit for the next level have no further appeal options.

e. Each appeal level will put your claim before an entirely new set of people. While you may submit additional documentation at any level, it is important that you do not delete any previously submitted material. It is also in your best interest to personally verify that all previously reviewed information is transferred to the next level.

2. **Non-Covered Services:** Medicare has excluded these items from its list of covered services. No appeals process is available.

3. **Incomplete Information:** Many claims are returned for missing information. The reason code on your Remittance Advice form will not identify what is missing, so you will need to pay very close attention to each detail to ensure that nothing is overlooked. Not Otherwise Specified (NOS) coding, used when a service is provided that cannot be described with an existing code, is another cause of claim denials. Adequate documentation

must be included with these codes so that Medicare can determine the appropriateness and reimbursement level for the procedure or device.

4. **Duplicate Submission:** Claims denied for this reason should be investigated immediately. Contact Medicare to determine why this reason was given. If the claim was indeed resubmitted, find out what happened to the original claim.

5. **Not Separately Payable:** Claims denied because the service was considered to be included in another code usually cannot be appealed. If you feel the interpretation is incorrect, you may present the case to your ombudsman, whose job is to assist you with difficult cases.

Your primary source of assistance with appeals and resubmission of denied claims will be your provider's administrative staff. It is in your best interest to have them do this for you. If necessary, you may want to ask them to do so. In order to provide this service for you, your provider will need your signature authorizing his staff to represent you in any needed claims review.

If you have questions about Social Security, call toll-free at 800-772-1213 or visit their local office search at https://secure.ssa.gov/apps6z/FOLO/fo001.jsp.

Medicaid

Medicaid is a jointly funded, cooperative venture between the federal and state governments to assist states in providing adequate medical care to eligible individuals. Within broad national guidelines that the federal government provides, each of the states:

- establishes its own eligibility standards;
- determines the type, amount, duration, and scope of services;
- sets the rate of payment for services;
- administers its own program.

Thus, Medicaid eligibility and covered services vary considerably from state to state, as well as within each state over time. Unfortunately, coverage for prosthetic care is not mandated, and therefore ranges from reasonably good to nonexistent.

To be eligible for federal funds, states must provide Medicaid coverage for most individuals who receive federally assisted income maintenance payments, as well as for related groups not receiving cash payments. Some examples of the mandatory Medicaid eligibility groups are:

- low-income families with children;

- Supplemental Security Income (SSI) recipients;

- infants born to Medicaid-eligible pregnant women;

- children under age 6 and pregnant women whose family income is at or below 133 percent of the Federal poverty level (states are required to extend Medicaid eligibility until age 19 to all children born after September 30, 1983);

- recipients of adoption assistance and foster care;

- certain Medicare beneficiaries;

- special protected groups who may keep Medicaid for a period of time, including people who lose SSI payments due to earnings from work or increased Social Security benefits; and families who are provided 6 to 12 months of Medicaid coverage following loss of eligibility under Section 1931 due to earnings, or 4 months of Medicaid coverage following loss of eligibility under Section 1931 due to an increase in child or spousal support.

For people who may have too much income to meet the mandatory eligibility requirements or those adopted by their state, many states have a "medically needy" program. This option allows them to "spend down" to Medicaid eligibility by incurring medical and/or remedial care expenses to offset their excess income, or by paying monthly premiums to the state in an amount equal to the difference between family income and the eligibility standard.

For information about your state's version of the Medicaid program, contact your state's administering agency, usually the Department of Human Health and Social Services, the Department of Human Services, or the Department of Medical Assistance. Phone numbers for these agencies can be found in the Blue Pages of your telephone directory. You may also want to visit cms.hhs.gov/RegionalOffices for a regional listing of Medicaid offices.

Help to Pay Your Healthcare Costs

Most of your healthcare costs are covered if you have Medicare and you qualify for Medicaid. States also have programs that pay some or all of Medicare's premiums and may also pay Medicare deductibles and coinsurance for certain people who have Medicare and a low income. To qualify, you must have:

- Part A (Hospital Insurance);

- assets such as bank accounts, stocks, and bonds that are not more than $4,000 for a single person, or $6,000 for a couple;

- a monthly income that is below certain limits.

There are also prescription drug assistance programs available. These programs offer discounts or free medications to individuals in need. For more information on these programs, call your nearest medical assistance office. You can find the number in the phone book under Medicaid, Social Services, Medical Assistance, Human Services, or Community Services. Or you can call the Medicare information line at 800-633-4227; a Medicare customer service representative can help you find the right office in your state.

Veterans Administration

The Veterans Health Administration (VHA) provides a broad spectrum of rehabilitative care to its beneficiaries, including a fairly wide array of prostheses, mobility devices such as wheelchairs, and adaptive driving equipment. In addition to coverage for veterans themselves, the VA provides needed healthcare benefits, including prosthetic devices, medical equipment, and supplies to certain children of Vietnam veterans (i.e., children suffering from spina bifida or an associated disability). Veterans may also receive VA healthcare benefits including prosthetics and medical equipment through participation in the VA's vocational rehabilitation program. Veterans outside of the United States, with certain exceptions, are only eligible for prosthetics, medical equipment, and supplies for a service-connected disability.

In order to be eligible for enrollment for healthcare, you must have:

- been discharged from active military service under honorable conditions;

- served a minimum of 2 years if discharged after September 7, 1980 (prior to this date, there is no time limit);

- served as a National Guard member or reservist for the entire period for which you were called to active duty, other than for training purposes only.

VA healthcare enrollment is a new system providing access to a comprehensive package of services. If you want to use the VA healthcare system, you must fill out the VA form 10-10EZ unless:

- the VA rates you as having a service-connected disability of 50 percent or more;

- it has been less than 1 year since you were discharged from military service for a disability that the military determined was incurred or aggravated in the line of duty, and have not yet been rated by VA;

- you are seeking care from VA for a service-connected disability only.

The 10-10EZ form may be obtained by visiting, calling, or writing any VA healthcare facility or veterans' benefits office, or by calling toll-free 877-222-8387. You can also access the form on the internet at www.va.gov/vaforms.

The form should be forwarded to your nearest VA healthcare facility for processing. Once you apply for enrollment and your application eligibility is verified, you will be assigned a priority group (ranging from 1 to 7, with 1 being the highest priority for enrollment) based on your specific eligibility status. Enrollment will be reviewed and renewed each year depending upon your priority group and available resources. If sufficient funding is not available for the VA to renew enrollment for your priority group for another year, you will be notified in writing before your enrollment period expires. Under the Uniform Benefits Package, the same services are generally available to all enrolled veterans, including treatment for both service-connected and non-service-connected disabilities.

Artificial limbs must be prescribed by a designated physician/podiatrist of the VA's Amputee Clinic Team or the prosthetic representative. Devices may then be fabricated and fitted by VA hospitals or clinics, private prosthetic facilities on contract with the VA, or, under certain circumstances, by non-contract prosthetists. While the VA prefers that patients use either VA facilities or private facilities under contract with the VA, veterans who have previously received artificial limbs from commercial sources may continue to receive services from their non-contract prosthetist, providing the prosthetist will accept the VA preferred provider rate for the geographic area. Veterans may also receive services from non-contract vendors when a prescribed limb or component is not available through VA or contract facilities.

Recreational artificial limbs, which allow an amputee to participate in a specific recreational or athletic activity, may be provided. The following are general guidelines regarding the issue of recreational prosthetic appliances:

- The physician or podiatrist of the Amputee Clinic Team must prescribe the prosthesis.

- The prescription must indicate the therapeutic, rehabilitative, or psychological benefit to be expected or achieved through participation in this specialized activity. The prescription must indicate that a conventional prosthesis that is worn daily is unsuitable for use in the recreational activity, either because of environmental factors that would affect the prosthesis or because a specialized function not available in the conventional limb is required in the activity.

For more information, call the VA Health Benefits Service Center toll-free at 877-222-8387 or visit the VA Website at www.va.gov/health.

TRICARE

TRICARE is the Department of Defense's worldwide healthcare program for active duty and retired uniformed service members and their families. TRICARE options include TRICARE Prime, a managed care option; TRICARE Extra, a preferred provider option; and TRICARE Standard (the old CHAMPUS program), a fee-for-service option. TRICARE for Life is also available for Medicare-eligible beneficiaries age 65 and over.

Eligible family members include:

- spouses and unmarried children, including stepchildren;

- those under age 21 (age 23 if full-time student) of active and retired service members;

- un-remarried spouses and unmarried children of deceased service members;

- spouses and unmarried children of reservists and retired reservists;

- Medal of Honor recipients and their family members;

- former spouses of active duty or retired service members, under certain circumstances.

Dependent parents and parents-in-law are only eligible for TRI-CARE Plus, a local military treatment facility (MTF)-based primary care enrollment program that may provide coverage for primary care services. They are also eligible for the Senior Pharmacy Program if they meet all of the requirements. The following is a brief overview of the available TRICARE programs.

TRICARE Prime is similar to a health maintenance organization (HMO). Prime enrollees choose a Primary Care Manager (PCM). The PCM becomes the beneficiary's primary physician for the duration of his or her enrollment in the program unless changed by the beneficiary by contacting a Beneficiary Service Representative at your TRICARE Service Center. Military retirees and their dependents pay an annual enrollment fee of $230 for an individual or $460 for a family. Active duty family members enroll for free. Active duty service members must enroll in Prime. Active duty family members, retirees, and their family members are encouraged, but not required, to enroll in Prime.

TRICARE Prime offers several benefits:

- No enrollment fees, deductibles, or co-payments for active duty members and their families

- $230 enrollment fee ($460 for families) and minimal copayments for retirees

- Limits on appointment wait time

- Limits on driving time from home to obtain care

- Limit on office waiting time of 30 minutes for non-emergency situations

Prime also offers a "point-of-service" option for care received outside the TRICARE Prime network; however, receiving care from a nonparticipating provider is not encouraged.

Members whose permanent duty assignment (and residence) is 50 miles or more from an MTF or other sources of military healthcare are eligible for TRICARE Prime Remote (TPR). TPR provides no-cost healthcare for active duty members. A new interim Waived Charges benefit for family members dispenses with out-of-pocket expenses. TPR is only available in the United States.

TRICARE Extra and TRICARE Standard are ideal for individuals who prefer greater flexibility in physician choice, since beneficiaries do not have to select a Primary Care Manager (PCM) physician and can be seen by any TRICARE authorized provider. No enrollment fees or forms are required for TRICARE Extra or Standard. Beneficiaries are responsible for annual deductibles and cost-shares. Deductibles are $50 or $100 per year for individuals and $150 or $300 for families, depending on the service member's grade. Maximum out-of-pocket expense is $3,000 per enrollment or fiscal year.

TRICARE Extra is a preferred provider option (PPO) in which beneficiaries choose medical providers within the TRICARE provider network. TRICARE Standard is a fee-for-service option, which allows you to see an authorized provider of your choice. People who are happy with service from a current civilian provider often choose this option. However, cost-shares are 5 percent more plus the difference between the TRICARE allowable charge and the doctor's billed charge.

TRICARE For Life (TFL) is for beneficiaries who have become eligible for Medicare. These beneficiaries are ineligible for TRICARE Prime but are eligible to use network and non-network providers under TRICARE Extra and Standard. There are no enrollment fees for TRICARE For Life. You are required to enroll in Medicare Part B and must pay Medicare Part B monthly fees. Enrollees also pay cost-shares for services not payable by Medicare.

The following groups are eligible to enroll in TFL:

- Medicare-eligible uniformed service retirees, including retired National Guard members and reservists

- Medicare-eligible family members, including widows/widowers

- Certain former spouses if they were eligible for TRICARE before age 65

The Continued Health Care Benefit Program (CHCBP) temporarily provides the same benefits as TRICARE Standard for military personnel who are discharged or released from active duty (under other than adverse conditions). Family members, emancipated children, and, in some cases, former spouses who have not remarried are also eligible. CHCBP coverage is available for 18 months. An unmarried dependent child or a former spouse who has not remarried may be eligible for coverage for 36 months. Typically, you must enroll during the 60-day period that begins at the time of discharge or loss of eligibility for care under the Military Health Services System in order to receive benefits. The premiums for this coverage are $933 per quarter for individuals and $1,996 per quarter for families. The CHCBP benefits are comparable to the TRICARE Standard benefit, which covers a majority of medical conditions, uses existing TRICARE providers, and follows most of the rules and procedures of TRICARE Standard. For more information about this program, you can visit www.humana-military.com/chcbp/main.htm or contact:

Humana Military Healthcare Services, Inc.

Attn: CHCBP
P.O. Box 740072
Louisville, KY 40201-7462
Toll-Free: 800-444-5445

For more information regarding any of the TRICARE programs, contact your TRICARE Service Center or visit the military's TRICARE Web page at www.tricare.mil or Palmetto Government Benefits Administrators' TRICARE page at www.mytricare.com.

Vocational Rehabilitation

Most states have vocational rehabilitation programs that provide assistance to people with limb loss or other disabilities in obtaining and keeping employment; or if a prosthesis or other adaptive device is designated as a daily living aid. These programs vary widely from state to state as to eligibility requirements and services. Some may fund prosthetic care if it is determined to be necessary for employment, or if the device allows for greater independence. Assistive devices such as wheelchairs, lifts, and adaptive driving equipment are often furnished to enable a person to get to the job site. Devices necessary for job performance also are usually provided.

The telephone number for your state's vocational rehabilitation office can be found in the Blue Pages of your local directory. You may also want to perform an internet search for contact information and links to your state vocational rehabilitation agency's website, which should provide an overview of their services. You can also locate your state's vocational rehabilitation program information by accessing the following website: askjan.org/cgi-win/typequery.exe?902.

State Technology Assistance Projects

This program, originally funded under the Technology-Related Assistance for Individuals with Disabilities Act of 1988, supports statewide, comprehensive, technology-related assistance for individuals of all ages with disabilities. State projects typically provide assistance in choosing and acquiring equipment, whether acquired commercially off the shelf, modified or customized, that is used to increase, maintain, or improve functional capabilities of individuals with disabilities. Each state, within federal guidelines, determines what services it provides. Some services frequently provided are:

• information and referral;

- product demonstration;
- equipment recycling and loan programs;
- device modification;
- low-interest loan programs;
- advocacy in obtaining funding for devices.

A few states' programs provide direct financial assistance to individuals in need of various types of adaptive equipment, including prostheses, and some have loan programs; others provide no funding at all to individuals. Most do have information and referral services, and may be able to direct you to local sources of financial assistance for which you qualify. The telephone number for your state's program may be found in the Blue Pages of your local directory. A listing of state assistive technology projects, complete with contact information and links to Web pages, may be found on the Rehabilitation Engineering and Assistive Technology Society of North America (RESNA) Web site at www.resna.org.

Protection and Advocacy (P&A)/Client Assistance Program (CAP)

In an effort to address public outcry in response to the abuse, neglect, and lack of programming in institutions for people with disabilities, Congress created a system in each state and territory that provides protection of the rights of people with disabilities through legally based advocacy. The governor in each state designated an agency to be the Protection & Advocacy (P&A) system and provided assurance that the system was and would remain independent of any service provider. This federally mandated system includes several programs. Those most likely to be of assistance to people with limb loss are:

- The Protection and Advocacy for Individual Rights (PAIR) Program: Established to protect and advocate for the legal and human rights of all people with disabilities;

- The Protection & Advocacy for Assistive Technology (PAAT) Program: Created to assist individuals with disabilities and their family members, guardians, advocates, and authorized representatives in accessing technology devices and assistive technology services through case management, legal representation, and self-advocacy training.

The Client Assistance Program (CAP) was established by 1984 Amendments to the Rehabilitation Act as a condition for receiving allotments under Section 110. CAP services include assistance in pursuing administrative, legal, and other appropriate remedies to ensure the protection of people receiving or seeking services under the Rehabilitation Act.

If you have received unsatisfactory services or have been denied services to which you believe you are entitled under federally funded programs, your state's P&A or CAP should provide assistance. Telephone listings for these agencies may not be available in your local directory. Call the Rehabilitation Services Administration at 202-245-7488 or visit their website at www.ed.gov/about/offices/list/osers/rsa.

Private Insurance

Coverage for prosthetic care and DME varies widely from one insurance company to another and can also differ with various policies offered by a given company. Coverage can range from all medically necessary devices for life to no coverage at all. While it is impossible to provide specific information about the many health insurance companies currently in business, there are some basic things to consider when selecting an insurance policy. You should ask about:

- eligibility requirements;
- preexisting condition clauses;
- devices that are covered (get something in writing to ensure that artificial limbs are covered);
- coverage limits;
- limits on the number of items per year or per lifetime;
- the rate of payment (should be at least comparable to Medicare rates);
- the Preferred Provider Network (is your current prosthetist included?).

The Georgetown University Health Policy Institute provides Health-InsuranceInfo.net, with information on insurance regulations for every state (www.healthinsuranceinfo.net).

Many health insurance companies have their own websites that offer specific information about their policies. In addition, there are several websites that inform consumers and help them compare health insurance companies and policies. Some of these are:

- www.insure.com/health;
- www.insweb.com;
- www.netquote.com.

Insurance Problems

If you have problems getting the coverage to which you are entitled from your insurance company, the most valuable source of assistance is your state department of insurance. This office is located in the capital city of each state and the telephone number should be in the Blue Pages of your local directory. Insurance commissioners can take action against insurance companies, agents, and brokers. They are empowered to conduct investigations, acquire records relevant to your case, issue orders, hold hearings, and suspend and revoke licenses. Contact information for your state's department of insurance may also be found on the National Association of Insurance Commissioners Web site at www.naic.org/state_web_map.htm.

Medical Discount Programs

Medical discount programs are relatively new on the healthcare scene. These companies negotiate with PPO providers for their members to receive discounts on medical goods and services ranging from prescription drugs to office visits to nursing home care. While DME is often included in the benefits packages provided in the programs, prosthetic care is not usually specifically mentioned.

The programs' advantages to the provider are immediate payment, less paperwork, and no "red tape" in getting approval for services provided. Advantages to the patient are discounted medical fees, no deductibles and no preexisting condition clauses, unlimited use of services, no claim forms to fill out, and relatively low "premiums" or fees.

Most of the companies stress that this is not insurance and should not replace existing insurance. However, for those who are uninsurable or cannot afford insurance coverage, this may be an alternative worth investigating. Since all of these companies are relatively new and have not established an extensive track record, it would be wise to thoroughly check out any company before making a commitment. Read all the fine print, make sure all of your questions are answered to your satisfaction, and consider consulting the Better Business Bureau to see if complaints have been registered.

Nonprofit Organizations

The following organizations provide assistance to people who otherwise are unable to afford prosthetic care. Some provide other services as well. Each organization has its own method of providing services and requirements for eligibility. If you do not qualify for one program, you may be eligible for another, so don't give up.

Barr Foundation
136 NE Olive Way
Boca Raton, FL 33432
Phone: 561-391-7601
Website: www.oandp.com/resources/organizations/barr
E-mail: t-barr@t-barr.com

This fund pays for materials and fitting of a new prosthesis after the prosthetist has established that there are no other sources of funding available. The Barr Foundation also accepts used prosthetic devices. Please call the Barr Foundation for further information.

Bowman Limb Bank Foundation
100 Spanish Oak Road
Weatherford, TX 76087
Phone: 817-597-1826
Website: www.danabowman.com/bank_foundation.php
E-mail: danabowman@aol.com

The Bowman Limb Bank Foundation acts as a ready resource for artificial limbs for those in need. It is a nonprofit organization seeking to fulfill the need for artificial limbs in underdeveloped nations and here in the United States where traditional funding is unavailable.

Challenged Athletes Foundation
9591 Waples Street
San Diego, CA 92121
Phone: 858-866-0959
Website: www.challengedathletes.org
E-mail: caf@challengedathletes.org

The Challenged Athletes Foundation raises money to help people with physical disabilities pursue an active lifestyle through physical fitness and competitive athletics.

Limbs for Life Foundation
218 E. Main Street
Oklahoma City, OK 73104
Toll-Free: 888-235-5462
Phone: 405-843-5174
Website: www.limbsforlife.org
E-mail: admin@limbsforlife.org

Each qualified applicant will be provided with partial or complete funding for an advanced prosthesis, fitted by a highly qualified prosthetist.

Limbs of Love
1000 S Loop West, Suite 150
Houston, TX 77054
Phone: 713-747-7647
Website: www.limbsoflove.com

Limbs of Love uses the time, skills, and resources of medical professionals and manufacturers who receive no remuneration in an effort to improve the overall quality of life for amputees, primarily in Texas.

National Amputation Foundation
40 Church Street
Malverne, NY 11565
Phone: 516-887-3600
Website: www.nationalamputation.org
E-mail: amps76@aol.com

The National Amputation Foundation (NAF) has for over 80 years been offering valuable assistance to veterans of World War I, II, Korea, the Vietnam Conflict, Desert Storm, and Iraqi Freedom. Since then, the Foundation has expanded its facilities to include civilian amputees as well.

Local Service Clubs

Lions, Rotary, Elks, Shriners, or any other fraternity or special interest groups in your community could provide dollars or assistance in fundraising. Please contact the respective organization for further information.

Children's Services

Programs for Children with Special Healthcare Needs

In 1988, then-Surgeon General Dr. C. Everett Koop introduced a National Agenda for Children with Special Health Care Needs (CSHCN).

In 1989, this agenda was translated into legislation through Title V of the Social Security Act, which requires state CSHCN programs to provide and promote family-centered, community-based, coordinated care for children with special healthcare needs and to facilitate the development of community-based systems of services for such children and their families.

Each state has a Title V CSHCN program administered through the Department of Health and Human Services by agencies called Children's Special Needs Services, Children's Medical Services, or similar names. Under the Title V legislation, children with special healthcare needs include all children who have or are at increased risk for chronic physical, developmental, behavioral, or emotional conditions, and who also require health and related services of a type or amount beyond that generally required by children. A directory of state Title V CSHCN programs, along with information regarding eligibility and services is available online at https://perfdata.hrsa .gov/mchb/TVISReports.

State Children's Insurance Program

The State Children's Health Insurance Program (SCHIP) is the largest expansion of health insurance coverage for children in over 30 years. SCHIP enables states to insure children at little or no cost to working families with incomes too high to qualify for Medicaid, but too low to afford private coverage. The initiative is a partnership between the federal and state governments that will help provide children with the health coverage they need to grow up healthy and strong. You can get information about this program by calling 877-543-7669 or by visiting www.insurekidsnow.gov.

Administration for Children and Families (ACF)

The Administration for Children and Families (ACF), within the Department of Health and Human Services (DHHS), is responsible for federal programs that promote the economic and social well-being of families, children, individuals, and communities. Among these is the Temporary Assistance for Needy Families (TANF) program, which replaced the Aid to Families with Dependent Children and the Job Opportunities and Basic Skills Training programs. States, territories, and tribes determine eligibility and benefit levels and services provided to needy families. For more information on ACF programs, contact your DHHS office or visit the ACF website at www.acf.hhs.gov.

Shriners Hospital

Shriners Hospitals for Children, a network of hospitals that provide expert, free orthopedic and burn care to children under 18, is the Shrine of North America's official philanthropy. Shriners Hospitals are open to all children without regard to race, religion, or relationship to a Shriner. Any child may be eligible for care at Shriners Hospitals if:

- the child is under the age of 18;

- there is a reasonable possibility the child's condition can be helped.

The service area of Shriners Hospitals includes the United States, Canada, and Mexico. Special procedures must be followed for those applying from outside one of these countries.

Application forms for admission to Shriners Hospitals may be obtained:

- from any Shrine Temple or Shrine Club;

- by calling the Shriners Hospitals toll-free referral line at 800-237-5055;

- from the Shriners website at www.shrinershospitalsforchildren. org/en/ReferAPatient.aspx.

St. Jude Children's Hospital

Children may receive prosthetic care at St. Jude's in conjunction with treatment of a catastrophic illness such as osteosarcoma. Acceptance for treatment is based solely on a patient's eligibility for an ongoing clinical trial at St. Jude Children's Research Hospital. To determine if your child is eligible, your child's physician must:

- call the referral line at 888-226-4343 (emergencies: 800-349-4334);

- fax relevant information to 901/495-4011;

- complete a referral online at hospital.stjude.org/apps/hospital forms/fb/physicianReferral.

Blue Cross/Blue Shield

Some Blue Cross/Blue Shield companies have established "Caring for Children Foundations" that provide free or low cost coverage to children who are not insurable through Medicaid or private insurance.

Some of these foundations work with the SCHIP programs in their states. Others work independently and accept no government funding. Services and eligibility requirements vary. Call your local Blue Cross/ Blue Shield office or visit the national website at www.bcbs.com to find out if such a program exists in your area.

Variety: The Children's Charity of the United States

Variety bills itself as the largest children's charity in the world, with 51 chapters in 13 countries. Dedicated to improving the quality of life of children who are less fortunate than others, the traditions of Variety are rooted in show business and the circus. The members, largely drawn from the world of entertainment, leisure, media and business, work to assist children who may be sick, handicapped, or disadvantaged by social circumstances. For more information, contact:

Variety of the United States
5757 Wilshire Boulevard, Suite 445
Los Angeles, CA 90036
Phone: 323-954-0820
Website: www.usvariety.org
E-mail: info@usvariety.org

Other Information Sources

AgrAbility Project

The AgrAbility Project assists agricultural and agribusiness workers who have physical and mental disabilities, including such disabilities as amputation, arthritis, spinal cord injury, and hearing impairments. Easter Seals and the University of Wisconsin administer a national program of education, outreach, and technical assistance to farmers with disabilities. State AgrAbility projects are a partnership between nonprofit disability service providers and the state U.S. Department of Agriculture (USDA) extension services. Staff from the state projects work with individual farmers and farm families to assess farm buildings and equipment to make recommendations on modifications that can help farmers with disabilities remain safely on the farm and help them find solutions to financing these modifications. To find out if your state has an AgrAbility program, call your local Easter Seals office or the National AgrAbility Project, toll-free, at 866-259-6280. See the website at fyi.uwex.edu/agrability.

Area Agencies on Aging

Area Agencies on Aging (AAAs) provide many services to enable seniors to continue living independently in their homes, including information and referral, insurance counseling, and care management. By making a range of options available, AAAs make it possible for seniors to choose the services and living arrangement that suit them best. You can find your local AAA in the White Pages of your telephone directory or call the toll-free Eldercare Locator at 800-677-1116. This service is funded by the U.S. Administration on Aging and administered in cooperation with the National Association of State Units on Aging. Individuals calling this service have access to over 4,800 state and local information and referral service providers, identified for every ZIP code in the country. The database also includes special purpose information and referral telephone numbers for Alzheimer's hotlines, adult day care and respite services, nursing home ombudsman assistance, consumer fraud, in-home care complaints, legal services, elder abuse/protective services, Medicare/Medicaid/Medigap information, tax assistance, and transportation.

National Association of Area Agencies on Aging
Website: www.n4a.org

Eldercare Locator
Website: www.eldercare.gov/Eldercare.NET

Independent Living Centers

Independent Living Centers (ILCs) are typically nonresidential, private, nonprofit, consumer-controlled, community-based organizations providing services and advocacy by and for people with all types of disabilities. Their purpose is to assist individuals with disabilities to achieve their maximum potential within their families and communities. ILCs are also good sources of information and referral. A listing of ILCs by state is available online at www.ilru.org/html/publications/directory. You may also call their information line at 713-520-0232, ext. 130.

Index

Index

Page numbers followed by 'n' indicate a footnote. Page numbers in *italics* indicate a table or illustration.

A

AAFP *see* American Academy of Family Physicians
AAPMR *see* American Academy of Physical Medicine and Rehabilitation
AARP, contact information 582
AbilityJobs, contact information 582
"Abuse of Children with Intellectual Disabilities" (Davis) 48n
ACB Radio, website address 275
access, defined 573
accessibility, defined 573
Access Living, housing publication 502n
Access Media Group LLC, publications computer users 282n
low vision 268n
Access to Sailing, contact information 599
Access World, website address 273, 276
accommodations
air travel 311–13
students 475–80
see also reasonable accommodations

accreditation
occupational therapists 289
physical therapists 291
Achilles International, contact information 599
acoustics, hearing assistance 250
acquired apraxia 124–25
activities of daily living (ADL)
defined 573
intellectual disabilities 232–33
statistics 12
ADA *see* Americans with Disabilities Act
"ADA Home" (Americans with Disabilities Act National Network) 577n
A.D.A.M., Inc., pressure sores publication 377n
"Adapting Motor Vehicles for People with Disabilities" (NHTSA) 306n
Adaptive Environments Center, contact information 582
Adaptive Sports Center, contact information 597
adaptive switches, described 207
addiction disorders, described 167

ADHD *see* attention deficit
hyperactivity disorder
ADL *see* activities of daily living
Administration for Children and
Families (ACF) 523
Administration on Aging (AOA)
contact information 577
publications
assistive technology 207n
older Americans 23n
Administration on Developmental
Disabilities (ADD), contact
information 577
adult day care
checklist 323–24
defined 573
described 425
overview 327–30
respite care 318
"Adult Day Care: One Form of
Respite for Older Adults"
(ARCH National Respite Network
and Resource Center) 327n
adult foster homes,
described 425–26
advance directives,
overview 548–57, 551–54
advance health care directive,
defined 573
affective disorders, described 167
Affordable Care Act
disabled Americans 392–94
insurance coverage 390–92
"Affordable Care Act for Americans
with Disabilities" (DHHS) 392n
age factor
disabilities 23–25
disability statistics *9, 10*
hearing loss 98–99
Agency for Healthcare Research
and Quality (AHRQ), contact
information 578
age-related macular degeneration
(AMD), described 103–4
AgingCare, LLC, bathing guidelines
publication 365n
AgrAbility Project 625
Air Carrier Access Act 491
air travel, accommodation 311–13

alcohol-related birth defects
(ARBD), described 131
alcohol-related neurodevelopmental
disorder (ARND), described 131
alcohol use
fetal alcohol
spectrum disorders 130–31
pain management 384
Alliance for Technology Access
(ATA), contact information 234
ALS *see* amyotrophic
lateral sclerosis
Alzheimer, Alois 170
Alzheimer care units, described 426
Alzheimer disease
bathing tips 365–67
overview 170–71
Alzheimer's Association
contact information 582
respite care guide
publication 316n
"Alzheimer's Disease Fact
Sheet" (NIA) 170n
Alzheimer's Foundation of America,
contact information 583
American Academy of Family
Physicians (AAFP)
contact information 583
inborn errors of metabolism
publication 81n
American Academy of Physical
Medicine and Rehabilitation
(AAPMR)
contact information 583
organizations directory
publication 597n
American Amputee Hockey
Association (AAHA), contact
information 599
American Amputee Soccer
Association, website address 599
American Blind Bowling Association
(ABBA), contact information 598
American Blind Skiing Foundation
(ABSF), contact information 598
American Camp Association,
website address 594
American Council of the Blind,
contact information 583

American Foundation for the Blind
contact information 583
publications
braille 277n
reading, vision loss 270n
American Geriatrics Society,
rehabilitation publication 407n
American Geriatrics Society
Foundation for Health in Aging,
contact information 583
American Health
Assistance Foundation,
contact information 583
American Heart Association,
contact information 583
American Medical Association
(AMA), contact information 584
American Parkinson Disease
Association, contact information 584
American Printing House for the
Blind, contact information 584
American Psychiatric Association,
contact information 584
American Psychological Association,
contact information 584
American Recovery and
Reinvestment Act (ARRA) 400
American Society on Aging,
contact information 584
American Speech-Language-Hearing
Association (ASHA)
contact information 584
publications
augmentative and alternative
communication 260n
hearing assistive
technology 249n
"Americans With Disabilities, 2005"
(US Census Bureau) 7n
Americans with Disabilities
Act (ADA; 1990)
captions 240
caregivers 32
described 7
dyslexia 142
home modifications 226
housing 510
overview 487–90, 495–99
service animals 301

Americans with Disabilities Act
National Network
network centers
contact information 591–92
network centers publication 577n
"Americans with Disabilities Act:
Questions and Answers"
(EEOC) 495n
American Wheelchair Bowling
Association (AWBA), contact
information 599
amnesia, traumatic brain injury 202
amputations
overview 190–92
rehabilitation 413–15
Amputee Coalition
contact information 192, 584
publications
financial assistance 603n
limb loss 190n
amyotrophic lateral sclerosis (ALS),
overview 172–74
Amyotrophic Lateral Sclerosis
Association, contact information 585
"Amyotrophic Lateral Sclerosis Fact
Sheet" (NINDS) 172n
analgesic medications, pain
management 381–82
antidepressant medications,
pain management 381–82
anxiety disorders
coping strategies 385–88
described 167
AOA *see* Administration on Aging
"Aphasia" (NIDCD) 122n
aphasia, overview 122–23
see also speech disorders
appointment of health care agent 549
apraxia, overview 124–25
see also speech disorders
"Apraxia of Speech" (NIDCD) 124n
The Arc
contact information 585
technology, intellectual
disabilities publication 231n
Architectural Barriers Act (ABA) 494
ARCH National Respite Network and
Resource Center, adult day care
publication 327n

Area Agencies on Aging
  described 626
  home modifications 229
arthritis, overview 175–78
Arthritis Foundation, contact
  information 585
articulation disorders
  described 256
  therapy 258
artificial nutrition and hydration,
  described 561–63
"Art Therapist: Making a
  Difference in the Lives of Children
  with Special Needs" (Council for
  Exceptional Children) 294n
art therapy, overview 294–96
asanas
  described 353–54
  exercises 358–59
ASHA *see* American Speech-
  Language-Hearing Association
assisted living facilities
  checklist 324–26
  described 426–27
Assisted Living Federation of
  America, contact information 585
assistive devices
  defined 574
  financial assistance 603–26
  hearing loss 100
  intellectual disabilities 231–35
  overview 207–9
  rehabilitation 420–21
  vision problems 107–8
  see also mobility aids
"Assistive Technology" (AOA) 207n
Associated Services for the
  Blind and Visually Impaired,
  contact information 585
Association of Assistive Technology
  Act Programs (ATAP),
  contact information 234
Association of Independent Camps,
  website address 594
Association of University
  Centers on Disabilities,
  contact information 585
athletes, organizations contact
  information 597–601

"Attention Deficit Hyperactivity
  Disorder (ADHD)" (NIMH) 161n
attention deficit hyperactivity
  disorder (ADHD), overview 161–64
Audible, website address 272
audiologists, hearing aids 248
"Augmentative and
  Alternative Communication
  (AAC)" (ASHA) 260n
augmentative and alternative
  communication (AAC),
  overview 260–65
Autism Society,
  contact information 585
autism spectrum disorders,
  overview 157–60
"Autism Spectrum Disorders
  (Pervasive Developmental
  Disorders)" (NIMH) 157n
autistic disorder, described 167
autonomic dysreflexia, spinal cord
  injury 198
axons, spinal cord injury 196

B

back pain, overview 193–95
"Balancing Academics and Serious
  Illness" (Nemours Foundation) 431n
Barbier, Charles 277
Barr Foundation,
  contact information 621
bathing, disabilities 365–67
"Bathing How-To's for Parents
  with Alzheimer's Disease"
  (AgingCare, LLC) 365n
Batiste, Linda Carter 299n
Beach Center on Disability,
  contact information 234
Becker muscular dystrophy 91
bedsores *see* pressure sores
behavior disorders
  child abuse 49–50
  traumatic brain injury 203
belly breathing, described 353
Birth Defect Research for Children,
  Inc., contact information 585
birth defects
  defined 574
  overview 61–64

"Birth Defects: Frequently Asked
    Questions (FAQs)" (NCBDDD) 61n
bladder disorders
    disabilities 372–75
    spinal cord injury 199
bladder management options *374*
blindness, communication
    tips 28–29
    see also vision impairment
blood clots
    rehabilitation 415
    spinal cord injury 198
blood pressure, defined 350
Blue Cross/Blue Shield 624–25
BMI *see* body mass index
body mass index (BMI),
    described 343–44
Book Courier, website address 276
Bookshare,
    website address 274, 275
bowel disorders
    disabilities 369–72
    spinal cord injury 199
"Bowel System: Common
    Problems" (Rehabilitation
    Institute of Chicago) 369n
Bowman Limb Bank Foundation,
    contact information 621
Bradykinesia, Parkinson disease 187
braille
    overview 277–79
    Web-Braille 280–82
Braille, Louis 277, 279
Braille Book Review,
    website address 281
Brain Injury Association of America,
    contact information 585
Brain Trauma Foundation,
    contact information 586
Brave Kids: Camps and Resources
    for Children with Chronic, Life-
    Threatening Illnesses or
    Disabilities, website address 594
breathing problems,
    spinal cord injury 197
Broca aphasia 122–23
bulging disks, back pain 193–94
bullying, overview 44–48
bursitis, described 177

C

caffeine, pain management 383
Camp Channel, website address 594
The CampPage Summer Camps
    Guide, website address 594
CampResource.com: Special Needs
    Camps, website address 595
Camps for Children with
    Diabetes, website address 594
Candlelighters Childhood Cancer
    Foundation, summer camps 593
canes
    described 214
    rehabilitation 416–17
captions, overview 238–41
"Captions for Deaf and Hard-of-
    Hearing Viewers" (NIDCD) 238n
cardiopulmonary
    resuscitation (CPR),
    end of life care 563–64
cardiovascular exercise,
    described 351
caregivers
    adult day care 328
    bathing tips 365–67
    defined 574
    end of life care 546–47
    hospital visits 403–6
    overview 31–42
    respite care 316–27
carriers, cystic fibrosis 78
cataracts
    described 105
    warning signs *103*
catheters
    described *374*
    urinary tract 373–75
CDC *see* Centers for Disease
    Control and Prevention
Centers for Disease Control
    and Prevention (CDC)
    contact information 578
    publications
        obesity 343n
        reasonable
            accommodations 528n
        shaken baby syndrome 132n
        statistics 7n
        travel assistance 311n

cerebral palsy, overview 65–68
"Cerebral Palsy: Hope Through
    Research" (NINDS) 65n
cerebrospinal fluid (CSF), inborn
    errors of metabolism 84
certified occupational therapy
    assistants (COTA) 289
Challenged Athletes Foundation,
    contact information 621
Charles Bonnet syndrome 103
Chiari II malformation 95
Child, Julia 238
child abuse,
    intellectual disabilities 48–53
Child Abuse Prevention and
    Treatment Act (CAPTA; 1974) 51
Child Find, described 462
child protective services,
    described 51
children
    academics 431–33
    Affordable Care Act 390, 392
    anxiety 386
    attention deficit hyperactivity
        disorder 161–64
    autism spectrum disorders 157–60
    bullying 44–48
    caregivers 36
    cerebral palsy 65–68
    deaf-blindness 111–13
    diet and nutrition 337
    disability evaluations 447–58
    disability statistics 15–18
    obesity 344
    spina bifida 93–96
    yoga 355–57
Children's Health Insurance Program
    (CHIP), Medicaid 399–402
Children's Health Insurance
    Program Reauthorization Act
    (CHIPRA) 399–400
Children's Hemiplegia and
    Stroke Association (CHASA),
    website address 595
Children's Oncology Camping
    Association International,
    website address 595
Children with Special Health Care
    Needs (CSHCN) program 622–23

CHIP see Children's Health
    Insurance Program
"Choosing a long-term care setting"
    (Oregon Department of Human
    Services) 425n
Civil Right Act (1968) 511
Civil Rights of Institutionalized
    Persons Act (CRIPA) 492
"Cleft Lip and Palate"
    (Nemours Foundation) 69n
clefts
    described 62
    overview 69–75
Cleveland Clinic,
    contact information 586
client assistance program (CAP),
    described 618–19
"Cochlear Implants" (NIDCD) 242n
cochlear implants, overview 242–44
cognitive impairment
    communication tips 30
    defined 574
    multiple sclerosis 180–81
    traumatic brain injury 201–2
cold therapy, rehabilitation 423
Coleman Institute for
    Cognitive Disabilities,
    contact information 234
"Commonly Asked Questions About
    Service Animals in Places of
    Business" (DOJ) 299n
"Communicating with and
    about People with Disabilities"
    (ODEP) 27n
communication
    caregivers 40–42
    deaf-blindness 114–17
    intellectual disabilities 232
    paralyzation 253–54
    people with disabilities 27–30
    traumatic brain injury 202–3
    see also augmentative and
        alternative communication
communication equipment,
    assistive technology 208
Communications Act (1934) 490
community development block grants,
    home modifications 230
Community First Choice plan 394

Community Living Assistance
Services and Supports (CLASS)
Program 391
comorbidity, defined 574
complementary and alternative
medicine (CAM),
Parkinson disease 187
comprehensive evaluation
report (CER) 471–73
computers
assistive technology 208
low vision 282–85
transitions 483
"Connections That Count: Brain-
Computer Interface Enables
the Profoundly Paralyzed to
Communicate" (Klose) 253n
constipation, described 369–70
constructional dyspraxia *148*
continuing care retirement
communities, described 427
Cooke, David A. 3n, 19n, 27n, 81n,
124n, 231n, 238n, 249n, 260n, 288n,
290n, 294n, 306n, 327n, 334n, 407n,
487n, 529n, 532n, 546n
Council for Exceptional Children,
art therapy publication 294n
Crime Victims with Disabilities
Awareness Act (1998) 51
crutches, described 214
"Cystic Fibrosis" (NHLBI) 77n
cystic fibrosis (CF), overview 77–80
Cystic Fibrosis Foundation,
contact information 586

D

DAISY (Digital Accessible
Information System),
website address 276
Dancing on Wheels,
contact information 599
Davis, Leigh Ann 48n, 53n
deaf-blindness, overview 111–19
deafness
captions 238–41
cochlear implants 242–44
communication tips 29
hearing aids 245–48
see also hearing disorders

dementia, respite care 322
dental abnormalities, clefts 71
dental care, overview 364–65
"Dental Care Every Day:
A Caregiver's Guide" (NIDCR) 364n
Department of Education (ED)
see US Department of Education
Department of Health and Human
Services (DHHS; HHS) *see* US
Department of Health
and Human Services
Department of Homeland Security,
disaster preparation publication 521n
Department of Housing and Urban
Development (HUD) *see* US
Department of Housing and
Urban Development
Department of Justice
see US Department of Justice
Department of State
see US Department of State
depression
bathing tips 367
coping strategies 385–88
multiple sclerosis 181
"Depression and Anxiety"
(Rehabilitation Institute
of Chicago) 385n
developmental disabilities
defined 574
statistics 15–18
"Developmental Disabilities
Increasing in US" (CDC) 7n
developmental disorders, described 167
development apraxia
of speech (DAS) 124–25
DHHS *see* US Department
of Health and Human Services
dhyana, described 354
diabetes mellitus, limb loss 190–92
diabetic retinopathy
described 105
warning signs *103*
diarrhea, described 371
diet and nutrition
disabilities 334–41
pain management 383–84
PKU 85
swallowing difficulties 341–43

dieticians, institutional settings 339
"Directory of Athletes with
   Disabilities Organizations"
   (American Academy of Physical
   Medicine and Rehabilitation) 597n
disabilities
   age factor *9, 10*
   child abuse 48–53
   defined 574
   disaster preparedness 521–24
   fire safety 519–20
   homelessness 517–18
   myths 19–21
   overview 3–6
   sexual violence 53–58
   statistics 7–18
   tax information 539–44
"Disability Among Older
   Americans Continues
   Significant Decline" (NIA) 23n
"Disability Benefits" (SSA) 535n
disability benefits, Medicare 605–6
Disability.gov, website address 578
Disabled Sports USA,
   contact information 597
disaster preparedness,
   disabled people 521–24
distraction, pain management 383
DME *see* durable medical equipment
DOJ *see* US Department of Justice
do-not-intubate order (DNI order),
   described 569
do-not-resuscitate order (DNR order),
   end of life care 564–69
dopamine,
   Parkinson disease 184, 187
Doubleday Large Print Book Club,
   website address 271
Down syndrome
   described 62
   overview 128–29
drooling, cerebral palsy 67–68
drug abuse, birth defects 64
dry macular degeneration 103–4
Duchenne muscular dystrophy 91
durable medical equipment (DME),
   financial assistance 603
durable power of attorney
   for health care 549

"Dyscalculia" (National Center
   for Learning Disabilities) 134n
dyscalculia, overview 134–37
dysgraphia, overview 142–46
dyslexia, overview 138–42
"Dyslexia Basics" (International
   Dyslexia Association) 138n
dysphagia disorders, described 257
dyspraxia, overview 147–49

E

early intervention
   glaucoma 104
   inborn errors of metabolism 87
   legislation 459–67
   macular degeneration 104
ear wax, described 99
Easter Seals
   contact information 586
      AgrAbility Project 625
      summer camps 593
   publications
      myths 19n
      occupational therapy 288n
      physical therapy 290n
ED *see* US Department of Education
education
   intellectual disabilities 233
   transitions 481–84
   see also individualized
      education program
education cycle, described 435–38
Education for all Handicapped
   Children Act (1975) 492
EEOC *see* Equal Employment
   Opportunity Commission
Eldercare Locator,
   contact information 229, 578, 626
emotional concerns
   clefts 74–75
   traumatic brain injury 203
   vision problems 109
emotional support,
   caregivers 38–40
employment
   Americans with Disabilities Act
      487–88, 495–99
   disability statistics 14
   intellectual disabilities 233

end of life care
  overview 546–47
  planning strategies 548–69
"End-of-Life Care: Questions
  and Answers" (NCI) 546n
"End-of-Life Decisions"
  (National Hospice and Palliative
  Care Organization) 548n
environmental control,
  intellectual disabilities 232
environmental hazards,
  home use medical devices 223–25
Epilepsy Foundation, contact
  information 586
Equal Employment Opportunity
  Commission (EEOC)
  Americans with Disabilities
    Act publication 495n
  contact information 581
ethnic factors, disabilities 11
"Evaluating Children for Disability"
  (NICHCY) 447n
"Executive Function and
  Learning Disabilities"
  (National Center for Learning
  Disabilities) 149n
executive function disabilities,
  overview 149–54
exercise
  guidelines overview 348–52
  pain management 383
"Exercise Guidelines for
  People with Disabilities"
  (NCPAD) 348n
expressive language disorders,
  described 257

F

"Facts about Down Syndrome"
  (NICHD) 128n
"Fact Sheet: Medicare and Nonelderly
  People with Disabilities" (Kaiser
  Family Foundation) 395n
failure to thrive, cerebral palsy 67
Fair Housing Amendments Act
  (FHAA; 1988)
  described 7, 490–91
  home modifications 226
  overview 511–16

Family Caregiver Alliance
  contact information 586
  vision loss publication 102n
family issues
  adult day care 327–30
  caregivers 36–37
  deaf-blindness 118–19
  depression 388
  disability evaluations 449–51
  disaster preparedness 524
  education process 435–38
  end of life decisions 550, 557
  residential care 324
  respite care 313–27
FDA *see* US Food and Drug
  Administration
Federal Communications Commission
  (FCC), contact information 578
festination, Parkinson disease 186
fetal alcohol spectrum disorders
  (FASD), overview 130–31
"Fetal Alcohol Spectrum Disorders
  (FASDs) (NCBDDD) 130n
fibromyalgia
  back pain 194
  described 176
"Financial Assistance for Prosthetic
  Services, Durable Medical
  Equipment, and Other Assistive
  Devices" (Amputee Coalition) 603n
financial considerations
  adult day care centers 330
  arthritis 175
  assistive devices 603–26
  caregivers 32–34
  early intervention services 467
  motor vehicle adaptations 306–7
  respite care 320–21
  traumatic brain injury 200
  vision problems 109
fire safety, disabled people 519–20
first aid, pressure sores 378–79
Fishing Has No Boundaries, Inc.,
  contact information 599
flexibility/functionality exercise,
  described 352
fluency disorders, described 256
fluent aphasia 122–23
FM systems, hearing assistance 250

Food and Drug Administration
(FDA) *see* US Food and Drug
Administration
food preparation, rehabilitation 421
fragile X syndrome,
autism spectrum disorders 159–60
free appropriate public education
(FAPE) 473
Freedom's Wings International
(FWI), contact information 599
"Frequently Asked Questions About
Home Use Devices" (FDA) 220n
Fullmer, Carmen 299n

G

gait problems,
Parkinson disease 186
galactosemia, described 86
Gaucher disease, described 86–87
Gehrig, Lou 172
genes
CFTR 77
muscular dystrophy 90
see also heredity
genetic factors, birth defects 63
glaucoma
described 104
warning signs *103*
global aphasia 123
Goodwill Industries, contact
information 586
gout, described 177
grief, *versus* depression 386
group home, defined 574
Grown-Up Camps,
website address 595
guardian, defined 574
"A Guide for Caregivers: Managing
Major Changes" (National
Multiple Sclerosis Society) 31n
"A Guide to Disability Rights Law"
(DOJ) 487n

H

hallucinations, macular degeneration
103
Handicapped Hunting Resource
Guide, website address 599

health care agents
described 549–50
overview 554–60
health care power of attorney,
described 549
Healthfinder, contact information 578
health insurance *see* insurance
coverage
hearing aids
depicted *246*
described 100
overview 245–48
"Hearing Assistive Technology"
(ASHA) 249n
hearing assistive technology systems
(HATS), overview 249–52
hearing disorders
cerebral palsy 67
overview 98–101
see also deafness
"Hearing Loss" (NIA) 98n
heart disorders
described 62
rehabilitation 415
spinal cord injury 197–98
heart rate, defined 349–50
heat therapy, rehabilitation 423
Heetderks, William J. 253–54
"Helping Kids Deal with Bullies"
(Nemours Foundation) 44n
hemorrhoids, described 371
heredity
amyotrophic lateral sclerosis 173
birth defects 63
cystic fibrosis 77–78
muscular dystrophy 89–90
Parkinson disease 183–85
herniated disks, back pain 193–94
HHS *see* US Department of Health
and Human Services
hip fractures, rehabilitation 412–13
Hodes, Richard J. 24
home-based rehabilitation,
described 410–11
home care providers, checklist 323
home health care
caregivers 33–34
defined 574
statistics 220

homelessness, disabled people 517–18
home medical equipment, defined 575
"Home Modification" (DHHS) 225n
home modifications
  assistive technology 208
  overview 225–30
  vision problems 106–407
"Home Use Devices" (FDA) 220n
home use medical devices,
  overview 220–25
Horowitz, Sheldon 149n
"Hospitalization Happens:
  A Guide to Hospital Visits for
  Individuals with Memory Loss"
  (NIA) 403n
hospitalizations
  children 432
  coping strategies 403–6
  depression 387
housing
  disability rights 507–10
  overview 502–7
  see also Fair Housing
    Amendments Act
"How To Live With Low Vision"
  (Access Media Group LLC) 268n
HUD *see* US Department of
  Housing and Urban Development
Humana Military
  Healthcare Services, Inc.,
  contact information 617
hypospadias, described 62

I

IADL *see* instrumental
  activities of daily living
"IDEA: The Individuals with
  Disabilities Education Act"
  (NICHCY) 440n
ideational dyspraxia *148*
ideomotor dyspraxia *148*
IEP *see* individualized
  education program
impairment, defined 575
inborn errors of metabolism,
  overview 81–88
"Inborn Errors of Metabolism in
  Infancy and Early Childhood:
  An Update" (AAFP) 81n

income levels,
  disability statistics 13–15
incontinence
  cerebral palsy 68
  described 372
independent educational
  evaluation (IEE) 456–57
Independent Living Centers (ILC),
  described 626
independent living facility, defined 575
individualized
  education program (IEP)
  accommodations 480
  deaf-blindness 117–18
  defined 575
  described 432, 436, 492–93
  modifications 479
  No Child Left Behind Act 443
  overview 469–74
  transitions 481
"Individualized Education Programs
  (IEPs)" (Nemours Foundation) 469n
individualized family service plan
  (IFSP) 461, 464–67
individualized treatment plans
  occupational therapy 289
  physical therapy 291–92
Individuals With Disabilities
  Education Act (IDEA; 2004)
  children 431, 447–58, 469–74
  described 7, 440, 492–93
  dyslexia 141
  early intervention services 459–67
  related services 478
  specially designed instruction 476
  supplementary aids
    and services 478–79
induction loop systems,
  hearing assistance 251
indwelling catheter, described *374*
infants
  head trauma 132
  inborn errors of metabolism 81–84
infectious arthritis, described 177
"Information Processing Disorders"
  (National Center for Learning
  Disabilities) 155n
information processing disorders,
  described 155–56

infrared systems,
  hearing assistance 250–51
instrumental activities
  of daily living (IADL), statistics 12
insurance coverage
  assistive devices 619–20
  life-sustaining treatments 563
  overview 390–92
  see also prescription
    drug coverage; Social Security
    Disability Insurance
intellectual and developmental
  disabilities (IDD), described 128
intellectual disabilities
  assistive technology 231–35
  sexual violence 54–57
interferons, multiple sclerosis 182
Internal Revenue Service (IRS),
  tax benefits publication 539n
International Association
  of Audio Information Services,
  website address 275
International Dyslexia Association
  contact information 586
  dyslexia publication 138n
International Wheelchair Aviators,
  contact information 600
International Wheelchair
  Basketball Federation (IWBF),
  website address 600
"Investing in People: Job
  Accommodation Situations
  and Solutions" (ODEP) 529n
IRS *see* Internal Revenue Service

J

Job Accommodation Network,
  contact information 586
joint problems,
  rehabilitation 415–16
"A Journalist's Guide to
  Shaken Baby Syndrome:
  A Preventable Tragedy"
  (CDC) 132n
Justice Department *see* US
  Department of Justice
justification statement, described 604
juvenile idiopathic arthritis,
  described 176

K

Henry J. Kaiser Family Foundation,
  publications
  Medicare, children 399n
  Medicare, nonelderly 395n
Kids' Camps, website address 595
Klose, Christopher 253n
K-Modifiers, described 606–7
Koop, C. Everett 622

L

language intervention activities,
  described 257
laughing/weeping syndrome,
  multiple sclerosis 181
L-Code system, described 606–7
learning disabilities
  defined 575
  evaluations 455
  executive functions 149–54
  information processing 155–56
  see also dyscalculia; dysgraphia;
    dyslexia; dyspraxia
Lewy bodies, Parkinson disease 184
Lezzonni, Lisa 212
Library of Congress (LOC)
  contact information 578
  Web-Braille publication 280n
life-sustaining treatments
  defined 575
  described 560–61
limb loss, overview 190–92
"Limb Loss FAQs" (Amputee
  Coalition) 190n
Limbs for Life Foundation,
  contact information 622
Limbs of Love,
  contact information 622
living trust, described 549
living will, described 548–49, 551
  see also advance directives
LOC *see* Library of Congress
long term care
  choices 425–28
  defined 575
Lou Gehrig disease *see* amyotrophic
  lateral sclerosis
low back pain, overview 193–95

"Low Back Pain Fact Sheet"
(NINDS) 193n
low blood pressure,
spinal cord injury 197–98
Low Income Home Energy Assistance
Program (LIHEAP) 229
low vision
computer users 282–85
coping strategies 109–10, 268–69
treatment 106
"Low Vision Aids for Computer Users"
(Access Media Group LLC) 282n
lung disorders, rehabilitation 416
lupus *see* systemic lupus
erythematosus

M

macular degeneration
described 103–4
warning signs *103*
magnifiers, vision problems 108
maintenance rehabilitation,
described 407
malnutrition, described 335–37
Manton, Kenneth G. 23
manual wheelchairs,
described 211, *215*
March of Dimes,
contact information 587
masked face, Parkinson disease 186
Maternal and Child Health Bureau
(MCHB), contact information 578
math learning disabilities *see*
dyscalculia
"Maximizing Productivity:
Accommodations for Employees
with Psychiatric Disabilities"
(ODEP) 532n
maximum heart rate, defined 350
MCAD deficiency, described 86
Meals-on-Wheels Association of
America, contact information 587
Medicaid
Affordable Care Act 391, 393–94
financial assistance 610–11
home modifications 230
MedicAlert bracelets 403
medical power of attorney
see health care power of attorney

Medicare
chronic disabilities 24
home-based rehabilitation 410–11
home modifications 230
limb loss 192
nonelderly disabled people 395–98
nursing facilities 410
prosthetic services 605–8
medications
attention deficit hyperactivity
disorder 163–64
back pain 195
disaster preparedness 522
multiple sclerosis 181–82
pain management 381–82
Parkinson disease 187
MedWatch,
contact information 222
Meltzer, Lynn 153
meningocele, described 93–94
mental disorders, overview 165–68
"Mental Disorders -
Adult" (SSA) 165n
mental illness, defined 575
mental retardation
autism spectrum disorders 159
cerebral palsy 66
described 167
methylmalonicaciduria disorders,
described 85–86
Miles, Barbara 111n
Milestone 311, website address 276
mitochondria, Parkinson disease 185
mobility
deaf-blindness 117
intellectual disabilities 232
mobility aids
assistive technology 208
overview 211–17
"Mobility Alternatives: From Cranes
to Wheelchairs" (United
Spinal Association) 211n
mobility impairments,
communication tips 29–30
modifications
housing 508–9, 513–15
students 475–80
Money Follows the
Person Program 393–94

money matters *see* financial
considerations
motor vehicles,
adaptations overview 306–10
Motor Voter Act 492
multidisciplinary evaluation and
assessment, described 462–64
multiple sclerosis (MS)
caregivers 31–42
overview 179–82
"Multiple Sclerosis:
Hope Through Research"
(NINDS) 179n
Murphy, Mary Brugger 327
muscular dystrophy, overview 89–91
Muscular Dystrophy Association,
contact information 587
"Muscular Dystrophy:
Hope Through Research"
(NINDS) 89n
music therapy, overview 296–98
"Music Therapy Helps
People with Disabilities"
(US Department of State) 296n
myelomeningocele, described 93–94
My Summer Camps,
website address 595
"Myths and Facts About
People with Disabilities"
(Easter Seals) 19n

N

National Adult Day
Services Association
contact information 587
described 327
National Alliance
for Accessible Golf,
contact information 600
National Alliance for Caregiving,
contact information 587
National Amputation Foundation,
contact information 622
National Amputee Golf Association
(NAGA), contact information 600
National Association of Area Agencies
on Aging, website address 626
National Association of the Deaf,
contact information 587

National Camp Association, Inc.,
summer camps 594
National Cancer Institute (NCI)
contact information 578
end-of-life care publication 546n
National Center for
Complementary and
Alternative Medicine (NCCAM),
contact information 579
National Center for
Health Statistics (NCHS),
contact information 579
National Center for Learning
Disabilities
contact information 587
publications
dyscalculia 134n
dysgraphia 142n
dyspraxia 147n
executive functioning
disabilities 149n
information processing
disorders 155n
No Child Left
Behind Act 441n
National Center of Physical
Activity and Disability,
contact information 587
National Center on Birth Defects
and Developmental Disabilities
(NCBDDD), publications
birth defects 61n
fetal alcohol
spectrum disorders 130n
National Center on
Physical Activity and
Disability (NCPAD)
Fun and Leisure:
Camp Resources,
website address 595
publications
exercise guidelines 348n
yoga 352n
summer camps 593
National Consortium
on Deaf-Blindness,
contact information 587
National Council on Disability (NCD),
contact information 579

National Dissemination
Center for Children with
Disabilities (NICHCY)
contact information 588
publications
children, disabilities 447n
early intervention 459n
IDEA 440n
student accommodations 475n
summer camps 577n
National Down Syndrome Society,
contact information 588
National Family Caregivers
Association,
contact information 588
National Federation of the Blind,
contact information 588
National Heart, Lung, and Blood
Institute (NHLBI)
contact information 579
cystic fibrosis publication 77n
National Highway Traffic Safety
Administration (NHTSA), motor
vehicle adaptions publication 306n
National Hospice and
Palliative Care Organization
advance planning publication 548n
contact information 588
National Institute of Arthritis
and Musculoskeletal and
Skin Diseases (NIAMS)
arthritis publication 175n
contact information 579
National Institute of Child Health
and Human Development (NICHD)
contact information 579
Down syndrome publication 128n
National Institute of Dental and
Craniofacial Research (NIDCR)
contact information 579
dental care publication 364n
National Institute
of Mental Health (NIMH)
contact information 580
publications
attention deficit
hyperactivity disorder 161n
autism spectrum
disorders 157n

National Institute of Neurological
Disorders and Stroke (NINDS)
contact information 580
publications
amyotrophic
lateral sclerosis 172n
cerebral palsy 65n
low back pain 193n
multiple sclerosis 179n
muscular dystrophy 89n
Parkinson disease 183n
spina bifida 93n
spinal cord injury 196n
traumatic brain injury 200n
National Institute on Aging (NIA)
contact information 580
publications
Alzheimer disease 170n
disabilities 23n
hearing loss 98n
hospital visits 403n
National Institute on Deafness
and Other Communication
Disorders (NIDCD)
contact information 580
publications
aphasia 122n
apraxia 124n
captions 238n
cochlear implants 242n
hearing aids 245n
National Institute on Disability and
Rehabilitation Research (NIDRR),
contact information 580
National Library of Medicine (NLM),
contact information 582
National Library Service (NLS)
contact information 271
International Union Catalog,
website address 281
National Multiple Sclerosis Society
caregivers publication 31n
contact information 588
National Organization for Rare
Disorders, contact information 588
National Parkinson Foundation, Inc.,
contact information 589
National Rehabilitation Information
Center, contact information 589

National Respite Network and
Resource Center, contact
information 589
National Rifle Association (NRA),
contact information 600
National Shooting Sports
Foundation (NSSF),
contact information 600
National Softball Association for
the Deaf, contact information 598
National Spinal Cord Injury
Association,
contact information 589
National Sports Center for the
Disabled (NSCD), contact
information 597
National Stroke Association,
contact information 589
National Technical Information
Service (NTIS),
contact information 580
National Voter Registration
Act (1993) 492
National Wheelchair Basketball
Association (NWBA),
contact information 600
National Wheelchair
Poolplayers Association (NWPA),
contact information 600
National Women's Health
Information Center (NWHIC),
contact information 581
NCBDDD *see* National Center
on Birth Defects and
Developmental Disabilities
NCI *see* National Cancer Institute
NCPAD *see* National Center on
Physical Activity and Disability
needs assessments, assistive
technology 208–9
Nemours Foundation
contact information 589
publications
academics, disabilities 431n
bullying 44n
clefts 69n
individualized education
programs 469n
speech-language therapy 256n

neural tube defects,
described 62, 93
newborn screening, described 81
The New York Times,
website address 270
NFB-Newsline, website address 274
NHLBI *see* National Heart,
Lung, and Blood Institute
NHTSA *see* National Highway
Traffic Safety Administration
NIA *see* National Institute on Aging
NIAMS *see* National Institute of
Arthritis and Musculoskeletal
and Skin Diseases
NICHCY
see National Dissemination
Center for Children
with Disabilities
NIDCD *see* National Institute on
Deafness and Other
Communication Disorders
NIDCR *see* National Institute of
Dental and Craniofacial Research
NIMH *see* National Institute
of Mental Health
NINDS *see* National Institute
of Neurological Disorders
and Stroke
NLS *see* National Library Service
No Child Left Behind Act
(NCLB; 2001) 441–44
"No Child Left Behind Act (NCLB)"
(National Center for Learning
Disabilities) 441n
non-fluent aphasia 122–23
norepinephrine,
Parkinson disease 184
nursing facilities
long term care 427
rehabilitation 410
nursing homes
checklist 324–26
defined 575
nutrition *see* diet and nutrition
"Nutrition and Disability"
(University of Montana) 334n
"Nutrition for Swallowing
Difficulties" (Rehabilitation
Institute of Chicago) 341n

O

obesity
  described 337–38
  overview 343–45
O'Brien, Dan 526n
occulta, described 94
occupational health services,
  defined 575–76
occupational therapy
  defined 576
  overview 288–89
ODEP *see* Office of Disability
  Employment Policy
Office of Disability
  Employment Policy (ODEP)
  contact information 581
  publications
    communication 27n
    job accommodation 529n
    psychiatric disabilities 532n
older adults
  assistive technology 207–9
  disabilities 23–25
  home modifications 225–26
  rehabilitation 421
oral clefts, described 69–70
oral motor therapy,
  described 258
Oregon Department of Human
  Services, long term care
  publication 425n
organic mental disorders,
  described 167
orientation, deaf-blindness 117
ornithine transcarbamylase
  deficiency, described 85
oromotor dyspraxia *148*
orthotic equipment
  assistive technology 208
  rehabilitation 417–19
osteoarthritis, described 176
osteoporosis
  back pain 194
  hip fractures 413
outpatient rehabilitation,
  described 410
Overdrive, website address 273
"Overview of Deaf-Blindness"
  (Miles) 111n

"Overview of Early Intervention"
  (NICHCY) 459n
overweight, overview 343–45
"Overweight and Obesity Among
  People with Disabilities"
  (CDC) 343n

P

pain management
  overview 381–84
  spinal cord injury 199
"Pain: Medications for Pain Relief"
  (Rehabilitation Institute
  of Chicago) 381n
"Pain: Non-Drug Pain Management
  Techniques" (Rehabilitation
  Institute of Chicago) 381n
paralyzation, communication 253–54
paranoid disorders, described 167
"Parent Role in the Education
  Process" (Walter Reed
  Army Medical Center) 431n
Parkinson disease, overview 183–87
Parkinson's Disease Foundation,
  contact information 589
"Parkinson's Disease: Hope
  Through Research" (NINDS) 183n
Partners for Access to the Woods
  (PAW), contact information 597
Patient Protection and Affordable
  Care Act (ACA; 2010) 399, 401
pensions, tax information 541–42
"People with Disabilities and
  Their Caregivers" (USFA) 519n
"People with Disabilities: Coming
  Improvements" (DHHS) 390n
"People with Disabilities: Recent
  Improvements" (DHHS) 390n
"People with Disabilities: Top 5
  Things to Know" (DHHS) 390n
"People with Intellectual Disabilities
  and Sexual Violence" (Davis) 53n
personal hygiene,
  rehabilitation 421–22
personality disorders, described 167
pervasive developmental disorders,
  described 167
Peterson's Summer Programs,
  summer camps 594

pets, home use medical devices 223
see also service animals
phenylalanine hydroxylase 85
Physically Challenged Bowhunters
of America, Inc. (PCBA),
contact information 600
Physical Therapist
Assistants (DPT) 291
physical therapy
defined 576
disabilities 290–92
overview 290–92
PKU, described 85
PlayAway Books,
website address 273
pneumonia, spinal cord injury 197
polymyalgia rheumatica,
described 177
polymyositis, described 177
Porter Sargent Handbooks,
summer camps 594
postconcussion syndrome (PCS) 201
posttraumatic amnesia (PTA) 202
postural instability,
Parkinson disease 187
posture, pain management 383
poverty status,
disability statistics 13
power assist devices, described 212
power wheelchairs,
described 212, *215*, 216–17
pranayama
described 353
exercises 357–58
pregnancy
birth defects 62
clefts 70
"Preparing Makes Sense for
People with Disabilities and
Special Needs" (Department of
Homeland Security) 521n
presbycusis, described 99
prescription drug coverage,
Medicare 397
prescriptions, home use
medical devices 222
pressure sores
overview 377–80
spinal cord injury 198–99

"Pressure Ulcer"
(A.D.A.M., Inc.) 377n
Prevent Child Abuse America,
contact information 52, 57
Professional Association of
Therapeutic Horsemanship
(PATH) International,
contact information 600
prosthetic equipment,
assistive technology 208
prosthetic services, financial
assistance 603–8
Protection and Advocacy
for Assistive Technology
(PAAT) Program 618
Protection and Advocacy of
Individual Rights (PAIR)
Program 618
protruding disks, back pain 193–94
psoriatic arthritis, described 177
PsychCentral, contact
information 589
psychiatric disabilities,
overview 165–68
psychotherapy, attention deficit
hyperactivity disorder 164
psychotic disorders, described 167
public assistance programs,
home modifications 229–30

Q

"Questions and Answers about
Arthritis and Degenerative
Diseases" (NIAMS) 175n
"Questions and Answers on
Special Education and
Homelessness" (ED) 517n

R

racial factor, disabilities 11
Random House Large Print,
website address 271
ratings of perceived exertion
(RPE), defined 350
Reader's Digest,
website address 270
"Reading and Vision Loss"
(American Foundation
for the Blind) 270n

reading options,
vision impairment 270–76
reasonable accommodations
Americans with Disabilities Act
489–90, 498–99
disabled employees 528–31
housing 508, 513–15
Rebuilding Together, Inc., contact
information 229
receptive language disorders,
described 257
Recording for the
Blind and Dyslexic (RFB&D),
website address 275
Regional Resource Center Program,
website address 589
regulations, captions 240–41
rehabilitation
defined 576
overview 407–23
"Rehabilitation" (American
Geriatrics Society) 407n
Rehabilitation Act (1973)
described 7, 493–94
dyslexia 141
Section 504 445–46, 448,
493–94, 511
Rehabilitation Institute of Chicago
contact information 590
publications
bowel problems 369n
depression, anxiety 385n
pain management 381n
swallowing difficulty 341n
relaxation
pain management 383
yoga 354, 359
residential care
checklist 324–26
defined 576
residential care facilities,
long term care 428
resonance disorders, described 257
Resources for Children with Special
Needs, summer camps 593
respite care
defined 576
long term care 428
overview 316–27

"Respite Care Guide"
(Alzheimer's Association) 316n
response to intervention (RTI),
dyslexia 140
restorative rehabilitation,
described 407
retirement homes,
long term care 428
rheumatic diseases, described 175–78
rheumatoid arthritis, described 176
rigidity, Parkinson disease 186–87
RPE *see* ratings of perceived exertion
ruptured disks, back pain 193–94

S

Sacks, Oliver 296
Safe Return bracelets 403
safety considerations
caregivers 37–38
home adaptations 34
St. Jude Children's Hospital 624
schizophrenic disorders,
described 167
sciatica, back pain 194
scleroderma, described 176
scooters, described 212, *215*
Section 504
see Rehabilitation Act (1973)
seizures
autism spectrum disorders 159
cerebral palsy 67
self-help groups, caregivers 42
self-image, dyslexia 139
sensory enhancements, assistive
technology 208
sensory problems, autism
spectrum disorders 158–59
service animals
air travel 313
overview 299–303
"Service Animals in the Workplace"
(Batiste; Fullmer) 299n
sexual function, spinal
cord injury 199–200
sexuality, caregivers 41–42
sexual violence, disabilities 53–58
shaken baby syndrome, described 132
Shriners Hospitals for Children 524
signal to noise ratio, described 249

Skating Athletes Bold at Heart
(SABAH), contact information 598
skeletal irregularities, back pain 194
Ski for Light, Inc.,
contact information 598
SLE
see systemic lupus erythematosus
social challenges, clefts 74–75
Social Security Administration (SSA)
contact information 582
publications
disability benefits 535n
mental disorders 165n
Social Security Disability (SSD)
assistive devices 605–6
overview 535–38
Social Security Disability
Insurance (SSDI), Medicare 395
somatoform disorders, described 167
spasm, spinal cord injury 198
special education
defined 576
described 476–78
Special Olympics,
contact information 597
speech disorders
cerebral palsy 67
clefts 71
communication tips 30
see also aphasia; apraxia
speech-language pathologists
aphasia 123
apraxia 125
augmentative and alternative
communication 264–65
described 257–59
"Speech-Language Therapy"
(Nemours Foundation) 256n
speech-language therapy,
overview 256–59
speech therapy
clefts 74
defined 576
spina bifida, overview 93–96
Spina Bifida Association,
contact information 590
"Spina Bifida Fact Sheet"
(NINDS) 93n
spinal cord injury, overview 196–200

"Spinal Cord Injury:
Hope Through Research"
(NINDS) 196n
spinal deformities, cerebral palsy 67
spinal degeneration, back pain 194
spinal stenosis, back pain 194
SPLORE (Special Populations
Learning Outdoor Recreation and
Education), contact information 597
spondylitis, back pain 195
spondyloarthropathies, described 177
sports activities, organizations contact
information 597–601
sports and recreation, intellectual
disabilities 233
SSA *see* Social Security
Administration
SSDI *see* Social Security
Disability Insurance
State Children's Health Insurance
Program (SCHIP) 623
State Department
see US Department of State
"The State of Housing for People with
Disabilities" (Access Living) 502n
state technology assistance projects,
described 617–18
statistics
adult day care centers 330
amyotrophic lateral sclerosis 173
augmentative and alternative
communication 261
birth defects 61–62
clefts 69
cystic fibrosis 78
disabilities 7–18
dyslexia 138–39
home health care services 220
limb loss 190–91
low vision 268
multiple sclerosis 179
nonelderly Medicare
beneficiaries 396
obesity 344
Parkinson disease 183
rheumatic diseases 178
spina bifida 93
traumatic brain injury 200–201
stereognosis, cerebral palsy 68

steroid medications,
multiple sclerosis 182
stool impaction, described 370
strength training, described 351
stress management, caregivers 38–40
stroke, rehabilitation 411–12
substance abuse, birth defects 64
substance addiction disorders,
described 167
summer camps,
contact information 593–95
"Summer Camps 2008"
(NICHCY) 577n
Summer Camp Search,
website address 595
Summer Camps for Amputees and
Children with Limb Differences,
website address 595
Summer Camps for Deaf and Hard
of Hearing Children and Teens,
website address 595
supplemental security income (SSI),
tax information 541
"Support Employees
with Disabilities" (CDC) 528n
support groups
defined 576
disaster preparedness 524
"Supports, Modifications, and
Accommodations for Students"
(NICHCY) 475n
supports, students 475–80
surgical procedures
back pain 195
clefts 72–73
Parkinson disease 187
Suzman, Richard 24
swallowing difficulties,
diet and nutrition 341–43
systemic lupus erythematosus
(SLE), described 176
systemic sclerosis 176

T

Talking Books,
website address 271, 275
target heart rate, defined 350
"Tax Highlights for Persons with
Disabilities" (IRS) 539n

tax information,
disabled people 539–44
TBI *see* traumatic brain injury
"Technology for People with
Intellectual Disabilities"
(The Arc of the United States) 231n
telecommunications, Americans
with Disabilities Act 490
Telecommunications Act (1996) 490
captions 241
described 7
tendonitis, described 178
TENS *see* transcutaneous
electrical nerve stimulation
tests, inborn errors
of metabolism 81–83
therapy, assistive technology 208
tinnitus, described 99
tobacco use, birth defects 64
toddlers, inborn errors
of metabolism 84
"To Improve the Health and Wellness
of Persons with Disabilities"
(DHHS) 3n
Tomaino, Concetta M. 296–97
transcutaneous electrical nerve
stimulation (TENS),
rehabilitation 422–23
transfers, rehabilitation 419–20
transitions, overview 481–84
transportation
Americans with Disabilities Act 489
rehabilitation 410
wheelchairs 214
traumatic brain injury (TBI),
overview 200–203
"Traumatic Brain Injury: Hope
Through Research" (NINDS) 200n
travel considerations
airlines 311–13
motor vehicle adaptations 306–10
"Travelers with Disabilities" (CDC)
311n
tremor, Parkinson disease 186
TRICARE, assistive devices 614–17
trisomy 21 *see* Down syndrome
tuberous sclerosis, autism spectrum
disorders 160
tyrosine 85

U

ultrasound, rehabilitation 423

"Understanding Occupational
Therapy" (Easter Seals) 288n

"Understanding Physical Therapy"
(Easter Seals) 290n

"Understanding the Fair Housing
Amendments Act" (United Spinal
Association) 511n

"Unique Considerations
in the Home" (FDA) 220n

United Cerebral Palsy, contact
information 590

United Foundation for Disabled
Archers (UFFDA), contact
information 600

United Spinal Association
contact information 590
publications
Fair Housing
Amendments Act 511n
mobility aids 211n

United States Association
of Blind Athletes (USABA),
contact information 598

United States Blind Golf Association
(USBGA), contact information 598

United States Deaf Cycling
Association (USDCA),
contact information 598

United States Deaf Ski and
Snowboard Association(USDSSA),
contact information 599

United States Electric Wheelchair
Hockey Association (U.S.EWHA),
contact information 600

United States Flag Football for the
Deaf (USFFD), website address 599

United States Handcycling,
contact information 601

United States Paralympic Team,
contact information 598

United States Rowing,
contact information 601

United States Sailing: Sailors with
Special Needs, website address 601

United States Tennis Wheelchair,
website address 601

University of Montana, nutrition,
disability publication 334n

urinary catheters *see* catheters

urinary system, described 372

USA Deaf Soccer Association,
website address 599

USA Deaf Sports
Federation (USADSF),
contact information 598, 599

USA Deaf Track and Field,
contact information 599

USA Swimming,
contact information 601

USA Water Ski,
contact information 601

US Census Bureau,
statistics publication 7n

US Department of Education (ED)
contact information 581
publications
higher education
transition 481n
homelessness 517n

US Department of Health
and Human Services
(DHHS; HHS), publications
Affordable Care Act 392n
disabilities 3n
health insurance 390n
home modifications 225n
Section 504,
Rehabilitation Act 445n

US Department of Housing and
Urban Development (HUD)
contact information 581
housing rights publication 507n

US Department of Justice (DOJ)
contact information 581
publications
disability rights 487n
service animals 299n

US Department of State,
music therapy publication 296n

US Department of Transportation
(DOT), contact information 581

US Department of
Veterans Affairs (VA),
contact information 581

USFA *see* US Fire Administration

US Fire Administration (USFA),
fire safety publication 519n
US Food and Drug
Administration (FDA)
contact information 582
home use medical devices
publication 220n
US Government Printing Office
(GPO), contact information 582

V

Variety of the United States,
contact information 625
Very Special Arts,
contact information 590
Veterans Health Administration
(VHA), assistive devices 612–14
Victor Reader Stream (VR Stream),
website address 275
viruses, Parkinson disease 185
vision impairment
cerebral palsy 67
communication tips 28–29
low vision 268–69
multiple sclerosis 180
overview 102–10
reading options 270–76
see also blindness
"Vision Loss" (Family Caregiver
Alliance) 102n
Visiting Nurses Associations of
America, contact information 590
vocational rehabilitation programs,
described 617
Voting Accessibility for
the Elderly and Handicapped
Act (1984) 491–92

W

walkers
described 214–15
rehabilitation 417
walking problems, rehabilitation
416–19
walking sticks, described 214

Walter Reed Army Medical
Center, education,
parents publication 431n
Weatherization Assistance Program
(WAP) 229
Web Accessibility Initiative
contact information 590
Web-Braille 280–82
"Web-Braille" (LOC) 280n
WE MOVE, contact information 590
wet macular degeneration 103–4
"What Is Braille?" (American
Foundation for the Blind) 277n
"What is Dysgraphia?"
(National Center for Learning
Disabilities) 142n
"What is Dyspraxia?"
(National Center for Learning
Disabilities) 147n
Wheelchair and Ambulatory Sports,
USA, contact information 598
wheelchairs
online information 217
overview 211–17
rehabilitation 418–20
"Why Work Matters for People
with Disabilities" (O'Brien) 526n
Wilderness Inquiry, contact
information 598
will, described 549
Wolpaw, Jonathan R. 253–54
workplace
disabilities 526–27
reasonable accommodations 528–31
service animals 299–303
World T.E.A.M. Sports, contact
information 598

Y

yoga, overview 352–62
"Yoga for Individuals with
Disabilities" (NCPAD) 352n
"Your Rights under Section 504
of The Rehabilitation Act"
(DHHS) 445n

Health Reference Series

Adolescent Health Sourcebook, 3rd Edition

Adult Health Concerns Sourcebook

AIDS Sourcebook, 5th Edition

Alcoholism Sourcebook, 3rd Edition

Allergies Sourcebook, 4th Edition

Alzheimer Disease Sourcebook, 5th Edition

Arthritis Sourcebook, 3rd Edition

Asthma Sourcebook, 3rd Edition

Attention Deficit Disorder Sourcebook

Autism & Pervasive Developmental Disorders Sourcebook, 2nd Edition

Back & Neck Sourcebook, 2nd Edition

Blood & Circulatory Disorders Sourcebook, 3rd Edition

Brain Disorders Sourcebook, 3rd Edition

Breast Cancer Sourcebook, 3rd Edition

Breastfeeding Sourcebook

Burns Sourcebook

Cancer Sourcebook for Women, 4th Edition

Cancer Sourcebook, 6th Edition

Cancer Survivorship Sourcebook

Cardiovascular Disorders Sourcebook, 4th Edition

Caregiving Sourcebook

Child Abuse Sourcebook, 2nd Edition

Childhood Diseases & Disorders Sourcebook, 2nd Edition

Colds, Flu & Other Common Ailments Sourcebook

Communication Disorders Sourcebook

Complementary & Alternative Medicine Sourcebook, 4th Edition

Congenital Disorders Sourcebook, 2nd Edition

Contagious Diseases Sourcebook, 2nd Edition

Cosmetic & Reconstructive Surgery Sourcebook, 2nd Edition

Death & Dying Sourcebook, 2nd Edition

Dental Care & Oral Health Sourcebook, 3rd Edition

Depression Sourcebook, 2nd Edition

Dermatological Disorders Sourcebook, 2nd Edition

Diabetes Sourcebook, 5th Edition

Diet & Nutrition Sourcebook, 4th Edition

Digestive Diseases & Disorder Sourcebook

Disabilities Sourcebook, 2nd Edition

Disease Management Sourcebook

Domestic Violence Sourcebook, 3rd Edition

Drug Abuse Sourcebook, 3rd Edition

Ear, Nose & Throat Disorders Sourcebook, 2nd Edition

Eating Disorders Sourcebook, 3rd Edition

Emergency Medical Services Sourcebook

Endocrine & Metabolic Disorders Sourcebook, 2nd Edition

Environmental Health Sourcebook, 3rd Edition

Ethnic Diseases Sourcebook

Eye Care Sourcebook, 4th Edition

Family Planning Sourcebook

Fitness & Exercise Sourcebook, 4th Edition

Food Safety Sourcebook

Forensic Medicine Sourcebook

Gastrointestinal Diseases & Disorders Sourcebook, 2nd Edition

Genetic Disorders Sourcebook, 4th Edition

Head Trauma Sourcebook

Headache Sourcebook

Health Insurance Sourcebook

Healthy Aging Sourcebook

Healthy Children Sourcebook

Healthy Heart Sourcebook for Women

Hepatitis Sourcebook

Household Safety Sourcebook

Hypertension Sourcebook

Immune System Disorders Sourcebook, 2nd Edition

Infant & Toddler Health Sourcebook

Infectious Diseases Sourcebook